FIRST AID FOR THE

MEDICINE clerkship

THE STUDENT TO STUDENT GUIDE

SERIES EDITORS:

LATHA G. STEAD, MD
Assistant Professor of Emergency Medicine
Mayo Medical School
Rochester, Minnesota

S. MATTHEW STEAD, MD, PhD
Class of 2001
State University of New York—Downstate Medical Center
Brooklyn, New York

MATTHEW S. KAUFMAN, MD
Resident in Internal Medicine
Long Island Jewish Medical Center
Albert Einstein College of Medicine
New Hyde Park, New York

TITLE EDITOR:

BARBARA G. LOCK, MD
Attending Physician in Emergency Medicine
Columbia Presbyterian Medical Center
New York, New York

SUPERVISING EDITOR AND CONTRIBUTING AUTHOR:

SAMY I. MCFARLANE, MD, FACE, CCD
Assistant Professor of Medicine and Radiology
Division of Endocrinology, Diabetes and Hypertension
Director, Fellowship Program in Endocrinology
Director for Education, Third Year Clerkship in Medicine
Department of Medicine
State University of New York Health Science Center—Brooklyn
Brooklyn, New York

McGraw-Hill
Medical Publishing Division

New York   Chicago   San Francisco   Lisbon   London   Madrid
Mexico City   Milan   New Delhi   San Juan   Seoul
Singapore   Sydney   Toronto

McGraw-Hill

A Division of The McGraw·Hill Companies

First Aid for the Medicine Clerkship

234567890 CUS/CUS 098765432

ISBN 0-07-136421-8

Notice

Medicine is an ever-changing science. As new research and clinical experience broaden our knowledge, changes in treatment and drug therapy are required. The authors and the publisher of this work have checked with sources believed to be reliable in their efforts to provide information that is complete and generally in accord with the standards accepted at the time of publication. However, in view of the possibility of human error or changes in medical sciences, neither the authors nor the publisher nor any other party who has been involved in the preparation or publication of this work warrants that the information contained herein is in every respect accurate or complete, and they disclaim all responsibility for any errors or omissions or for the results obtained from use of the information contained in this work. Readers are encouraged to confirm the information contained herein with other sources. For example and in particular, readers are advised to check the product information sheet included in the package of each drug they plan to administer to be certain that the information contained in this work is accurate and that changes have not been made in the recommended dose or in the contraindications for administration. This recommendation is of particular importance in connection with new or infrequently used drugs.

This book was set in Goudy by Rainbow Graphics.
The editor was Catherine A. Johnson.
The production supervisor was Lisa Mendez.
Project management was provided by Rainbow Graphics.
The index was prepared by Oneida Indexing.
Von Hoffman Graphics was the printer and binder.

This book is printed on acid-free paper.

Library of Congress Cataloging-in-Publication Data

First aid for the clinical clerkship. Medicine / editor, Barbara G. Lock ; supervising
editor and contributing author, Samy I. McFarlane.
    p. ; cm.
  Includes bibliographical references and index.
  ISBN 0-07-136421-8 (softcover)
   1. Clinical clerkship. I. Lock, Barbara G. II. McFarlane, Samy I.
  [DNLM: 1. Clinical Clerkship. 2. Career Choice. 3. Fellowships and Scholarships. 4.
Medicine. W 18 F527 2001]
  R839 .F57 2001
  610′.71′55–dc21

2001030091

Contributing Authors

ROBIN R. BLUM, MD
Resident in Dermatology
Mount Sinai School of Medicine
New York, New York
Dermatology

THOMAS M. BOYD, MD
Resident in Emergency Medicine
Jacobi-Montefiore EM Residency
Albert Einstein College of Medicine
Bronx, New York
Nephrology and Acid–Base, Endocrinology

ERIC MICHAEL FIELDS, DO
Resident in Emergency Medicine
Beth Israel Medical Center
Albert Einstein College of Medicine
New York, New York
Gastroenterology

BARBARA G. LOCK, MD
Attending Physician in Emergency Medicine
Columbia Presbyterian Medical Center
New York, New York
*Cardiology, Pulmonology, Gastroenterology, Health
    Promotion*

R. ANAND NARASIMHAN, MD
Resident in Internal Medicine
Mayo Graduate School of Medicine
Rochester, Minnesota
Neurology, Hematology—Oncology

JONATHAN POSNER, MD
Resident in Radiology
Cornell/New York Medical Center
New York, New York
Rheumatology

Contents

Introduction

This clinical study aid was designed in the tradition of the *First Aid* series of books, formatted in the same way as the other titles in this series. Topics are listed by bold headings to the left, while the "meat" of the topic comprises the middle column. The outside margins contain mnemonics, diagrams, summary or warning statements, "pearls," and other memory aids. These are further classified as "exam tip" noted by the ✎ symbol and "ward tip" noted by the ☤ symbol.

The content of this book is based on the Committee of Directors in Internal Medicine (www.im.org/cdim/) recommendations for the internal medicine curriculum for third-year medical students. Each of the chapters contain the major topics central to the practice of internal medicine and closely parallel CDIM's medical student learning objectives.

The Medicine clerkship can be an exciting hands-on learning experience. For some medical students, it may be the first opportunity for patient interaction during medical school. There are two keys to doing well in this clerkship: Treat all patients and staff with respect and kindness, and organize your learning. You will find that rather than simply preparing you for success on the clerkship exam, this book will also help guide you in the clinical diagnosis and treatment of the many interesting problems you will see during your medicine rotation.

Acknowledgments

We would like to thank the following faculty for their help in reviewing the manuscript for this book:

Anderson Spickard III, MD
Director of Medical Student Clerkships
Department of Medicine
Vanderbilt University School of Medicine
Nashville, Tennessee

Kevin D. Whittle, MD
Assistant Professor of Internal Medicine
Third-Year Clerkship Director
University of South Dakota School of Medicine
Sioux Falls, South Dakota

How to Succeed
in the Medicine Clerkship

Be on Time

Most medical ward teams begin rounding between 7 and 8 A.M. If you are expected to "pre-round," you should give yourself at least 10 minutes per patient that you are following to see the patient and learn about the events that occurred overnight. Like all working professionals, you will face occasional obstacles to punctuality, but make sure this is occasional. When you first start a rotation, try to show up at least 15 minutes early until you get the routine figured out.

Dress in a Professional Manner

Even if the resident wears scrubs and the attending wears stiletto heels, you must dress in a professional, conservative manner. Wear a *short* white coat over your clothes unless discouraged (as in pediatrics).

> **Men** should wear long pants, with cuffs covering the ankle, a long collared shirt, and a tie. No jeans, no sneakers, no short-sleeved shirts.
> **Women** should wear long pants or knee-length skirt and a blouse or dressy sweater. No jeans, no sneakers, no heels greater than 1½ inches, no open-toed shoes.
> **Both men and women** may wear scrubs occasionally, during overnight call or in the operating room. Do not make this your uniform.

Act in a Pleasant Manner

The medical rotation is often difficult, stressful, and tiring. Smooth out your experience by being nice to be around. Smile a lot and learn everyone's name. If you do not understand or disagree with a treatment plan or diagnosis, do not "challenge." Instead, say "I'm sorry, I don't quite understand, could you please explain. . . ." Be empathetic toward patients.

Be Aware of the Hierarchy

The way in which this will affect you will vary from hospital to hospital and team to team, but it is always present to some degree. In general, address your questions regarding ward functioning to interns or residents. Address your medical questions to attendings; make an effort to be somewhat informed on your subject prior to asking attendings medical questions.

Address Patients and Staff in a Respectful Way

Address patients as Sir, Ma'am, or Mr., Mrs., or Miss. Try not to address patients as "honey," "sweetie," and the like. Although you may feel these names are friendly, patients will think you have forgotten their name, that you are being inappropriately familiar, or both. Address all physicians as "doctor," unless told otherwise.

Take Responsibility for Your Patients

Know everything there is to know about your patients: their history, test results, details about their medical problem, and prognosis. Keep your intern or resident informed of new developments that they might not be aware of, and ask them for any updates you might not be aware of. Assist the team in developing a plan; speak to radiology, consultants, and family. Never give bad news to patients or family members without the assistance of your supervising resident or attending.

RESPECT PATIENTS' RIGHTS

1. All patients have the right to have their personal medical information kept private. This means do not discuss the patient's information with family members without that patient's consent, and do not discuss any patient in hallways, elevators, or cafeterias.
2. All patients have the right to refuse treatment. This means they can refuse treatment by a specific individual (you, the medical student), or of a specific type (no nasogastric tube). Patients can even refuse life-saving treatment. The only exceptions to this rule are if the patient is deemed to not have the capacity to make decisions or understand situations, in which case a health care proxy should be sought, or if the patient is suicidal or homicidal.
3. All patients should be informed of the right to seek advanced directives on admission. Often, this is done by the admissions staff, in a booklet. If your patient is chronically ill or has a life-threatening illness, address the subject of advanced directives with the assistance of your attending.

Volunteer

Be self-propelled, self-motivated. Volunteer to help with a procedure or a difficult task. Volunteer to give a 20-minute talk on a topic of your choice. Volunteer to take additional patients. Volunteer to stay late.

Be a Team Player

Help other medical students with their tasks; teach them information you have learned. Support your supervising intern or resident whenever possible. Never steal the spotlight, steal a procedure, or make a fellow medical student look bad.

Be Honest

If you don't understand, don't know, or didn't do it, make sure you always say that. Never say or document information that is false (a common example: "bowel sounds normal" when you did not listen).

Keep Patient Information Handy

Use a clipboard, notebook, or index cards to keep patient information, including a miniature history and physical, and lab and test results, at hand.

Present Patient Information in an Organized Manner

Here is a template for the "bullet" presentation:

> "This is a [age]-year-old [gender] with a history of [major history such as HTN, DM, coronary artery disease, CA, etc.] who presented on [date] with [major symptoms, such as cough, fever, and chills] and was found to have [working diagnosis]. [Tests done] showed [results]. Yesterday, the patient [state important changes, new plan, new tests, new medications]. This morning the patient feels [state the patient's words], and the physical exam is significant for [state major findings]. Plan is [state plan].

The newly admitted patient generally deserves a longer presentation following the complete history and physical format.

Some patients have extensive histories. The whole history should be present in the admission note, but in ward presentation, it is often too much to absorb. In these cases, it will be very much appreciated by your team if you can generate a **good summary** that maintains an accurate picture of the patient. This usually takes some thought, but it's worth it.

HOW TO PRESENT A CHEST RADIOGRAPH (CXR)

- First, confirm that the CXR belongs to your patient.
- If possible, compare to a previous film.

Then, present in a systematic manner:

1. *Technique:* Rotation, anteroposterior (AP) or posteroanterior (PA), penetration, inspiratory effort.
2. *Bony structures:* Look for rib, clavicle, scapula, and sternum fractures.
3. *Airway:* Look for tracheal deviation, pneumothorax, pneumomediastinum.
4. *Pleural space:* Look for fluid collections, which can represent hemothorax, chylothorax, pleural effusion.
5. *Lung parenchyma:* Look for infiltrates and consolidations: These can represent pneumonia, pulmonary contusions, hematoma, or aspiration. The location of an infiltrate can provide a clue to the location of a pneumonia:
   - Obscured right (R) costophrenic angle = Right lower lobe
   - Obscured left (L) costophrenic angle = Left lower lobe
   - Obscured R heart border = Right middle lobe
   - Obscured L heart border = Left upper lobe

6. *Mediastinum:* Look at size of mediastinum—a widened one (> 8 cm) goes with aortic dissection. Look for enlarged cardiac silhouette (> ½ thoracic width at base of heart), which may represent congestive heart failure (CHF), cardiomyopathy, or pericardial effusion.
7. *Diaphragm:* Look for free air under the right hemidiaphragm (suggests perforation). Look for stomach, bowel, or nasogastric tube (NGT) above diaphragm (suggests diaphragmatic rupture).
8. *Tubes and lines:*
   - Identify all tubes and lines.
   - An endotracheal tube should be 2 cm above the carina. A common mistake is right mainstem bronchus intubation.
   - A chest tube (including the most proximal hole) should be in the pleural space (not in the lung parenchyma).
   - An NGT should be in the stomach and uncoiled.
   - The tip of a central venous catheter (central line) should be in the superior vena cava (not in the right atrium).
   - The tip of a Swan–Ganz catheter should be in the pulmonary artery.
   - The tip of a transvenous pacemaker should be in the right atrium.

A sample CXR presentation may sound like:

This is the CXR of Mr. Jones. The film is an AP view with good inspiratory effort. There is an isolated fracture of the eighth rib on the right. There is no tracheal deviation or mediastinal shift. There is no pneumo- or hemothorax. The cardiac silhouette appears to be of normal size. The diaphragm and heart borders on both sides are clear; no infiltrates are noted. There is a central venous catheter present, the tip of which is in the superior vena cava.

HOW TO PRESENT AN ELECTROCARDIOGRAM (ECG)

- First, confirm that the ECG belongs to your patient.
- If possible, compare to a previous tracing.

Then, present in a systematic manner:

1. *Rate* (see Figure 1-1): The rate is [number of] beats per minute (bpm):
   - The ECG paper is scored so that one big box is .20 seconds. These big boxes consist of five little boxes, each of which is 0.04 seconds.

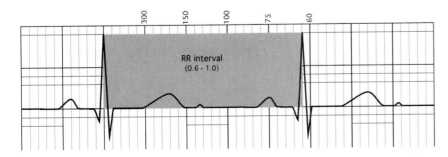

FIGURE 1-1. Calculating rate.

- A quick way to calculate rate when the rhythm is regular is the mantra: **300, 150, 100, 75, 60, 50** (= 300 / # large boxes), which is measured as the number of large boxes between two QRS complexes. Therefore, a distance of one large box between two adjacent QRS complexes would be a rate of 300, while a distance of five large boxes between two adjacent QRS complexes would be a rate of 60.
- For irregular rhythms, count the number of complexes that occur in a 6-second interval (30 large boxes) and multiply by 10 to get a rate in bpm.

2. *Rhythm:* The rhythm is [sinus]/[atrial fibrillation]/[atrial flutter] or other:
   - If p waves are present in all leads and upright in leads I and aVF, then the rhythm is sinus. Lack of p waves suggests a disorganized atrial rhythm, a junctional rhythm, or a ventricular rhythm. A ventricular rhythm (V Fib or V Tach) is an unstable one (could spell imminent death), and you should be getting ready for advanced cardiac life support (ACLS).
   - Normal sinus rhythm is usually a regular narrow-complex rhythm with each QRS complex preceded by a p wave.

3. *Axis* (see Figure 1-2): The axis is [normal]/[deviated to the right]/[deviated to the left]:
   - If I and aVF are both upright or positive, then the axis is normal.
   - If I is upright and aVF is upside down, then there is left axis deviation (LAD).

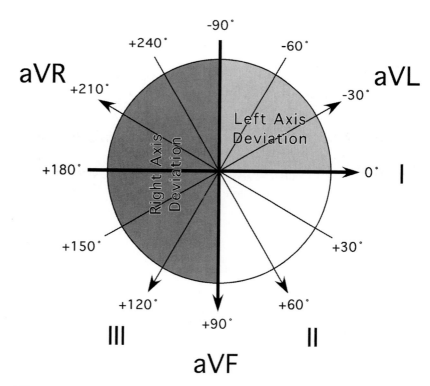

FIGURE 1-2. ECG axes.

- If I is upside down and aVF is upright, then there is right axis deviation (RAD).
- If I and aVF are both upside down or negative, then there is extreme RAD.

4. *Intervals* (see Figure 1-3): The [PR]/[QRS] intervals are [normal]/[shortened]/[widened]:
   - Normal PR interval = .12 to .20 seconds:
     - Short PR is associated with Wolff–Parkinson–White syndrome (WPW).
     - WPW syndrome is characterized by a "delta" wave, or slurred upstroke of QRS complex.
     - Long PR interval is associated with heart block of which there are three types:
       - First-degree block: PR interval > .20 seconds (one big box)
       - Second-degree (Mobitz type I or Wenckebach) block: PR interval lengthens progressively until a QRS is dropped.
       - Second-degree (Mobitz type II) block: PR interval is constant, but one QRS is dropped at a fixed interval.
       - Third-degree heart block: Complete AV dissociation
   - Normal QRS interval ≤ .12 seconds:
     - Prolonged QRS is seen when the beat is initiated in the ventricle rather than the sinoatrial node, when there is a bundle branch block, and when the heart is artificially paced with longer QRS intervals. Prolonged QRS is also noted in tricyclic overdose and Wolfe–Parkinson–White syndrome.

5. *Wave morphology* (see Figure 1-4):
   a. *Ventricular hypertrophy:* There [is/is no] [left/right] [ventricular/atrial] hypertrophy:
      - There are multiple criteria for determining right (RVH) and left ventricular hypertrophy (LVH). A few are listed here:
        - *Clues for LVH:*
          - $R_I > 15$ mm
          - $R_{I, II \text{ or } aVF} > 20$ mm
          - $R_{aVL} > 11$ mm

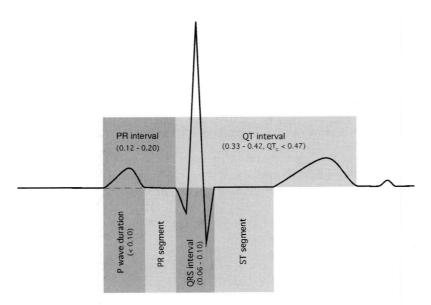

FIGURE 1-3. ECG intervals.

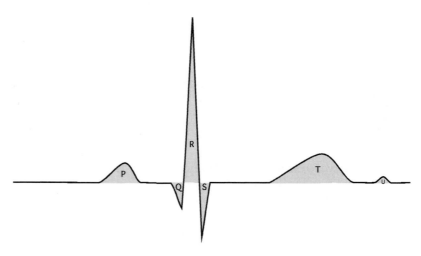

FIGURE 1-4. ECG wave morphology.

- R_{V5} or $R_{V6} > 26$ mm
- $R_I + S_{III} > 25$ mm
- $R + S$ in V lead > 45 mm
- $S_{V1} + R_{V5}$ or $R_{V6} > 35$ mm
- *Clues for RVH:*
- $R_{V1} > 7$ mm
- $S_{V1} < 2$ mm
- R/S ratio in $V_1 > 1$
- RAD of $110°$ or more

b. *Atrial hypertrophy:*
- Right atrial hypertrophy: tall or peaked p waves in limb or precordial leads
- Left atrial hypertrophy: broad or notched p waves in limb leads

c. *Ischemic changes:* There [are/are no] S-T wave [depressions/elevations] or [flattened/inverted] T waves. Presence of Q wave indicates an old infarct.

d. *Bundle branch block:* There [is/is no] [left/right] bundle branch block. Clues:
- Presence of RSR′ wave in leads V_1–V_3 with ST depression and T wave inversion goes with RBBB.
- Presence of notched R wave in leads I, aVL, and V_4–V_6 goes with LBBB.

Document Information in an Organized Manner

A complete medical student initial History and Physical is neat, legible, organized, and usually two to three pages long. Major topics should include: chief complaint, history of present illness, medical history, surgical history, medications, allergies, sexual history, smoking and alcohol history, occupation, travel, review of systems, vital signs, physical exam, lab results, test results, assessment or problem list, and plan.

The main advantage to doing the medical clerkship is that you get to see patients. The patient is the key to learning medicine, and the source of most satisfaction and frustration on the wards. Plan your learning before the rotation starts as follows:

Make a List of Core Material to Learn

This list should reflect common symptoms, illnesses, and areas in which you have particular interest, or in which you feel particularly weak. Do not try to learn every possible topic. The Committee of Directors in Internal Medicine (*www.im.org/cdim/*) publishes a list of core content, on which this book is based. The CDIM emphasizes:

Symptoms and Lab Tests
- Abdominal pain
- Altered mental status
- Anemia
- Back pain
- Chest pain
- Cough
- Dysuria
- Fluid, electrolyte, and acid–base disorders

Common Illnesses
- Chronic obstructive pulmonary disease (COPD)
- Congestive heart failure
- Depression
- Diabetes mellitus
- Dyslipidemia
- Human immunodeficiency virus (HIV) infection
- Hypertension
- Smoking cessation
- Substance abuse
- Common cancers

We Also Recommend
- Adult vaccinations
- Domestic violence
- Dysrhythmias
- Nutritional disorders

Select Your Study Material

We recommend:
- This review book, *First Aid for the Clinical Clerkship in Medicine*
- A major medicine textbook such as *Harrison's Principles of Internal Medicine* (costs about $140)
- A full-text online journal database, such as *www.mdconsult.com* (subscription is $99/year for students)

- A small pocket reference book to look up lab values, clinical pathways, and the like, such as *Maxwell Quick Medical Reference* (costs $7)
- A small book to look up drugs, such as *Pocket Pharmacopoeia* (Tarascon Publishers, $8)

Make a Schedule to Learn the Illness-Based Topics

This schedule should reflect the rotation you are doing. For example, for the time you are going to be rotating in a clinic or office, make a schedule to study smoking cessation, dyslipidemia, depression, and diabetes. First, read this review book on each topic, then read the major textbook, taking notes. Make sure to include all chosen topics in your schedule, but leave room at least two weeks before the clerkship exam for review.

As You See Patients, Note Their Major Symptoms and Diagnosis for Review

Your reading on the symptom-based topics above should be done with a specific patient in mind. For example, if a patient comes to the office with cough, fever, and night sweats and is thought to have tuberculosis, read about chronic and acute cough, postnasal drip, asthma, gastroesophageal reflux disease (GERD), pneumonia, and tuberculosis in this review book that night.

Prepare a Talk on a Topic

You may be asked to give a small talk once or twice during your rotation. If not, you should volunteer! Feel free to choose a topic that is on your list; however, realize that this may be considered dull by the people who hear the lecture. The ideal topic is slightly uncommon but not rare, for example, cardiomyopathy. To prepare a talk on a topic, read about it in a major textbook and a review article not more than 2 years old, and then search online or in the library for recent developments or changes in treatment.

HOW TO PREPARE FOR THE CLINICAL CLERKSHIP EXAM

If you have read about your core illnesses and core symptoms, you will know a great deal about medicine. To study for the clerkship exam, we recommend:

2 to 3 weeks before exam: Read this entire review book, taking notes.
10 days before exam: Read the notes you took during the rotation on your core content list and the corresponding review book sections.
5 days before exam: Read this entire review book, concentrating on lists and mnemonics.
2 days before exam: Exercise, eat well, skim the book, and go to bed early.
1 day before exam: Exercise, eat well, review your notes and the mnemonics, and go to bed on time. Do not have any caffeine after 2 P.M.

Other helpful studying strategies include:

Study with Friends

Group studying can be very helpful. Other people may point out areas that you have not studied enough and may help you focus on the goal. If you tend to get distracted by other people in the room, limit this to less than half of your study time.

Study in a Bright Room

Find the room in your house or in your library that has the best, brightest light. This will help prevent you from falling asleep. If you don't have a bright light, get a halogen desk lamp or a light that simulates sunlight (not a tanning lamp).

Eat Light, Balanced Meals

Make sure your meals are balanced, with lean protein, fruits and vegetables, and fiber. A high-sugar, high-carbohydrate meal will give you an initial burst of energy for 1 to 2 hours, but then you'll drop.

Take Practice Exams

The point of practice exams is not so much the content that is contained in the questions, but the training of sitting still for 3 hours and trying to pick the best answer for each and every question.

Tips for Answering Questions

All questions are intended to have one best answer. When answering questions, follow these guidelines:

Read the answers first. For all questions longer than two sentences, reading the answers first can help you sift through the question for the key information.

Look for the words "EXCEPT, MOST, LEAST, NOT, BEST, WORST, TRUE, FALSE, CORRECT, INCORRECT, ALWAYS, and NEVER." If you find one of these words, circle or underline it for later comparison with the answer.

Evaluate each answer as being either true or false. Example:

Which of the following is *least* likely to be associated with pulmonary embolism?
A. Tachycardia **T**
B. Tachypnea **T**
C. Chest pain **? F not always**
D. Deep venous thrombosis **? T not always**
E. Back pain **F ? aortic dissection**

By comparing the question, noting LEAST, to the answers, "E" is the best answer.

As the boy scouts say, "BE PREPARED."

NOTES

High-Yield Facts

Cardiology
Pulmonology
Neurology
Gastroenterology
Hematology—Oncology
Rheumatology
Nephrology and Acid–Base
Endocrinology
Urology
Immunology
Dermatology
Health Promotion

Cardiology

Barbara G. Lock

LEADING CAUSES OF DEATH IN THE UNITED STATES

1. Heart disease
2. Cancer
3. Stroke
4. Chronic obstructive pulmonary disease (COPD)
5. Accidents/trauma
6. Pneumonia, influenza
7. Diabetes mellitus
8. Suicide
9. Kidney disease
10. Liver disease

CAUSES OF CHEST PAIN

- **Costochondritis/musculoskeletal:** Sharp, localized pain and reproducible tenderness, often exacerbated by exercise
- **Myocardial infarction/angina:** Chest heaviness, pressure, or pain, often radiating to left arm, shoulder, or jaw
- **Pericarditis:** Chest pain radiating to shoulder, neck, or back, worse with deep breathing or cough, relieved by sitting up/leaning forward
- **Aortic dissection:** Severe chest pain radiating to the back, can be associated with unequal pulses or unequal blood pressure in right and left arms
- **Abscess/mass:** Often sharp, localized pain, worse with deep breathing (pleuritic)
- **Pulmonary embolism:** Often worse with deep breathing or cough (pleuritic). Frequently associated with tachypnea and tachycardia
- **Pneumonia:** Often worse with deep breathing or cough (pleuritic)
- **GERD/esophageal spasm/tear:** Burning pain, dysphagia, may be similar to pain of myocardial infarction (MI)
- **Other causes:** Peptic ulcer disease, biliary disease, herpes zoster, anxiety, pneumothorax

Myocardial infarction can be *silent*, with no symptoms or atypical symptoms, especially in diabetics (due to neuropathy).

RISK FACTORS FOR CORONARY HEART DISEASE

Criteria for **family history** of coronary artery disease:
- MI before age 40 in men
- MI before age 55 in women

- Smoking
- High low-density lipoprotein (LDL)
- Low high-density lipoprotein (HDL)
- Hypertension
- Obesity (apple-shaped)
- Diabetes mellitus
- Postmenopausal without hormone replacement therapy
- Hyperhomocystinemia
- Family history
- Less common risk factors include high C-reactive protein and increased circulating fibrinogen.

DYSLIPIDEMIA

- About half of all cases of coronary artery disease are associated with disorders of lipid metabolism.

A level of HDL > 60 is cardioprotective.

Major Lipoproteins

- Chylomicrons: Transport cholesterol from the gut in the bloodstream
- Chylomicron remnants: Left over after lipoprotein lipase liberates free fatty acids from chylomicrons for use in tissues
- Very low-density lipoprotein (VLDL): Secreted from the liver; carries cholesterol in the bloodstream
- Intermediate-density lipoprotein (IDL): Metabolized from VLDL
- LDL: Metabolized from IDL, it carries cholesterol in the bloodstream to tissues
- HDL: Uptakes free cholesterol secreted by tissues and transports it to the liver

Isolated Hypercholesterolemia

All isolated hypercholesterolemia is type IIa.

- Familial hypercholesterolemia: Elevated LDL (type IIa)
- Familial defective apo B100: Elevated LDL (type IIa)
- Polygenic hypercholesterolemia: Elevated LDL (type IIa)

Isolated Hypertriglyceridemia

- Familial hypertriglyceridemia: Elevated VLDL (type IV)
- Familial lipoprotein lipase deficiency: Elevated chylomicrons (type I, V)
- Familial apo CII deficiency: Elevated chylomicrons (type I, V)

Combined Hypertriglyceridemia and Hypercholesterolemia

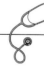

Patients with very high triglyceride levels (> 1,000) are at risk of developing pancreatitis.

- Combined hyperlipidemia: Elevated VLDL, LDL (type IIb)
- Dysbetalipoproteinemia: Elevated VLDL, IDL (type III)

HIGH-YIELD FACTS

Cardiology

Signs and Symptoms

Certain physical findings are associated with hypercholesterolemia:
- Xanthelasma: Painless, nonpruritic raised yellow plaques that occur on eyelids near inner canthi
- Xanthoma: Reddish brown papules on scalp, face, trunk, and flexor surfaces of limbs

Diagnosis

Serum lipoprotein analysis is done after a 12-hour fast. One-time sample cholesterol levels may not represent true levels in the following circumstances:
- Weight loss
- Pregnancy
- Major surgery
- Severe illness

Note: In patients who have MI, lipoprotein levels obtained within the first 24 hours will more closely approximate true pre-MI levels than later levels, which may not return to baseline for several weeks.

For cholesterol levels, see Table 2-1.

Treatment of Hypercholesterolemia

Goals of treatment:
- For a patient with no risk factors, keep LDL ≤ 160.
- For a patient with risk factors but no known heart disease, keep LDL ≤ 130.
- For a patient with known atherosclerotic heart disease, keep LDL ≤ 100.

For treatment strategies, see Table 2-2.

Formulae for calculating lipid levels:
LDL = TC − HDL − VLDL
VLDL = Trig/5
Total cholesterol (TC):
Normal: < 200
Borderline: 200–240
High: > 240
Normal HDL: 30–100

HIGH-YIELD FACTS

Cardiology

	Type	Total Cholesterol Level (mg/dL)	LDL Level	VLDL	Chylomicrons
Familial hypercholesterolemia	IIa	275–500	High	Normal	Normal
Familial defective apo B100	IIa	275–500	High	Normal	Normal
Polygenic hypercholesterolemia	IIa	240–350	High	Normal	Normal
Familial hypertriglyceridemia	IV	250–750	Normal/High	High	Normal/High
Familial lipoprotein lipase deficiency	I, (I,V)	> 750	Normal/High	Normal/High	High
Familial apoprotein CII deficiency	I, (I,V)	> 750	Normal/High	Normal/High	High
Familial combined hyperlipidemia	IIb	250–500	High	High	Normal/High
Dysbetalipoproteinemia	III	250–500	Normal	High	Normal/High

TABLE 2-1. Cholesterol Levels Associated with Familial Disease

TABLE 2-2. Treatment of Hypercholesterolemia

Treatment	Mechanism	Results
Diet therapy	Step 1 diet: Months 1–3 ■ Total fat < 30% total calories ■ Saturated fat < 10% ■ Dietary cholesterol < 300 mg/day Step 2 diet: Months 4–6 if step 1 diet fails ■ Total fat < 30% of total calories ■ Saturated fat < 7% ■ Dietary cholesterol < 200 mg/dL	Step 2 diet reduces total cholesterol by 10–12%. Exercise variably raises HDL. If diet therapy and exercise fail by 6 months, progress to medications.
Statins	Statins are HMG-CoA reductase inhibitors and act to reduce LDL and increase HDL.	Can lower LDL cholesterol by 35% and raise HDL by ~8%
Bile acid sequestrants	Cholestyramine and colestipol bind bile acids in the gut.	Reduces LDL cholesterol by 15–20%
Nicotinic acid	Reduces lipolysis in adipose tissue, inhibits hepatic synthesis of cholesterol	Can reduce LDL cholesterol by ~20% over 6 months. Side effects include cutaneous flushing, abdominal pain, nausea.
Fibrinates	Best for reducing triglycerides (in VLDL and chylomicrons)	Increases HDL by 5–30%

CORONARY ARTERY DISEASE

ACUTE CORONARY SYNDROME

A syndrome of atherosclerotic plaque rupture, thrombosis, and occlusion, presenting clinically as unstable angina or acute myocardial infarction

MYOCARDIAL INFARCTION

Definition

Myocardial infarction is myocardial cell death caused by inadequate oxygen supply.

Epidemiology

MI most commonly occurs in men over age 55 and postmenopausal women, although it can occur in any age group under certain circumstances.

Etiology

- Ruptured plaque with local thrombus
- Coronary vasospasm

- Embolized thrombus
- Poor coronary perfusion due to shock

Pathophysiology

MI usually occurs in patients with coronary artery disease (see above). A cholesterol plaque in a coronary artery ruptures, and local thrombus blocks blood flow to the myocardium.

Signs and Symptoms

- Left-sided chest pain, heaviness, or squeezing sensation ("crushing pain")
- Radiation of pain to left arm, shoulder, or jaw
- Diaphoresis
- Sense of impending doom
- Often begin a few hours after awakening
- May present with syncope
- May be "silent" especially in the elderly and in diabetics

Electrocardiogram Diagnosis

ECG Findings
- Q wave MI: New Q waves or loss of R waves, indicating a transmural infarct. Most MIs with ST elevation progress to Q wave MIs.

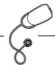

Inferior wall MI:
ST elevation in II, III, aVF
(cor pulmonale: ST *depression* in II, III, aVF)
(see Figure 2-1)
Anteroseptal MI:
ST elevation in V_1, V_2, V_3
(see Figure 2-2)
Lateral wall MI:
ST elevation in V_4, V_5, V_6
Posterior wall MI:
ST depression in V_1, V_2

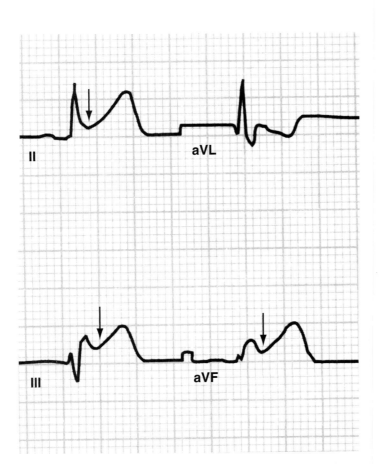

FIGURE 2-1. ECG of inferior wall MI demonstrating ST elevation in leads II, III, and aVF.

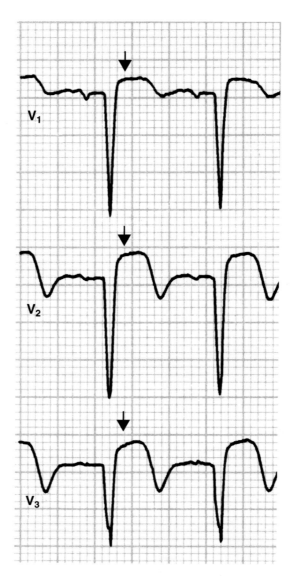

FIGURE 2-2. ECG of anteroseptal MI demonstrating ST elevation in leads V_1, V_2, and V_3.

- Non–Q wave MI: Infarct through the subendocardial zone of the heart. ECG typically shows ST/T segment flattening or depression.

Other Diagnostic Tests

Cardiac Markers
- Myoglobin: Elevated within 1 hour of MI but is nonspecific
- CPK: Elevated within 4 to 8 hours of MI, also nonspecific
- CK MB isoenzyme: More specific marker for myocardial tissue damage
- Troponin T or I: Very sensitive markers for cardiac muscle injury, can be used to detect microinfarcts that CK MB fails to detect. Elevated within 3 hours, can stay elevated for more than a week.
- "Serial enzymes" consist of the above every 6 to 8 hours in a 24-hour period. ECG should be done simultaneously.

Emergent Treatment

Aspirin
- Reduces death from myocardial infarction by 25%
- Irreversibly inhibits platelets, decreasing clot formation

Oxygen
- Maximizes oxygen saturation

Nitroglycerin
- Sublingual or intravenous, dilates coronary arteries, reduces preload

Morphine
- Reduces pain, anxiety, and myocardial oxygen consumption

Beta Blockade
- Intravenous therapy, usually metoprolol 5 mg Q 5–15 minutes for three doses, or until a heart rate of 60
- Shown to decrease mortality

Absolute Contraindications
- Heart rate < 60/min
- Systolic blood pressure < 100 mm Hg
- 2nd- or 3rd-degree heart block
- Moderate to severe LV dysfunction
- Severe COPD
- Signs of peripheral hypoperfusion

Relative Contraindications
- Concurrent use of calcium channel blockers
- Brittle diabetes (difficult to control)
- 1st-degree heart block
- Severe peripheral vascular disease
- Asthma

Heparin
- Standard or low molecular weight, to prevent further thrombosis
- Standard heparin given as loading dose of 80 U/kg followed by infusion at 18 U/kg/hr
- aPTT is monitored every 6 hours. Keep it between 60 and 80 seconds, or 1.5 to 2.0 times patient's normal value.

Thrombolytics
- Agents include streptokinase, urokinase, anistreplase, alteplase, and reteplase.
- Work by breaking up clots
- Should be given to selected patients within 12 hours

Indications
- > 0.1 mV ST elevation in at least two contiguous leads
- New LBBB

Absolute Contraindications
- Systolic blood pressure > 180
- History of hemorrhagic stroke
- Any stroke within past 1 year
- Suspected aortic dissection
- Active bleeding

Heparin does not dissolve already-present clots; rather, it prevents future ones from forming.

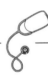

Low-molecular-weight heparin is given sub-Q every 12 hours. PT/PTT does not need to be checked.

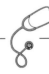

The thrombolytic *streptokinase* is highly immunogenic and cannot be used in the same patient twice within a 6-month period.

Relative Contraindications
- Recent surgery
- Cardiopulmonary resuscitation (CPR)
- Bleeding disorder
- Active peptic ulcer disease

Percutaneous Transluminal Coronary Angioplasty (PTCA)
- Procedure whereby occluding clot and plaque is physically broken up with a balloon catheter in order to restore coronary flow
- Should be done within 90 minutes of diagnosis

Indications
- For patients who meet thrombolysis criteria but in whom it is contraindicated or thrombolysis is not available
- Can also be used as an adjunct to thrombolysis
- For patients with recurrent ischemia with single- or double-vessel disease

Typical scenario:
A 58-year-old man who was discharged from the hospital after MI 2 weeks ago presents with fever, chest pain, and generalized malaise. ECG shows diffuse ST-T wave changes. *Think: Dressler's syndrome.* Treat with nonsteroidal anti-inflammatory drugs (NSAIDs).

Postinfarction Complications

- Heart failure
- Free wall rupture
- New ventricular septal defect (VSD)
- Mitral regurgitation
- Ventricular dysrhythmias
- Supraventricular dysrhythmias
- Bradycardia
- AV block
- Pericarditis (Dressler's syndrome)
- Thromboembolism
- Left ventricular aneurysm

Care of Patients After MI

- Pre-discharge stress test
- MUGA (Multi Gated Acquisition scan) or echo to assess left ventricular function
- Continue ASA and beta-blocker therapy
- Angiotensin-converting enzyme (ACE) inhibitor therapy for patients with ejection fraction < 40% (see below)
- Aggressive management of conditions associated with increased risk of coronary artery disease such as diabetes mellitus, hypertension, and hyperlipidemia
- Reinforce adherence to good lifestyle habits such as quitting smoking, eating a heart-healthy diet, and daily moderate exercise.
- Consider cardiac catheterization and/or CABG (coronary artery bypass graft) for patients with low EF, ventricular dysrhythmias, or continued ischemia.

ACE Inhibitor Therapy

- Actions: Reduces mortality, slows the rate of progression to symptomatic HF, improves exercise performance, and enhances overall quality of life

- Absolute contraindications: Pregnancy, bilateral renal artery stenosis and severe renal disease

ANGINA

Definition

Unstable angina: An acute coronary syndrome diagnosed by the following history:
- New-onset angina
- Angina that changes or accelerates in pattern, location, or severity
- Angina at rest

Stable angina: A chronic, episodic pain syndrome due to temporary myocardial ischemia. Pattern of pain is similar to that of acute MI, but resolves with rest or medication.

Prinzmetal's angina: Angina due to coronary vasospasm, not linked to exertion. Distinguished from unstable angina by chronic, intermittent nature. Pain usually occurs at a specific hour in the early morning. Coronary vessels are angiographically normal.

Etiology

Temporary myocardial ischemia

Diagnosis

ECG
- ST segment depression or elevation
- T wave inversion
- May be normal

Treatment

For Unstable Angina
- Most patients should be admitted to the cardiac care unit (CCU), to monitor for impending MI.
- Heparin or LMWH to prevent propagation of clot

For Stable and Unstable Angina
- Beta blockade: Reduces myocardial oxygen demand
- Aspirin: Reduces risk of MI in asymptomatic patients

For Prinzmetal's Angina
- Calcium channel blockers and nitrates to reduce vasospasm

For All Angina
- Modify risk factors for coronary heart disease.
- Sublingual nitroglycerin for episodic pain
- Consider coronary revascularization: Percutaneous transluminal coronary angioplasty (PTCA) or CABG.

Typical scenario:
A 62-year-old smoker presents complaining of three episodes of severe heavy chest pain this morning. Each episode lasted 3 to 5 minutes, but he has no pain now. He has never had this type of pain before.
Think: Unstable angina.

Typical scenario:
A 62-year-old man presents with frequent episodes of dull chest pain on and off for 8 months. He says the pain wakes him from sleep.
Think: Prinzmetal's angina.

HIGH-YIELD FACTS

Cardiology

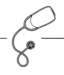

The maximum heart rate is estimated as: [220 – patient's age].

Exercise Stress Testing

- Patients are asked to walk on a treadmill at increasing levels of difficulty to reach a heart rate that is 85% of predicted maximum for age.
- Alternatively, pharmacologic agents such as dobutamine may be administered IV to stimulate myocardial function in a patient who cannot exercise.
- ECG monitoring during the procedure detects changes.
- A test is considered positive for coronary artery disease if the patient develops:
  - Early ST depression
  - ST depression > 2 mm in multiple leads
  - ST elevation
  - Decreased BP
  - Failure to exercise more than 2 minutes due to symptoms
- Failure to complete the test due to reasons other than cardiac symptoms (i.e., arthritis) is not diagnostic.

Stress Myocardial Perfusion Imaging

Patients are injected with a radioisotope (thallium 201 or technetium 99m sestamibi) and stressed (with exercise or pharmacologic agent). Nuclear imaging is obtained immediately after exercise and in 4 hours. The test can detect:
- Myocardial perfusion
- Ventricular volume
- Ejection fraction

Echocardiography

- Echocardiography, or ultrasound of the heart, is used to evaluate many different types of heart disease.
- Transthoracic echo is best done in thin patients. Transesophageal echo is used to see more detail and to assess great vessels.
- For specific uses of echocardiography, see Table 2-3.

Cardiac Catheterization

- Cardiac catheterization is used for diagnosis and treatment of many different types of heart disease.
- The right heart is accessed by the femoral, brachial, or internal jugular vein.
- The left heart is accessed by the femoral artery, brachial artery, or the transseptal approach (from the right heart).
- For specific uses of cardiac catheterization, see Table 2-4.

TABLE 2-3. Uses of Echocardiography

Myocardial infarction	Assess wall motion abnormalities.
Heart failure	Assess ventricular function, ejection fraction.
Heart murmur	Identify and evaluate valvular disease.
Pericardial effusion	Assess volume and early tamponade.
Aortic dissection	Identify presence of tear.
Pulmonary embolism	Identify saddle emboli or evidence of increased right-sided pressure.
Patent foramen ovale	Assess bubbles traversing PFO (air administered through peripheral IV).
Congenital heart disease	Identify coarctation of the aorta, pulmonary stenosis, tetralogy of Fallot, VSD, ASD.

Definition

Congestive heart failure (CHF) is the failure of the heart to pump blood effectively to the tissues. Left heart failure (LHF) causes pulmonary venous congestion (blood flow back-up into the lungs) and compromised systemic circulation. Right heart failure (RHF) causes systemic venous congestion.

Risk Factors

- Valvular disease
- Congenital heart disease
- Restrictive cardiomyopathy
- Constrictive pericarditis

Cardiac output is a measure of blood pumped by the left ventricle and is the product of stroke volume and heart rate.

The most common cause of RHF is LHF.

TABLE 2-4. Uses of Cardiac Catheterization

Myocardial infarction and unstable angina	Coronary artery angiography, balloon dilatation of stenoses, stent placement, laser techniques
Valvular heart disease	Balloon valvuloplasty of mitral stenosis, pulmonary stenosis, aortic stenosis
Dysrhythmias	Electrophysiologic mapping of bypass tracts, radiofrequency ablation
Myocardial disease	Biopsy of myocardium for cardiomyopathies, glycogen storage disease
Congenital heart disease	Cardiac and pulmonary angiography to identify abnormality, transcatheter closure of some types of ASDs, VSDs, PFOs

Etiology

Can be precipitated by:
- MI
- Pulmonary embolus
- Dysrhythmias
- Anemia
- Pneumonia
- Thyrotoxicosis
- Wet beriberi

Signs and Symptoms

LHF
Orthopnea
Paroxysmal nocturnal dyspnea (PND)
Rales
Dyspnea on exertion (DOE)
Cough
Nocturia
S_3 gallop
Diaphoresis
Tachycardia

RHF
RUQ pain (due to hepatic congestion)
Hepatomegaly
Hepatojugular reflex
Jugular venous distention (JVD)
Ascites
Cyanosis
Peripheral edema

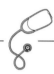
Diagnosis

Chest film: Enlargement of cardiac silhouette, pulmonary vascular congestion with redistribution to upper lobes
Urinalysis: Oliguria, proteinuria, hyalin casts, increased specific gravity

Treatment

Preload Reduction
- Restrict Na to < 2 g day, or 4 g "salt" (NaCl)
- Diuresis with furosemide PO (chronic) or IV (acute)
- Nitrates cause venodilation.

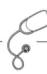
Afterload Reduction
- ACE inhibitor (decreases mortality; see contraindications in MI section)

Increase Inotropy
- Digoxin

Treatment Based on Ethnicity
- Blacks respond best to Ca^{2+} channel blockers.
- Whites and diabetics respond to ACE inhibitors and beta blockers.
- Thiazide diuretics—black and elderly

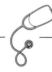
Acute Pulmonary Edema

Acute pulmonary edema (APE) is caused by rapid decompensation of left ventricular function, due to:

- Dysrhythmias
- MI
- Noncompliance with medications
- Increased dietary or intravenous sodium load
- Drugs that cause decreased inotropy
- Strain

Paroxysmal Nocturnal Dyspnea

- Also called cardiac asthma
- A brief episode of breathlessness that awakens patient from sleep
- Is due to increased volume load on heart when lying in the horizontal position or sudden decrease in myocardial contractility, which results in pulmonary edema, impairing the exchange of oxygen
- Distinguished from true asthma by improvement with walking a few steps, and lack of improvement with bronchodilators

RHEUMATIC FEVER

Definition

- Rheumatic fever (RF) is a systemic immune process that occurs due to streptococcal pharyngeal infection.
- Rheumatic heart disease (RHD) is the occurrence of valvular abnormalities due to immune complex deposition in valve leaflets generated by rheumatic fever.

Etiology

Recent streptococcal infection of pharynx

Diagnosis

Laboratory Findings
- Positive ASLO (antistreptolysin-O) antibody titers
- Elevated erythrocyte sedimentation rate (ESR)

Diagnosis of rheumatic fever requires presence of two major criteria or one major and two minor criteria.

Major Criteria
- Arthritis (migratory, multiple joints)
- Carditis (endo-, myo-, peri-)
- Erythema marginatum rash
- Subcutaneous nodules
- Sydenham's chorea

Minor Criteria
- Fever
- Arthralgias
- Elevated ESR
- Prolonged PR interval
- Recent streptococcal pharyngitis

First-line therapy for APE:
NOMAD
Nitroglycerin
Oxygen
Morphine
Aspirin
Diuretic

Other therapy: **ADD**
- **A**mrinone increases inotropy with vasodilation.
- **D**obutamine increases inotropy without vasoconstriction.
- **D**opamine increases inotropy with vasoconstriction.

Most common valve affected by RHD is mitral, followed by aortic, then tricuspid.

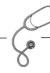

The reason for treating strep throat is to prevent the complication of rheumatic fever, not due to worry of the pharyngitis itself, which would resolve without antibiotics.

Treatment

Acute
- Course of penicillin to eradicate throat carriage of group A streptococci
- ASA for arthritis
- Steroids for carditis

Chronic
- Monthly doses of benzathine penicillin to prevent recurrences
- Follow-up with cardiologist in severe cases

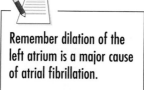

Patients with history of RF require endocarditis prophylaxis when undergoing invasive dental or gastrointestinal/ genitourinary procedures.

VALVULAR HEART DISEASE (VHD)

MITRAL STENOSIS

Etiology

Rheumatic heart disease (most common), congenital (rare)

Epidemiology

Most cases occur in women.

Signs and Symptoms

- Dyspnea on exertion (DOE)
- Rales
- Cough
- Hemoptysis
- Systemic embolism (due to stagnation of blood in enlarged left atrium)
- Accentuated right ventricle precordial thrust
- Signs of right ventricular failure
- Hoarse voice (due to enlarged left atrium impinging on recurrent laryngeal nerve)

Remember dilation of the left atrium is a major cause of atrial fibrillation.

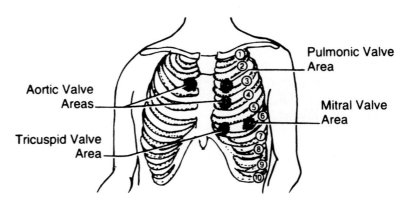

FIGURE 2-3. Cardiac auscultation sites.

(Reproduced, with permission, from DeGowin and DeGowin, *Diagnostic Examination,* 6th ed. New York: McGraw-Hill, 1994: 359.)

Diagnosis

- Murmur is mid-diastolic with opening snap, low-pitched rumble.
- Best heard over left sternal border between 2nd to 4th interspace (see Figure 2-3)
- CXR may show straight left heart border due to enlarged left atrium and Kerley B lines from pulmonary effusion.
- ECG may show left atrial enlargement, right ventricular hypertrophy, atrial fibrillation.
- Echocardiography demonstrates diseased valve.

Treatment

- Endocarditis prophylaxis
- Treat for heart failure (diuretics, digitalis) and dysrhythmias as needed.
- Anticoagulation for atrial thrombus/fibrillation if present
- Surgical repair or balloon valvuloplasty in symptomatic patients with orifice ≤ to 1.2 cm^2

Balloon valvuloplasty in mitral stenosis is an effective intervention; it has a low incidence of restenosis, in contrast to aortic stenosis.

MITRAL REGURGITATION

Etiology

- Papillary muscle dysfunction from either ischemia or infarction (post-MI papillary muscle rupture causes massive regurgitation)
- Rupture of chordae tendineae (can happen spontaneously in otherwise healthy individuals)
- Valve destruction—scarring from rheumatic heart disease or destruction from endocarditis
- Prolapse frequently progresses to valvular incompetence.

Endocarditis prophylaxis is given to patients with VHD and those with previous history of endocarditis 30 minutes prior to:
- Dental procedures
- GI procedures
- Urologic procedures

Signs and Symptoms

- Dyspnea
- Fatigue
- Weakness
- Cough
- Atrial fibrillation
- Systemic emboli

Diagnosis

- Murmur is loud, holosystolic, high-pitched, apical radiating to the axilla
- Wide splitting of S$_2$ with inspiration (widening occurs in severe cases due to premature emptying of LV)
- S$_3$ due to rapid filling of LV by blood regurgitated during systole
- ECG shows enlarged left atrium.
- Echocardiography demonstrating diseased/prolapsed valve

Atrial septal defects also have a wide, fixed split S$_2$.

Treatment

- Medical therapy: Not definitive but used until surgery, or in poor surgical candidates

Patient has a good prognosis if LV function is preserved.

- Diuretics to reduce volume load
- Vasodilators to reduce afterload favoring aortic exit
- Anticoagulation for atrial fibrillation
- Surgical therapy: Valve replacement or repair

MITRAL VALVE PROLAPSE

Etiology

- Idiopathic, rheumatic heart disease, ischemic heart disease, ASD, or Marfan's syndrome
- More common in women (90% of cases)
- Genetic predisposition (can be inherited as an autosomal dominant trait)

Signs and Symptoms

- Mostly asymptomatic
- Atypical chest pain
- Shortness of breath (SOB)
- Fatigue

Diagnosis

- Mid-systolic click followed by late-systolic, high-pitched murmur (if mild regurgitation is present)
- Best heard at apex
- S_3 sometimes present
- Wide splitting of S_2
- Echocardiography demonstrates diseased valve.

Treatment

- Prophylaxis for endocarditis
- Vigilant follow-up

AORTIC STENOSIS

Etiology

Degenerative calcific disease (idiopathic, older population), congenital stenosis, bicuspid aortic valve, or rheumatic heart disease

Signs and Symptoms

- Usually asymptomatic early in course
- Dyspnea

Typical scenario:
A young woman with atypical chest pain and mid-systolic click. *Think: Mitral valve prolapse.*

Prognosis:
Mean survival for patients with AS and:
Angina = 5 years
Syncope = 2–3 years
Heart failure = 1–2 years

- Angina and syncope: Particularly during exercise—peripheral resistance falls, LV pressure remains the same due to stenotic valve, CO cannot maintain BP causing syncope, low BP to coronary arteries causes angina
- Heart failure

Diagnosis

- Forceful apex beat with normally located PMI
- Loud systolic ejection murmur, crescendo–decrescendo, medium pitched loudest at 2nd R interspace, radiates to carotids
- S_4 (presystolic gallop) frequently present due to reduced LV compliance
- Paradoxical splitting of S_2
- Narrow pulse pressure
- Best heard over right 2nd interspace, transmitted to carotid arteries
- ECG may show left ventricular strain pattern.
- Echocardiography demonstrates diseased valve.
- Calcification of aortic valve may be seen on CXR.

Treatment

- Avoid strenuous activity.
- Avoid afterload reduction.
- Valve replacement is definitive therapy.
- Valvuloplasty produces only temporary improvement as rate of restenosis is very high.

AORTIC REGURGITATION

Etiology

- Aortic root dilatation: Idiopathic (correlates with hypertension [HTN] and age), collagen vascular disease, Marfan's syndrome
- Valvular disease: Rheumatic heart disease, endocarditis
- Proximal aortic root dissection: Cystic medial necrosis (Marfan's syndrome), syphilis, HTN, Ehlers–Danlos, Turner's syndrome, 3rd trimester pregnancy

Signs and Symptoms

- Dyspnea, orthopnea, paroxysmal nocturnal dyspnea
- Angina (due to reduced diastolic coronary blood flow due to low pressure in aortic root)
- Left ventricular failure
- Wide pulse pressure
- Bounding "Corrigan" pulse, "pistol shot" femorals, pulsus bisferiens (dicrotic pulse with two palpable waves in systole)
- Duroziez sign: Presence of diastolic femoral bruit when femoral artery is compressed enough to hear a systolic bruit
- Hill's sign: Systolic pressure in the legs > 20 mm Hg higher than in the arms
- Quincke's sign: Alternating blushing and blanching of the fingernails when gentle pressure is applied
- De Musset's sign: Bobbing of head with heartbeat

Left ventricular strain pattern is ST segment depression and T wave inversion in I, aVL, and left precordial leads.

Patients with aortic stenosis should be considered for valve replacement for:
- persistent symptoms
- aortic orifice <0.5 cm²/m² body surface area

Other conditions with wide pulse pressure:
- Hyperthyroidism
- Anemia
- Wet beriberi
- Hypertrophic subaortic stenosis
- Hypertension

Diagnosis

- High-pitched, blowing, decrescendo diastolic murmur best heard over 2nd right interspace or 3rd left interspace, accentuated by leaning forward
- Austin Flint murmur: Observed in severe regurgitation, low-pitched diastolic rumble due to regurgitated blood striking the anterior mitral leaflet (similar sound to mitral regurgitation)
- A2 accentuated (due to high pulse pressure in the aorta at the beginning of ventricular diastole)
- Hyperdynamic down and laterally displaced PMI due to LV enlargement
- ECG shows left ventricular hypertrophy (see Figure 2-4).
- Echocardiography demonstrates regurgitant valve.

Treatment

- Treat left ventricular failure.
- Endocarditis prophylaxis
- Valve replacement is necessary for severe cases and is the only definitive treatment.

TRICUSPID STENOSIS

Etiology

Rheumatic heart disease, congenital, carcinoid

Signs and Symptoms

- Peripheral edema
- JVD
- Hepatomegaly, ascites, jaundice

Diagnosis

- Murmur is diastolic, rumbling, low pitched
- Murmur accentuated with inspiration
- Accentuated precordial thrust of right ventricle
- Diastolic thrill at lower left sternal border
- Best heard over left sternal border between 4th to 5th interspace
- Echocardiography demonstrates diseased valve.

Treatment

Surgical repair

A rumbling diastolic murmur can be due to mitral stenosis (MS) or tricuspid stenosis (TS). TS will increase with inspiration.

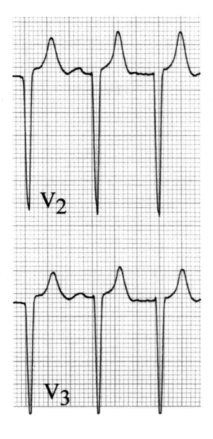

FIGURE 2-4. Left ventricular hypertrophy.

TRICUSPID REGURGITATION

Etiology

- Increased pulmonary artery pressure (e.g., from left-sided failure or mitral regurgitation/stenosis)
- Right ventricular dilation stretching the outflow tract (e.g., from right heart failure, infarction, or tricuspid regurgitation itself)
- Right papillary muscle rupture from infarction
- Tricuspid valvular lesions (e.g., from rheumatic heart disease or bacterial endocarditis)

Signs and Symptoms

- Signs of right heart failure: Prominent JVD, pulsatile liver

Right-sided bacterial endocarditis is most frequently associated with nonsterile technique in IV drug abusers.

A holosystolic murmur can be due to mitral regurgitation, tricuspid regurgitation, or ventricular septal defect.

Diagnosis

- Holosystolic, blowing, medium-pitched murmur heard best along the left sternal border in the 5th interspace, accentuated with inspiration
- ECG shows right ventricular enlargement.
- Atrial fibrillation is common.
- Echocardiography demonstrates diseased valve.

Treatment

- Treat left heart failure, if applicable.
- Diuresis to reduce volume load
- Surgical repair and endocarditis prophylaxis if valve defective

DILATED CARDIOMYOPATHY

Definition

Left or right ventricular enlargement with loss of contractile function causing congestive heart failure, dysrhythmias, or thrombus formation

Etiology

Infectious
- Irreversible—viral myocarditis

Toxic
- Reversible—prolonged EtOH abuse
- Irreversible—doxorubicin (Adriamycin), cocaine, heavy metals (Pb, Hg, Cb)

Endocrine
- Reversible—thyroid disease (hypo or hyper)
- Irreversible—acromegaly, pheochromocytoma

Metabolic
- Reversible—hypocalcemia, hypophosphatemia, thiamine deficiency (wet beriberi), selenium deficiency
- Genetic: 20% of cases have positive family histories
- Other: Pregnancy (reversible), neuromuscular disease (usually irreversible), idiopathic (usually irreversible)

Pathophysiology

- Dilatation and stiffening of ventricles
- Valvular dilatation, tricuspid and mitral regurgitation due to misalignment of papillary muscles
- Dysrhythmias
- Mural thrombi

Signs and Symptoms

- Symptoms similar to that of heart failure
- Angina due to increased O_2 demands of enlarged ventricles
- Neurologic deficits from thrombus emboli

Diagnosis

- Auscultation—S_3/S_4 gallop murmurs (stiffened ventricular walls), regurgitant valves, rales
- ECG—ventricular hypertrophy, bundle branch blocks (see Figure 2-5), nonspecific ST segment/T wave changes, dysrhythmias (atrial fibrillation most common)
- CXR—enlarged cardiac silhouette, pulmonary venous congestion
- Echocardiography—enlarged ventricles/atria, regurgitant valves, low ejection fractions

Treatment

- Address any reversible causes (e.g., discontinue toxic agent)
- Supportive care—medical management of heart failure (ACE inhibitors reduce mortality)
- Implanted automatic defibrillator for patients with life-threatening dysrhythmias
- Heart transplant

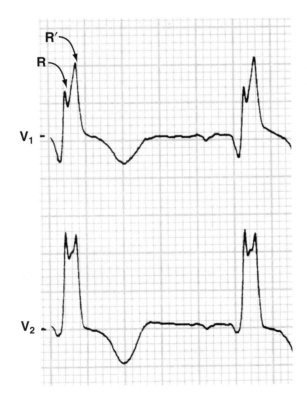

FIGURE 2-5. Right bundle branch block.

Definition

Scarring and infiltration of the myocardium causing decreased right or left ventricular filling

Etiology

- Endomyocardial fibroelastosis
- Eosinophilic endomyocardial disease (hypereosinophilic syndrome)
- Primary amyloidosis
- Hemochromatosis
- Sarcoidosis
- Carcinoid syndrome

Signs and Symptoms

- Signs of left/right heart failure, right failure usually predominates
- Exercise intolerance is common presenting symptom

Diagnosis

- Auscultation—S_3/S_4 gallop murmurs, mitral/tricuspid regurgitation
- ECG—low voltages, conduction abnormalities, nonspecific ST segment/T wave changes
- CXR—normal cardiac silhouette or enlarged atria, pulmonary venous congestion
- Echocardiography—normal-sized ventricles, large atria, thickened ventricular walls, mitral/tricuspid regurgitation
- Endomyocardial biopsy

Restrictive cardiomyopathy is often difficult to distinguish from constrictive pericarditis—biopsy can usually confirm.

Treatment

- Treatment is generally ineffective.
- In hemochromatosis, phlebotomy and desferrioxamine permit some recovery.

HYPERTROPHIC CARDIOMYOPATHY

Definition

Hypertrophy of the interventricular septum narrows the LV outflow tract. High-velocity systolic flow draws the anterior leaflet of the mitral valve into the tract (via the Bernoulli effect) causing a dynamic left ventricular outflow tract obstruction.

Hypertrophic cardiomyopathy is sometimes called idiopathic hypertrophic subaortic stenosis, or IHSS.

Etiology

- ~50% idiopathic, ~50% familial (autosomal dominant, with variable penetrance)
- Conditions that increase the LV end diastolic volume decrease the obstruction (e.g., increased blood volume, negative inotropic drugs, rest, increased peripheral resistance)
- Outflow obstruction can result in left atrial dilatation, atrial fibrillation, CHF, right heart failure, etc.

Signs and Symptoms

Angina
- Not well understood in terms of known pathophysiology
- Occurs at rest and during exercise
- Frequently unresponsive to nitroglycerin
- May respond to recumbent position (pathognomonic but rare)

Syncope
- Most often occurs following exercise
- Arrhythmias: Atrial fibrillation, ventricular tachycardia
- Palpitations due to arrhythmias
- Signs of CHF
- Sudden death is usually due to an arrhythmia rather than obstruction.

Diagnosis

- Systolic ejection murmur heard best along the left sternal border, decreases with increased LV blood volume (squatting), increases with increased blood velocities (exercise), and decreased LV end-diastolic volume (Valsalva)
- Paradoxical splitting of S_2
- ECG: LVH, PVCs, atrial fibrillation, septal Q waves, nonspecific ST segment and T wave abnormalities
- Echocardiography: Septal hypertrophy, LVH, small LV

Treatment

- Amiodarone may reduce the incidence of life-threatening dysrhythmias.
- Beta blockers reduce heart rate, increasing LV filling time and decreasing inotropy; calcium channel blockers considered second-line agents.
- Septal myomectomy for severely symptomatic patients
- Mitral valve replacement can reduce obstruction.
- Permanent pacemaker to change pattern of ventricular contraction, reducing obstruction
- Implanted automatic defibrillator should be considered.
- Patient should refrain from vigorous exercise.

Causes of paradoxical splitting of S_2:
- Hypertrophic cardiomyopathy
- Aortic stenosis
- LBBB

Typical scenario:
A 25-year-old man becomes severely dyspneic and collapses while running laps. His father had died suddenly at an early age. *Think: Hypertrophic cardiomyopathy.*

Splitting of S_2:
Normal physiologic: Aortic before pulmonic valve closure. Split widened by inspiration as increasingly negative intrathoracic pressure augments R heart filling, resulting in longer ventricular emptying times.
Paradoxical: Pulmonic before aortic valve due to a delay in aortic valve closure. Inspiration still delays pulmonic closure but now brings it closer to aortic closure, *paradoxically* narrowing the split.

Very few murmurs *decrease* with squatting (this one does).

Definition

Inflammation of the myocardium

Coxsackie B is the most common viral cause of myocarditis.

Etiology

- Viral—coxsackie A or B, echovirus, HIV, cytomegalovirus (CMV), influenza, Epstein–Barr, hepatitis B virus (HBV), adenovirus
- Bacterial—group A beta-hemolytic strep (rheumatic fever), *Corynebacterium, Meningococcus, B. burgdorferi* (Lyme), *Mycoplasma pneumoniae*
- Parasitic—*Trypanosoma cruzi* (Chagas'), *Toxoplasma, Trichinella, Echinococcus*
- Systemic disease—Kawasaki's, systemic lupus erythematosus (SLE), sarcoidosis, inflammatory conditions
- Drug allergies—sulfonamides, penicillins
- Cocaine
- Idiopathic—common

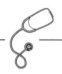

Symptoms prior to 30 years of age correlate with increased risk of sudden death, but severity of symptoms (whenever they occur) does not.

Signs and Symptoms

Spectrum of disease ranges from asymptomatic to fulminant cardiac failure and death. Findings may include:
- Retrosternal or precordial chest pain
- Fever, fatigue
- Preceding upper respiratory infection (URI)
- Palpitations, syncope
- Signs of CHF (dyspnea, rales, peripheral edema, JVD)

Diagnosis

- Auscultation—S_3/S_4, mitral or tricuspid regurgitation, friction rub (if pericardium involved)
- ECG—ST segment changes, low voltage, dysrhythmias, conduction disturbances
- CXR—often normal, cardiomegaly, pulmonary venous congestion
- Echocardiography—hypokinetic wall movements, dilated ventricles/atria, pericardial effusion
- Labs—leukocytosis, elevated ESR, elevated cardiac enzymes (slower rise and fall than acute MI, troponin I is most sensitive)
- Myocardial biopsy

Myocarditis often is associated with acute pericarditis.

Treatment

- Primarily supportive—admit to ICU, limit activity
- Treat heart failure, dysrhythmias—ACE inhibitors reduce necrosis and inflammation, digoxin should be used cautiously as its effects may be exaggerated by the inflamed myocardium.
- Address etiology if known/applicable (e.g., antivirals, antibiotics, diptheria—antitoxin).

- Immunosuppressive agents are contraindicated (steroids, cyclosporine, NSAIDs).
- IV immunoglobulin G (IgG) may be of benefit.

BACTERIAL ENDOCARDITIS

Bacterial endocarditis is a localized infection of the endocardium characterized by vegetations involving the valve leaflets or walls. It is best categorized by the infecting organism, which determines the course of the disease. It can also be classified as acute (ABE) or subacute (SBE).

ABE
- Infection of **healthy valves** by high-virulence organisms
- Produces metastatic foci
- Usually fatal if not treated within 6 weeks
- Most common organism is *S. aureus*

SBE
- Seeding of **previously damaged valves** (rheumatic heart disease, congenital valve defects: mitral valve prolapse) by low-virulence organisms
- Does not produce metastatic foci
- Most common organism is *Streptococcus viridans*
- Mitral valve is most often affected

Etiology
- Acute: *S. aureus*
- Subacute: *Streptococcus viridans*, other oral flora, group A beta-hemolytic strep, enterococci
- IV drug users: *S. aureus*, streptococci, enterococci, *Candida*
- Prosthetic valves (10 to 20% of cases): *S. aureus*, *Streptococcus viridans*, gram negative bacilli, fungi
- Nosocomial infections: Indwelling venous catheters, hemodialysis, CT surgery

There is a strong association between *Streptococcus bovis* endocarditis and colonic neoplasms.

Signs and Symptoms

ABE
- Acute onset of fever, chills, rigors
- New cardiac murmur
- Metastatic infections—meningitis, pneumonia

SBE
- Gradual onset of fever, sweats, weakness, arthralgia, anorexia, weight loss, and cutaneous lesions
- New cardiac murmur
- Splenomegaly

IV drug users: Right-sided ABE most often affects the tricuspid valve, septic pulmonary emboli are common.

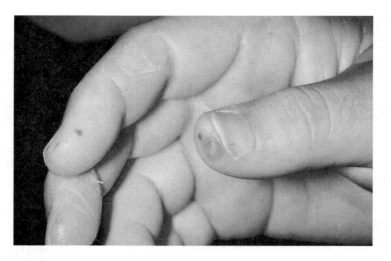

FIGURE 2-6. Osler's node.

(Courtesy of the Armed Forces Institute of Pathology, Bethesda, Maryland. Reproduced, with permission, from Knoop, Stack, and Storrow. *Atlas of Emergency Medicine.* New York: McGraw-Hill, 1997: 349.)

- Petechiae: Multiple nonblanching red macules on upper chest and mucous membranes
- **Osler's nodes:** Tender violaceous subcutaneous nodules on fingers and toes (see Figure 2-6)
- **Splinter hemorrhages:** Fine linear hemorrhages in middle of nailbed (see Figure 2-7)
- **Janeway lesions:** Multiple hemorrhagic nontender macules or nodules on palms and soles (see Figure 2-8)
- **Roth's spots:** Retinal hemorrhages seen on funduscopy
- Conjunctival hemorrhages

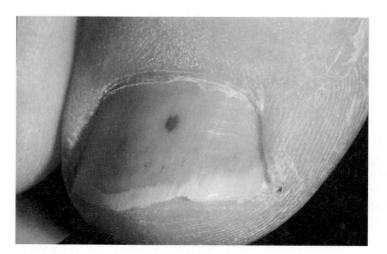

FIGURE 2-7. Splinter hemorrhage.

(Courtesy of the Armed Forces Institute of Pathology, Bethesda, Maryland. Reproduced, with permission, from Knoop, Stack, and Storrow. *Atlas of Emergency Medicine.* New York: McGraw-Hill, 1997: 349.)

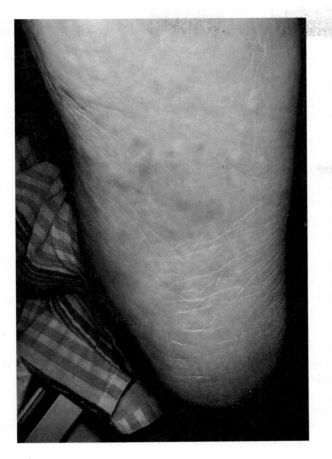

FIGURE 2-8. Janeway lesion.
(Courtesy of the Department of Dermatology, Wilford Hall USAF Medical Center and Brooke Army Medical Center, San Antonio, Texas. Reproduced, with permission, from Knoop, Stack, and Storrow. *Atlas of Emergency Medicine.* New York: McGraw-Hill, 1997: 348.)

Diagnosis

- Two positive blood cultures taken at least 12 hours apart, or 3+ positive cultures taken at least 1 hour apart
- Echocardiography—vegetations are pathognomonic but their absence does not rule out endocarditis; transesophageal echo is more sensitive.
- Labs—urinalysis may show hematuria, elevated ESR/C-reactive protein, leukocytosis

Treatment

- Streptococci: Penicillin G or ceftriaxone × 4 weeks
- Staphylococci: Nafcillin or oxacillin × 4 weeks
- MRSA: Vancomycin × 4 weeks

Definition

Inflammation of the pericardium

Etiology

Common Causes of Pericarditis

- Viral—pericarditis frequently occurs following a recent viral URI, though a definitive cause is not known.
- Bacterial—TB, streptococci, staphylococci
- Metastases—1° tumors usually breast or lung
- Acute myocardial infarction:
  - Immediate post-MI pericarditis—occurs within 24 hours of a *transmural* infarction due to direct pericardial irritation
  - Dressler's syndrome—pericarditis occurring one week to months after an MI due to an autoimmune response to infarcted myocardium, can progress to chronic condition
- Uremia—chronic renal failure, mental status changes
- Radiation—radiotherapy, occupational/environmental exposure
- Drug reaction—hydralazine, procainamide, isoniazid
- Collagen vascular tissue—SLE, scleroderma
- Myxedema
- Trauma—postpericardiotomy syndrome following CT surgery (usually brief clinical course)
- Idiopathic

Signs and Symptoms

- Chest pain, often pleuritic (inspiratory), radiating to left trapezial ridge
- Pain often relieved by sitting up and leaning forward
- Pain does not respond to nitroglycerin.

Diagnosis

- Auscultation—pericardial friction rub on expiration, pathognomonic but variably present
- ECG—*diffuse* ST elevations and PR depressions, low voltage (see Figure 2-9)
- CXR—possibly enlarged cardiac silhouette 2° to pericardial effusion
- Echocardiography—possible pericardial effusion

Treatment

- Address underlying cause if known/applicable.
- NSAIDs to relieve pain and reduce inflammation (ASA, indomethacin, ibuprofen)
- Steroids for intractable cases (e.g., Dressler's)

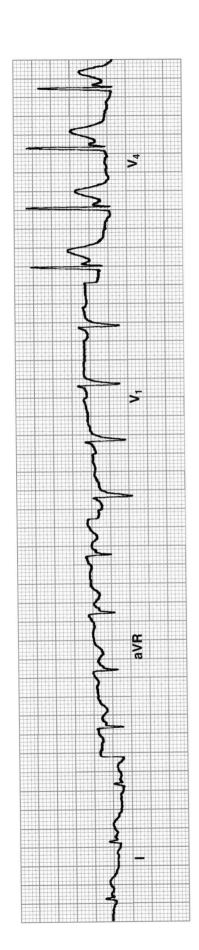
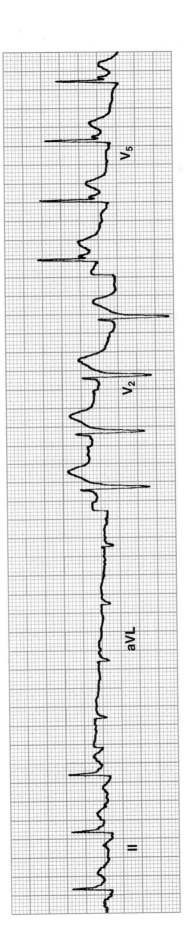
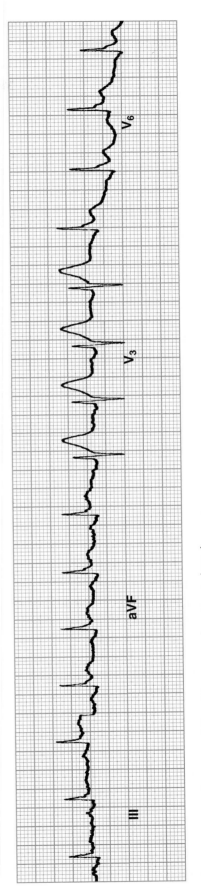

FIGURE 2-9. Pericarditis. Note *diffuse* ST segment elevation and PR depression.

PERICARDIAL TAMPONADE

Definition

Tamponade is the physiologic result of rapid accumulation of fluid in the in-elastic pericardial sac. Pericardial tamponade impairs cardiac filling and reduces cardiac output.

Etiology

- Pericarditis
- Trauma (accidental or iatrogenic)
- Ruptured ventricular wall (post MI)
- Aortic dissection with rupture into pericardium

Pulsus paradoxus is a transient fall in measured blood pressure > 10 mm Hg associated with inspiration (due to reduced stroke volume during inspiration).

Signs and Symptoms

Beck's Triad
- Hypotension
- Muffled heart sounds
- JVD

Other Symptoms
- Dyspnea
- Tachycardia
- Pulsus paradoxus
- Narrow pulse pressure

Diagnosis

- Auscultation may demonstrate distant heart sounds.
- ECG may show low voltage or electrical alternans.
- CXR may show enlarged cardiac silhouette.
- Echocardiogram will show large pericardial effusion.

Tamponade physiology:
During inspiration, venous return to the right atrium increases. In tamponade, the transiently enlarged right atrium bulges leftward, reducing left ventricular volume and output, causing BP to fall with inspiration.

Treatment

- Immediate pericardiocentesis for unstable patients
- Infuse fluids to expand volume.
- Pericardial window (surgery) for meta-stable and stable patients

CONSTRICTIVE PERICARDITIS

Pericardiocentesis yielding clotting blood probably came from the right ventricle, not the pericardial sac.

Definition

Granulation and scarring of the pericardium due to acute pericarditis. Cardiac output is limited.

Signs and Symptoms

- Dyspnea
- Fatigue
- Tachycardia
- JVD with patient upright
- Kussmaul's sign
- Left ventricular failure
- Peripheral edema

Kussmaul's sign is failure of jugular venous pressure to fall during inspiration.

Diagnosis

- Auscultation may demonstrate distant heart sounds.
- CXR may show pericardial calcification.
- ECG may show low voltage, T wave flattening or inversion in V_1 and V_2, notched P waves.
- Echocardiogram may show pericardial thickening.

Treatment

- Pericardiectomy

DYSRHYTHMIAS

VENTRICULAR FIBRILLATION AND PULSELESS VENTRICULAR TACHYCARDIA

Definition

- Ventricular fibrillation (see Figure 2-10) is disorganized electrical activity of the ventricular myocardium. Because the myocardium depolarizes in an irregular, disorganized fashion, regular myocardial contraction does not occur.
- Ventricular tachycardia is organized but inefficient depolarization of the myocardium (see Figure 2-11). It may degenerate into V-fib.

Ventricular fibrillation usually occurs after ventricular tachycardia.

Etiology

- Ischemic heart disease
- Myocardial infarction
- Prolonged QT syndrome
- Torsade de pointes
- Wolff–Parkinson–White (WPW) with A-fib and rapid ventricular response
- Administration of antidysrhythmic drugs

Signs and Symptoms

- Ventricular fibrillation is not compatible with life. A patient with V-fib lasting more than 5 to 6 seconds will lose consciousness.

HIGH-YIELD FACTS

Cardiology

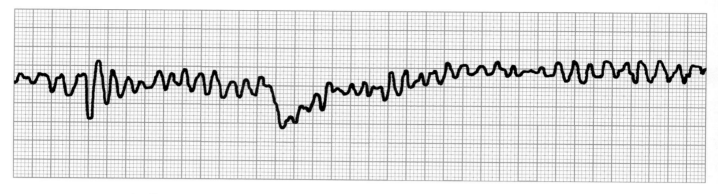

FIGURE 2-10. Ventricular fibrillation.

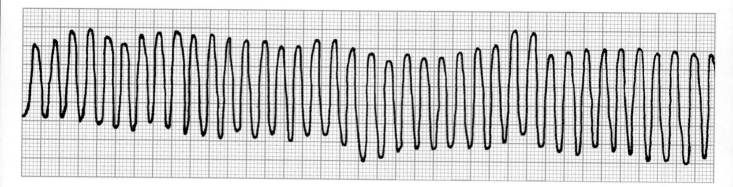

FIGURE 2-11. Ventricular tachycardia.

Causes of
prolonged QT:
"QT WIDTH"
QT: Prolonged QT
    syndrome
W: WPW
  I: Infarction
D: Drugs
T: Torsade
H: Heart disease
    (ischemic)

Treatment

- Bedside emergent DC cardioversion 200J, followed by 300J, then 360J if not successful
- Follow with epinephrine or vasopressin; shock again.
- If still no response, give amiodarone, lidocaine, magnesium, and procainamide with one shock between each drug (see Table 2-6 for clinical uses of cardiac medications).

For Prevention
- Cardiac pacemaker
- Implanted cardioverter/defibrillator (ICD)
- Electrophysiologic testing and radiofrequency ablation for accessory bypass tracts, AV nodal reentrant SVT, and others

TORSADE DE POINTES

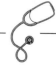

Cause of short QT:
Hypercalcemia

Definition

Arrhythmia with rotating axis and prolonged QT (see Figure 2-12)

Etiology

- Hypokalemia
- Hypomagnesemia

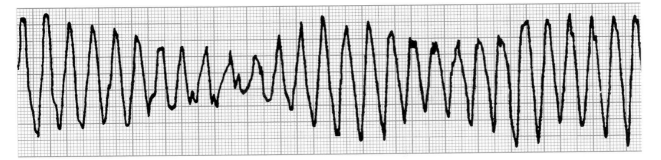

FIGURE 2-12. Torsade de pointes. Note bizarre, twisted point of QRS complexes and varying amplitude.

- Phenothiazines
- Tricyclic antidepressants
- Intracranial bleed
- Congenital prolonged QT syndrome
- Idiopathic
- Type I antidysrhythmics: Quinidine and procainamide

Signs and Symptoms

- Polymorphic ventricular tachycardia
- QT prolongation
- Often associated with syncope
- May degenerate into V-fib

Treatment

- Magnesium IV
- Overdrive pacing
- Beta blockers for prolonged QT syndrome

Causes of Torsade:
POINTES
Phenothiazines
Other meds (tricyclic antidepressants)
Intracranial bleed
No known cause (idiopathic)
Type I antidysrhythmics
Electrolyte abnormalities
Syndrome of prolonged QT

ATRIAL FIBRILLATION

Definition

- Disorganized electrical activity of the atrial myocardium, causing ineffective atrial contractions

Etiology

Seen often in patients with dilated atria, related to heart failure or valvular disease

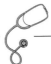

Atrial flutter may be confused with atrial fibrillation at high rates. Atrial flutter is distinguished by regular, distinct P waves in a sawtooth pattern.

Signs and Symptoms

- Sensation of palpitations or skipped beats
- Light-headedness, fatigue
- May develop chest pain
- May develop transient ischemic attack (TIA) or stroke

Causes of atrial fibrillation:
PIRATES
Pulmonary disease
Ischemia
Rheumatic heart disease
Anemia, atrial myxoma
Thyrotoxicosis
Ethanol
Sepsis

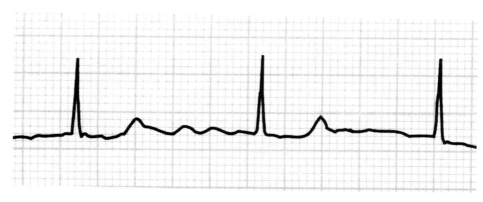

FIGURE 2-13. Atrial fibrillation. Note lack of P wave.

The ineffective atrial contractions of A-fib permit clot formation in the left atrium, which may embolize to the systemic circulation. Unless a patient is unstable, anticoagulate for 3 days prior to conversion to sinus rhythm.

Rapid atrial fibrillation is often difficult to identify. Adenosine can be used to temporarily slow a rapid supraventricular rhythm.

Diagnosis

- Pulse is irregularly irregular.
- ECG: P waves are irregular or difficult to identify; R-R interval is variable (see Figure 2-13).
- Echo: May be used to identify presence of clot in the left atrium

Treatment

For Stable Patients with Rate < 100 bpm
- Anticoagulate with heparin, followed by warfarin when therapeutic, unless contraindicated.

For Stable Patients with Rate > 100 bpm
- Obtain history of WPW or accessory bypass tract. (See next section for management.)
- Slow rhythm with an IV push of a calcium channel blocker (diltiazem) or a beta blocker (esmolol), followed by a drip of the medication that worked.
- Load patients with digoxin in divided doses and titrate to a therapeutic level.
- Anticoagulate.

For Unstable Patients with Any Rate
- Immediate synchronized cardioversion

WOLFF–PARKINSON–WHITE SYNDROME

Definition

- **WPW** is a ventricular preexcitation syndrome: An abnormal bundle of fast-conducting fibers connects the atria and ventricles and allow electrical impulse generated by the sinus node to bypass the normal anatomic conduction pathways.
- Anterograde conduction occurs down the His–Purkinje system and back up the accessory bypass tract (narrow-complex).
- Retrograde conduction occurs down the accessory bypass tract and up the His–Purkinje system (wide-complex).

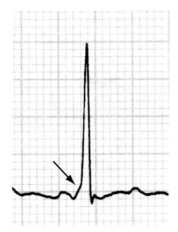

FIGURE 2-14. Wolff–Parkinson–White syndrome. Note slurred upstroke of QRS (arrow) known as the "delta" wave.

Diagnosis

- ECG: Shows a "delta" wave, a slurred upstroke of the QRS complex (see Figure 2-14)
- Patients with suspected WPW should have electrophysiologic testing in the cardiac catheterization lab and radiofrequency ablation of the detected bypass tract.

Treatment

- Patients with WPW, rapid atrial fibrillation, and rapid ventricular response require emergent synchronized cardioversion.
- Stable patients with WPW and atrial fibrillation or wide-complex SVT are treated with amiodarone, flecanide, procainamide, propafenone, or sotalol.
- Adenosine, beta blockers, calcium channel blockers, and digoxin are *contraindicated* because they preferentially block conduction at the AV node, allowing unopposed conduction down the accessory bypass tract.

Don't give ABCD (adenosine, beta blockers, calcium channel blocker, or digoxin) to someone with WPW.

HEART BLOCK

First-Degree Heart Block

- Prolonged PR interval (> 0.20 s) (see Figure 2-15)

Second-Degree Heart Block

Mobitz I (Wenckebach) (see Figure 2-16)
- Progressive PR prolongation with progressive shortening of the R-R interval until a beat is dropped
- For inadequate perfusion, treat with atropine or temporary pacing.

Mobitz II (see Figure 2-17)
- Fixed prolonged PR interval followed by a non-conducted beat at a regular interval
- Treat with atropine, temporary pacing, and permanent pacemaker.

Causes of Mobitz I:
- Inferior wall MI
- Digitalis toxicity
- Increased vagal tone

Causes of Mobitz II:
- Inferior wall or septal MI
- Conduction system disease

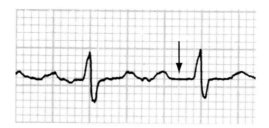

FIGURE 2-15. 1st-degree AV block. Note pause (arrow) before QRS complex.

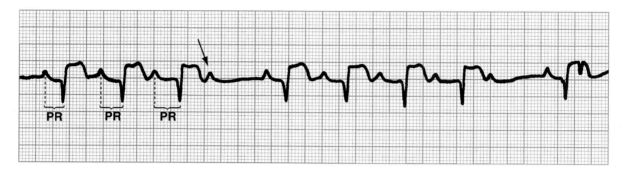

FIGURE 2-16. Wenckebach 2nd-degree AV block (Mobitz I). Note progressive lengthening of PR segment until a QRS complex is dropped. Arrow denotes nonconducted P wave.

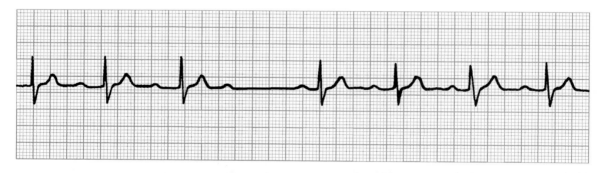

FIGURE 2-17. Mobitz II 2nd-degree AV block. Note constant PR interval followed by a non-conducted P at a regular interval.

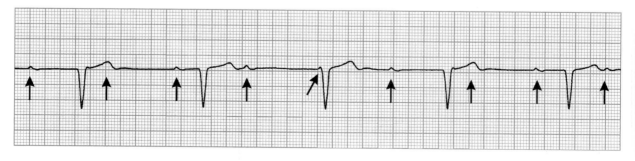

FIGURE 2-18. Complete (3rd-degree) AV block. Note dissociation between atrial and ventricular rhythms. Arrows denote P waves.

Third-Degree Heart Block (Complete Heart Block)

- Independent atrial and ventricular activity (see Figure 2-18)
- Treat symptomatic patients with atropine, temporary pacing, and permanent pacemaker.

SINUS BRADYCARDIA

Definition

- Rate below 60
- Normal P waves, PR intervals

Etiology

- Overmedication
- Inferior wall MI
- Increased intracranial pressure
- Hypothyroidism
- Carotid sinus hypersensitivity
- Normal variant: Well-trained athletes can have very low resting heart rates.

Signs and Symptoms

Often asymptomatic

Treatment

- Asymptomatic patients do not require immediate treatment: Look for underlying cause.
- Symptomatic patients: Atropine
- External or transvenous pacing
- Consider dopamine drip.

HYPERTENSION

Definition

Defined as an sBP > 140 or dBP > 90 on two separate occasions (see Table 2-5)

Epidemiology

- 25 to 35% of adults have hypertension

Etiology

- Essential hypertension (primary, idiopathic)
- Secondary causes:

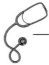

Causes of third-degree heart block:
- Inferior wall MI
- Digitalis toxicity
- Conduction system disease

"One INCH"
If the R-R distance is at least one inch, consider:
O: Overmedication
I: Inferior wall MI
Increased intracranial pressure
N: Normal variant
C: Carotid sinus hypersensitivity
H: Hypothyroidism

Over 90% of hypertension is essential, or idiopathic.

Hypertension due to **Pheochromocytoma** is characterized by ectopic production of epinephrine and norepinephrine, causing wide swings in blood pressure.

- Renal parenchymal disease (chronic pyelonephritis)
- Renal artery stenosis
- Primary hyperaldosteronism (Cushing's and Conn's syndromes)
- Pheochromocytoma
- Eclampsia and preeclampsia
- Coarctation of the aorta (congenital)

TABLE 2-5. Definition of Hypertension

Hypertension	Systolic Blood Pressure	Diastolic Blood Pressure
Stage 1	140–159	90–99
Stage 2	160–179	100–109
Stage 3	180–209	110–119
Stage 4	> 210	> 120

If patients do not fit into a discrete category, use the highest (worst) one.

Pathophysiology

Usual mechanism is a normal cardiac output with increased peripheral vascular resistance.

Risk Factors

- Diabetes
- High-sodium diet
- Obesity
- Tobacco use
- Family history of hypertension
- Black race
- Male gender

Signs and Symptoms

Most patients with hypertension have no symptoms. Patients with stage 3 or 4 hypertension (severe) may present with:
- Light-headedness
- Morning occipital headaches
- Epistaxis
- Hematuria
- Blurred vision
- Angina
- Congestive heart failure

Diagnosis

- Blood pressure in both arms, repeated if abnormal
- Funduscopic examination to look for AV nicking, hemorrhage, papilledema

- Auscultation for renal artery bruits
- ECG
- Urinalysis to look for active sediment, hematuria
- Blood urea nitrogen (BUN)/creatinine, serum potassium (evidence of renal insufficiency)

Treatment

For repeated elevated blood pressure measurements:
- Dietary changes: High fruits, vegetables, and low-fat dairy products, low total and saturated fats, low salt
- Weight loss, physical exercise
- Low-dose thiazide diuretics or beta blockers have proven mortality benefit.
- Low-dose ACE inhibitor or calcium channel blockers are also effective.
- Two- or three-drug therapy for patients not initially controlled (see Table 2–6 for commonly used cardiac medications)

Complications of Hypertension

Increases risk of:
- Stroke
- MI
- Atrial fibrillation
- Heart failure
- Peripheral vascular disease
- Renal disease

An active urinary sediment contains blood, protein, and red and white cell casts.

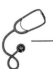

- ACE inhibitors are more effective in whites and diabetics.
- Calcium channel blockers are more effective in blacks.
- Beta blockers can cause hypertriglyceridemia via their actions on the pancreas.

HYPERTENSIVE EMERGENCY

Definition

Malignant hypertension is characterized by severely elevated blood pressure accompanied by end-organ damage. New-onset neurologic signs, papilledema, chest pain or heart failure, and renal failure should alert the physician to the need for rapid blood pressure reduction.

Diagnosis

- Presence of end-organ damage (ECG changes, new-onset renal failure, active urinary sediment, intracranial bleed, etc.)

Treatment

Reduce the mean arterial pressure by no more than 1/3. Common intravenous agents include:
- Nitroglycerin
- Nitroprusside
- Labetalol
- Phentolamine for pheochromocytoma
- Hydralazine or magnesium for preeclampsia-related hypertension

Use parenteral blood pressure–lowering agents only if end-organ damage is found, due to the risk of rapid reduction in coronary and cerebral perfusion.

The **mean arterial pressure** is: $(2dBP + sBP)/3$

Nitroprusside can cause cyanide toxicity.

Definition

- Usually associated with a transverse tear through the intima and internal media of the aortic wall
- Can lead to death by extension of the intimal tear to a full-thickness tear with hemorrhage into the extravascular space, dissection into the pericardium with tamponade, or extension into the branch arteries, including coronary arteries, carotids, mesenteric, renal, and iliac arteries

Classification

DeBakey
Type I: Ascending plus part of distal aorta (most common)
Type II: Ascending aorta only
Type III: Distal aorta only

Stanford
Type A: Ascending aorta
Type B: Descending aorta

Etiology

- Hypertension
- Congenital heart disease
- Connective tissue disease (Marfan's and Ehlers–Danlos syndromes)
- Trauma
- Pregnancy (3rd trimester)
- Aortic coarctation (Turner's syndrome, idiopathic)
- Cocaine use

Signs and Symptoms

- Severe "tearing" chest pain, may radiate to back
- Hypertension
- Unequal pulses distally for descending aortic dissection
- Aortic regurgitation murmur transmitted down right sternal border with ascending aortic dissection

Diagnosis

- CXR: Can be normal but often shows widened mediastinum, apical pleural capping, and loss of the aortic knob
- Helical CT with IV contrast *or* transesophageal echocardiography: May show dissection with extravasation of blood, intimal flap
- If aortic dissection is strongly suspected despite negative studies, the gold standard is angiogram.

Type A involves the Ascending aorta and can extend to descending aorta. **Type B** involves only the descending aorta.

Aortic dissection due to syphilis occurs because the treponema infect the vasa vasorum of the aorta.

Causes of aortic dissection:
PATC³H
Pregnancy
Aortic coarctation
Trauma
Cocaine, congential, connective tissue
Hypertension

HIGH-YIELD FACTS

Cardiology

Treatment

- Keep systolic blood pressure below 120, as long as the patient can maintain organ perfusion.
- Immediate surgical repair for type A dissection (ascending aorta)
- Medical stabilization for type B dissection (descending aorta)

Complications

- Myocardial infarction (dissection or obstruction of coronary arteries)
- Stroke (dissection or obstruction of carotids)
- Aortic regurgitation (dissection through aortic root)
- Cardiac tamponade (dissection into pericardium)

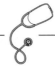

Always get a chest film when you suspect MI: Some of these patients will have aortic dissection, and thrombolysis may kill them.

HIGH-YIELD FACTS

Cardiology

AORTIC ANEURYSM

Definition

- The term *aortic aneurysm* generally refers to aneurysm of the abdominal aorta.
- **True aneurysm:** Disruption of all three layers of the aortic wall
- **Pseudoaneurysm:** Disruption of intima and media

Etiology

- Atherosclerosis
- Cystic medial necrosis
- Syphilis
- Mycotic infection
- Trauma
- Aortitis

Signs and Symptoms

- Most patients are asymptomatic.
- Back pain or abdominal pain radiating to the back
- Syncope
- Pulsatile abdominal mass
- Unequal pulses in upper and lower extremities

Diagnosis

- Abdominal ultrasound
- Computed tomograph (CT) of abdomen with IV contrast

The unstable patient with signs and symptoms suggestive of ruptured aortic aneurysm should be evaluated by a surgeon, without delay, before imaging.

Treatment

- Surgical repair for rapidly expanding aneurysms or those > 6.5 cm
- Control blood pressure.
- Blood transfusion, if necessary

TABLE 2-6. Commonly Used Cardiac Medications

	Medication	Main Clinical Uses	Adverse Effects
Class I: Sodium channel blockers	Lidocaine	Suppresses ventricular dysrhythmias	Mild: drowsiness, confusion, ataxia Severe: psychosis, seizures, AV block, respiratory depression
	Quinidine	Suppresses ventricular dysrhythmias, atrial premature beats, A-fib	Cinchonism: tinnitus, hearing loss, visual changes, delirium, psychosis. Also causes GI upset, promotes torsade de pointes (prodysrhythmic). Potentates many other medications.
	Procainamide	Suppresses ventricular dysrhythmias and A-fib, A-flutter, WPW	Myocardial depression, prolonged QT and QRS, torsade de pointes, V-fib
Class II: Beta blockers	Propranolol	SVT, thyrotoxicosis, acute MI, HTN	All beta blockers can cause bronchoconstriction; use with caution in asthmatics. Hypotension, light-headedness, fatigue, depression, and elevation of triglycerides can occur.
	Metoprolol	SVT, acute MI, HTN	
	Esmolol	SVT, thyrotoxicosis	
	Labetalol	Hypertension	
Class III: Prolongs action potentials	Amiodarone	VT, VF, A-Fib, WPW	Bradycardia, AV block, peripheral neuropathy, pulmonary fibrosis, corneal deposits, skin discoloration
	Bretylium	Ventricular dysrhythmias	Transient hypertension, hypotension
	Sotalol	AV reentry SVT, WPW	Bradycardia, CHF, peripheral edema
Class IV: Calcium channel blockers	Verapamil	Mild to moderate HTN	All calcium channel blockers reduce inotropy and are contraindicated in patients with heart failure, 2nd- or 3rd-degree heart block.
	Diltiazem	Mild to moderate HTN	
	Nifedipine	Mild to moderate HTN	
Other antidysrhythmic agents	Adenosine	Supraventricular tachycardia	Transient asystole, hypotension, flushing
	Digoxin	Rate control of atrial tachydysrhythmia, increased inotropy for CHF	Toxicity can occur in therapeutic range. Vomiting, anorexia, confusion, visual changes, AV block, PVCs, VT, VF. Hyperkalemia is seen with acute poisoning. Hypokalemia lowers threshold for toxicity (remember many drugs used for CHF can cause hypokalemia). Chronic therapy can cause gynecomastia.
	Magnesium	HTN due to preeclampsia, torsade de pointes	Hypotension, flushing, CNS changes, decreased reflexes, respiratory collapse
	Epinephrine	Asystole, anaphylaxis, pressor	May cause ischemia

TABLE 2-6. Commonly Used Cardiac Medications

Inotropic agents	Dopamine	Increases inotropy, chronotropic, pressor	Increases peripheral vasoconstriction at doses greater than 5–10 µg/kg/min
	Dobutamine	Increases inotropy	Associated with reflex arterial vasodilatation and tachycardia
	Atropine	Asystole, symptomatic bradycardia	Anticholinergic
	Nitroglycerin	Venous and coronary artery dilator, can be used for malignant hypertension	Hypotension, headache
Antihypertensive agents	Nitroprusside	Malignant hypertension	Can cause hypotension, cyanide toxicity, methemoglobinemia
	Minoxidil	Severe hypertension	Can cause hypotension, tachycardia, hair growth
	Hydralazine	Moderate to severe HTN, particularly in the setting of preeclampsia and eclampsia. Hydralazine is a direct vasodilator.	Can cause tachycardia, angina, lupuslike syndrome with a malar rash that disappears after discontinuing the drug
	Clonidine	Central-acting agent for HTN	Hypotension, rebound hypertension after halting medication
	Phentolamine	Parenteral alpha blocker used for HTN due to pheochromocytoma, cocaine	Hypotension, tachycardia, light-headedness
	Prazosin	PO alpha-blocker used for mild to moderate HTN	
	ACE inhibitors	Hypertension (decrease preload and afterload), nephroprotective CHF	All ACE inhibitors are variably associated with cough and angioedema and can cause acute renal failure in patients with bilateral renal artery stenosis. Captopril is associated with leukopenia and pancytopenia.
Antiplatelet agents	Aspirin	Used to prevent MI in patients with risk factors, can improve mortality from MI by about 25%	Associated with GI bleed. Some patients can have hypersensitivity reaction to aspirin.
	2b,3a inhibitors	Intravenous adjunct to heparin and thrombolysis in setting of acute MI; best use still being investigated	Can be associated with excessive bleeding
Antithrombotic agents	Warfarins	Long-term prevention of clots in deep vein thrombosis (DVT), A-fib, stroke, and others	Warfarins have an initial *procoagulant* effect. When anticoagulating as an inpatient, use heparin coverage initially. For outpatients, start at very low doses and raise gradually.
	Heparins	Myocardial infarction, pulmonary embolism, deep venous thrombosis	Both low-molecular-weight and unfractionated heparins can be associated with excessive bleeding.

(continues)

HIGH-YIELD FACTS

Cardiology

| TABLE 2-6. **Commonly Used Cardiac Medications (continued)** |

| Thrombolytic agents | Streptokinase | Myocardial infarction, pulmonary embolism, embolic cerebrovascular accident (CVA) | Relatively low cost. Cannot be used more than once within a 6-month period. Associated with hemorrhage at various sites. |
| | Tissue plasminogen activator | Myocardial infarction, pulmonary embolism, embolic CVA | High cost. Associated with hemorrhage at various sites. |

Pulmonology

Barbara G. Lock

HYPOXIA

- **Respiratory:** Due to V-Q mismatch, which is perfusion of poorly ventilated alveoli; or due to hypoventilation, both temporarily improved by supplemental oxygen
- **Right to left shunt:** Intrapulmonary due to perfusion of nonventilated lung, or extrapulmonary, such as congenital heart disease
- **Anemia:** Decreased hemoglobin decreases oxygen carrying capacity, has a normal PaO_2, decreased PvO_2
- **Circulatory hypoxia:** Poor perfusion due to heart failure or shock
- **Increased oxygen requirements:** Due to fever, thyrotoxicosis, exercise
- **Improper oxygen utilization:** Cytochrome impairment due to cyanide poisoning, diptheria toxin, etc.
- **Low inspired oxygen:** At high altitude or other low-oxygen environment
- **Carbon monoxide poisoning:** CO-Hgb "carboxy-Hgb" is unavailable for oxygen transport, O_2 unloaded at lower oxygen tensions. CO poisoning does not cause cyanosis. At highly toxic levels, it can cause a "cherry red" discoloration of lips and nails.

The most important determinant of the amount of oxygen delivery to tissues is *hemoglobin*.

Arterial oxygen content = $PaO_2 \times 0.0031 + 1.38 \times Hb \times SaO_2$

Typical scenario:
A married couple comes to the hospital complaining of "flulike" symptoms, including headache, nausea, vomiting, and disorientation. The wife thinks they caught the virus from a neighbor when they borrowed his home generator. *Think: Carbon monoxide poisoning.*

ACUTE COUGH

Definition

Cough is a common presenting complaint of patients. Acute cough, or cough of less than 3 weeks' duration, is most commonly caused by the postnasal drip associated with the common cold. See Table 3-1 for causes of acute cough.

POSTNASAL DRIP SYNDROME

Definition

Postnasal drip is thought to be the single most common cause of both acute and chronic cough.

TABLE 3-1. Causes of Acute Cough

Prevalence	Cause
Very common	Postnasal drip (due to common cold, acute bacterial sinusitis, allergic rhinitis, environmental irritant rhinitis)
Common	Pertussis Chronic obstructive pulmonary disease (COPD) exacerbation
Less common	Asthma Congestive heart failure Pneumonia Aspiration syndromes Pulmonary embolism

Etiology

All causes of rhinitis can cause postnasal drip and cough.

Pathophysiology

The mechanical action of secretions dripping into the hypopharynx triggers the cough reflex.

Signs and Symptoms

- Cough
- Nasal discharge or nasal obstruction
- Dripping sensation or tickle in the throat
- Drainage may be present on the posterior pharyngeal wall.

Treatment

Postnasal drip syndrome (PNDS) due to the common cold is treated with a first-generation antihistamine and a decongestant. Nonsedating antihistamines have been shown to be ineffective in this case.

PNDS due to allergic rhinitis is treated with nasal corticosteroids, nasal cromolyn, or nonsedating antihistamines.

Treatment of PNDS due to sinusitis is addressed below.

SINUSITIS

Definition

- Sinusitis is a common cause of PNDS and cough.
- Acute sinusitis is a bacterial infection that usually involves an obstructed maxillary sinus. Chronic sinusitis is the persistence of sinus inflammation for 3 or more months.
- Also associated with:
- Allergic rhinitis

- Dental infections
- Foreign body or tumor
- Cystic fibrosis
- Asthma

Signs and Symptoms

- Purulent nasal discharge
- Sinus pain worse on bending forward
- Fever
- Tenderness to percussion over sinuses

Diagnosis

- Transillumination findings are inconsistent.
- Computed tomography (CT) scan is extremely sensitive but is not specific to sinusitis, and many false positives occur. CT scan should be reserved for hospitalized patients, or for the diagnosis of chronic sinusitis.

Treatment

- Acute sinusitis: Amoxicillin or trimethoprim–sulfamethoxazole (TMP-SMX) or amoxicillin–clavulanic acid for 1 to 2 weeks, although some evidence suggests that a 3-day course of TMP-SMX produces the same results
- Persistent chronic sinusitis: May require subspecialist involvement

Complications of Untreated Chronic Sinusitis

- Preseptal or periorbital cellulitis
- Orbital cellulitis
- Epidural, subdural, or cerebral abscess
- Meningitis
- Dural sinus venous thrombosis

PERTUSSIS (WHOOPING COUGH)

Definition

Caused by *Bordetella pertussis*, a gram-negative coccobacillus

Epidemiology

Whooping cough is thought to be a common cause of cough in adults. Although only about 4,000 cases of pertussis are reported each year, seroprevalence studies indicate that pertussis is the cause of persistent cough in adults in 12 to 30% of cases.

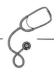

The classic "whoop" caused by rapid air inspiration against a closed glottis is rarely seen in adults.

Typical scenario:
A 27-year-old patient has pneumonia, bullous myringitis, and a chest film that looks worse than expected. *Think:* Mycoplasma pneumoniae.

Immunization

- Before routine immunization, whooping cough was a common cause of infant death.
- DTP (killed whole-cell) or DTaP (acellular) at 2, 4, 6, 18 months, and 4 to 6 years

Signs and Symptoms

Catarrhal Stage
- Lasts 1 to 2 weeks
- Characterized by mild upper respiratory infection (URI) symptoms

Paroxysmal Stage
- Lasts 2 to 4 weeks
- Characterized by prolonged paroxysmal cough
- Often worse at night

Convalescent Stage
- Characterized by gradual improvement of symptoms

Diagnosis

Nasopharyngeal swab and culture

Treatment

Macrolide antibiotics, such as erythromycin, will reduce the severity of the disease if started within 8 days. Identification and treatment of adult patients is important to help prevent transmission to unimmunized or incompletely immunized children.

PNEUMONIA

Definition

Infection of the lung parenchyma by any microorganism

Etiology

See Table 3-2 for organisms affecting immunocompetent host and Table 3-3 for those affecting immunocompromised hosts.

Pathophysiology

- Aspiration of nasopharyngeal, oral, or gastric contents
- Hematogenous spread
- Direct inoculation (stab wounds, endotracheal tube)

TABLE 3-2. Likely Organisms Causing Pneumonia

Community acquired, typical
1. S. pneumoniae
2. H. influenzae

Community acquired, atypical
1. Chlamydia pneumoniae
2. Legionella pneumophila
3. Mycoplasma pneumoniae

Hospital acquired
1. Pseudomonas aeruginosa
2. S. aureus
3. Enteric organisms

Signs and Symptoms

Patients with pneumonia may have few signs or symptoms, or may be extremely ill.

Typical Symptoms
- Fever
- Cough with sputum production
- Pleuritic chest pain

TABLE 3-3. Causes of Pneumonia in Immunocompromised Hosts

Immunocompromised hosts, HIV	CD4 count/dL
M. tuberculosis	< 500
Pneumocystis carinii	< 200
Histoplasma capsulatum	< 200
Cryptococcus neoformans	< 200
M. avium-intracellulare	< 50
Cytomegalovirus	< 50

Immunocompromised hosts, neutropenia
1. P. aeruginosa
2. Enterobacteriaceae
3. S. aureus
4. Aspergillus

Immunocompromised hosts, splenectomy, sickle cell anemia
Encapsulated organisms

Immunocompromised hosts, chronic steroid use
1. M. tuberculosis
2. Nocardia

Alcoholics
1. S. pneumoniae
2. H. influenzae
3. Klebsiella pneumoniae
4. M. tuberculosis

Typical scenario:
A patient with HIV who has a CD4 count of 52 does not take antiretroviral medications or TMP-SMX, is hypoxic on room air, and has a diffuse bilateral infiltrate on chest film. *Think:* Pneumocystis carinii *pneumonia* (PCP).

Typical scenario:
An elderly man presents with pneumonia, gastrointestinal symptoms, bradycardia, and hyponatremia. *Think: Legionella.*

If you see *currant jelly sputum*, think *Klebsiella.*

If you see *rusty sputum*, think *Pneumococcus.*

If a patient develops a *post-influenza pneumonia*, think *Pneumococcus.*

If you see *bulging fissure* on film, think *Klebsiella.*

Pulmonology

If there are no bacteria on Gram stain, consider *Legionella* and *Mycoplasma*.

If *serum LDH* is high, think PCP.

If you see *small gram-negative rods with a halo* on Gram stain, think *H. flu.*

Loeffler's pneumonia is idiopathic eosinophilic pneumonia.

Pneumonias causing relative bradycardia (slower than expected heart rate for temperature or disease, but above 60 bpm):
- *Legionella*
- *Salmonella*
- *Chlamydia psittaci*

Atypical Symptoms
- Dry cough
- Headache
- Malaise
- Gastrointestinal (GI) symptoms

Physical Exam
- Dullness to percussion
- Rales
- Tactile fremitus
- Egophony (E to A changes) with stethoscope

Diagnosis

Chest X-ray
Most patients with pneumonia will have an infiltrate on film corresponding to a lobe or segment. More specific findings may include:
- Upper lobe (*Mycobacterium tuberculosis*, *Klebsiella*)
- Small cavities without air-fluid levels (*M. tuberculosis*)
- Large cavities with air-fluid levels (*Staph* sp., anaerobes, gram-negatives, coccidioidomycosis, nocardiosis)
- Diffuse bilateral infiltrate (PCP, *Mycoplasma*)

Gram Stain
An adequate sputum sample should contain:
- < 10 epithelial cells per low-power field
- > 25 leucocytes per low-power field

Encapsulated organisms will appear to be surrounded by a halo (Quellung reaction):
Streptococcus pneumoniae
Hemophilus influenzae
Klebsiella sp.
Neisseria meningitidis

Criteria for Admission

Most patients with community-acquired pneumonia do well as outpatients. Those who may require admission include:
- Age > 50
- Nursing home residents
- Underlying chronic disease
- Change in mental status
- Tachypnea, tachycardia, or hypotension
- PaO$_2$ < 60
- Pleural effusion

Treatment

Many antibiotics treat community-acquired pneumonia. The best choices for initial use until cultures are completed are:

Typical pneumonia:
- Penicillins
- 2nd- or 3rd-generation cephalosporins
- Broad-spectrum fluoroquinolones

Atypical pneumonia: Expanded-spectrum macrolides
Hospital-acquired: Add *Pseudomonas* coverage
Immunocompromised: Add PCP coverage

Steroid administration in PCP prevents respiratory failure and improves survival.
Give for:
- A-a gradient > 35
- PaO$_2$ < 75

ADULT RESPIRATORY DISTRESS SYNDROME (ARDS)

- Condition that results from increased permeability of alveolar capillaries causing fluid to fill alveoli
- O$_2$ treatment does not improve condition due to effective AV shunting.
- Etiologies include shock, DIC, septicemia, trauma, and near drowning.
- Chest x-ray shows diffuse bilateral fluffy infiltrates.
- Treatment usually involves mechanical ventilation.
- Should resolve within 48 hours with appropriate management

CHRONIC COUGH

Definition

Cough of greater than 3 weeks' duration

Etiology

- Postnasal drip (PND)
- Asthma
- Gastroesophageal reflux disease (GERD)
- See Table 3-4 for a complete list of causes.

Postnasal drip syndrome, asthma, and GERD account for nearly 100% of causes of chronic cough in nonsmokers with normal chest films, who are not on angiotensin-converting enzyme (ACE) inhibitors.

TABLE 3-4. Causes of Chronic Cough

Prevalence	Causes
Common	Postnasal drip syndrome (PNDS)
	Asthma
	Gastroesophageal reflux disease (GERD)
Less common	Chronic bronchitis
	Bronchiectasis
	Postinfectious cough (pertussis)
Uncommon	Bronchogenic carcinoma
	ACE inhibitors
Rare in adults	Psychogenic cough

HIGH-YIELD FACTS

Pulmonology

Intrinsic asthma is associated with exercise and respiratory infections.

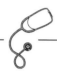

Extrinsic asthma is characterized by elevated **I**g**E** levels and **E**osinophilia.

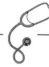

Cough-variant asthma: Cough is the patient's only symptom. The diagnosis of asthma is demonstrated by response to asthma-specific treatment.

A patient with a peak flow < 70% of expected should receive a course of steroids.

A patient with a peak flow < 40% expected is usually best cared for in hospital.

Definition

A chronic condition characterized by airway inflammation, bronchoconstriction, and hypersecretion

Pathophysiology

- The early phase of asthma is immunoglobulin **E** (IgE) mediated, associated with histamine release from mast cells.
- The late phase is associated with cytokine release and is improved by steroids.

History

- Exposure to pets, dust, smoke, carpets
- Aggravation by exercise, hot or cold weather
- Seasonal changes
- Past hospital admission or intubation

Signs and Symptoms

The airflow obstruction associated with asthma that produces expiratory wheezing in mild disease progresses to both inspiratory and expiratory wheezing in moderate disease, and then diminished breath sounds and no wheezing in severe disease:

- Chest tightness
- Wheezing
- Shortness of breath
- Cough (especially at night)

Other causes of wheezing include:

- Reactive airways disease (usually from postnasal drip syndrome)
- Congestive heart failure (CHF)
- Foreign body aspiration (most often in children)

Physical Exam

- Wheezing on exhalation
- Decreased air entry
- Decreased peak flow and FEV_1
- Retractions of sternocleidomastoids
- Intercostal muscle use for breathing
- Oxygen saturation < 95%
- Inability to speak full sentences

Treatment

Beta-2 Agonists
- Delivered by metered dose inhaler (MDI) or nebulizer
- Promote bronchodilation
- *Note:* Beta-2 agonists cause an intracellular shift of potassium and can be used as temporary treatment of hyperkalemia.

Ipratropium Bromide
- Delivered by nebulizer or MDI
- Dry up bronchial secretions
- Effects of beta agonists and ipratropium bromide are additive.

Steroids
- Reduce inflammation
- Delivered by MDI for asthma prevention
- Oral or IV use for acute exacerbations

Preventative Medications
- Leukotriene modifiers such as zafirlukast
- Mast cell stabilizers such as cromolyn

Methylxanthines such as theophylline are no longer regularly used for asthma due to the narrow therapeutic window and the frequency of adverse effects, including nausea, vomiting, headache, and, in severe toxicity, seizures and arrhythmias.

Allergen removal: Common environmental triggers should be addressed, including smoking, dust, pets, carpets, cockroaches and seasonal allergens.

Frequent visits to the PMD with review of medications and teaching can prevent acute attacks.

Intubation of Asthmatics

Patients with asthma may need to be electively or emergently intubated. The key indicator for intubation is the declining clinical status of the patient, including:
- Severe tachypnea
- Dyspnea
- Hypoxia
- Mental status changes or inability to communicate

Arterial blood gases **(ABGs)** can aid assessment of how sick the patient is but should never delay intubation in a patient who requires respiratory assistance.

Ventilation techniques in an intubated asthmatic include:
- Keep respiratory rate at 12 to 14/min.
- Keep tidal volume at 6 to 8 mL/kg.
- Prolong expiratory time to prevent stacking breaths.
- Do not try to overventilate to "blow off" CO_2 (this can lead to barotrauma).

MDIs deliver smaller particles than nebulizers and therefore reach the smallest airways better. Nebulizers are favored for hospital treatment because of ease of use.

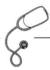

Permissive hypercapnia is the practice of allowing a patient to have high CO_2 while intubated.

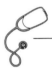

CO_2 is reduced by raising the patient's minute ventilation (tidal volume × respiratory rate).

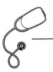

High tidal volumes and high rates can lead to barotrauma and are thought to contribute to ARDS.

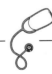

To interpret metabolic acid–base disturbances, you need a measured HCO_3 from a serum chemistry panel.

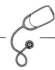
Interpretation of Arterial Blood Gases in Asthma

The notation for arterial blood gases is: $pH/PCO_2/PO_2$/calculated HCO_3/calculated SaO_2

Sample ABGs
- Normal: 7.4/40/98
- Mild asthma: 7.48/30/60 (acute respiratory alkalosis)
- Severe asthma: 7.40/40/55 (mixed acid–base disturbance: Respiratory alkalosis and metabolic acidosis; the "normalization" of the pH and PCO_2 in the presence of continued symptoms and hypoxia indicate that the patient is getting fatigued)

CHRONIC BRONCHITIS AND EMPHYSEMA

Definition

Chronic bronchitis and emphysema are forms of chronic obstructive pulmonary disease (COPD). COPD is defined by a chronic obstruction to expiratory airflow, accompanied by a decrease in FEV_1.

Chronic bronchitis: Chronic expiratory airflow obstruction accompanied by chronic productive cough for 3 or more months in each of 2 successive years

Emphysema: Chronic expiratory airflow obstruction accompanied by permanent enlargement of the airspace distal to the terminal bronchioles

Pathophysiology of Emphysema

- **Centrilobular** emphysema affects the respiratory bronchioles.
- **Panlobular or panacinar emphysema** occurs in patients with alpha-1-antitrypsin deficiency. Alpha-1-antitrypsin protects against the degradation of lung elastin.
- **Distal acinar emphysema** is associated with spontaneous pneumothorax.

Epidemiology

- Higher prevalence in men
- Mortality rates are higher in whites.

Risk Factors

- Smoking
- Alpha-1-antitrypsin deficiency (autosomal recessive inheritance, more common in Mediterraneans)
- Inhalation of coal dust, potash, and particulate matter
- Chronic exposure to sulfur dioxide and nitrogen dioxide
- Pneumonia before age 2

Symptoms

- Cough
- Dyspnea on exertion
- CO_2 retention (chronic bronchitis)
- Weight loss (emphysema)
- Tachypnea
- Depression

Treatment of COPD

- Smoking cessation
- Maintain vaccination against influenza and *S. pneumoniae*.
- Theophylline improves FEV_1 by 5 to 15% by bronchodilation and improved diaphragmatic contractility
- Beta agonists and ipratropium bromide improve FEV_1 modestly.
- Steroids improve FEV_1 by > 20% in about 11% of patients.
- Antibiotics for COPD exacerbations reduce the duration of COPD exacerbation symptoms by 20% and decrease hospital admissions by 50%.
- Oxygen has also been shown to improve COPDer's IQ and exercise tolerance. Oxygen should be given to:
  - Patients with a resting PaO_2 of < 55 mm Hg
  - Patients with PaO_2 of 55 to 59 who have cor pulmonale, erythrocytosis, or who desaturate during exercise
- Lung reduction surgery improves FEV_1 by 100% and decreases residual volume by 40%.

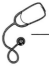

Supplemental oxygen is the only therapy for COPD proven to extend life.

BRONCHIECTASIS

Definition

Bronchiectasis is a chronic condition characterized by pathological dilatation of the medium-sized airways. It is usually caused by an abnormal inflammatory response to an initial infectious or toxic insult.

Etiology

- Cystic fibrosis
- Tuberculosis
- Aspiration or inhalation of toxins
- Retained foreign body
- Severe pneumonia

Pathophysiology

The resulting airway damage allows bacterial colonization, build-up of secretions, and continued bronchial destruction. Bronchiectasis is the cause of chronic cough in about 4% of cases.

Most common organisms to colonize bronchiectatic lung:
H. influenzae
S. aureus
Pseudomonas aeruginosa

Bronchiectasis is the most common cause of **hemoptysis.**

Signs and Symptoms

- Chronic cough
- Hemoptysis
- Wheezing
- Failure to thrive

Diagnosis

High-resolution CT scan will detect bronchial dilatation and destruction in 60 to 100% of cases. Patients with cystic fibrosis will have abnormal pancreatic function and an abnormal sweat test.

Treatment

- Chest physiotherapy
- Antibiotics
- Bronchodilators
- Uncommon treatments: Local resection, bronchial artery embolization for hemoptysis, lung transplantation

Typical scenario:
A patient with hemoptysis, sinusitis, and glomerulonephritis. *Think: Wegener's granulomatosis.*

HEMOPTYSIS

Definition

Coughing up of blood due to bleeding from the lower respiratory tract. See Table 3-5 for a list of causes.

Massive hemoptysis is bleeding > 600 mL in 48 hours, or bleeding causing clinical impairment of respiratory function.

TABLE 3-5. Causes of Hemoptysis

Incidence	Cause
Common	Bronchiectasis
	Lung cancer
	Bronchitis
	Pneumonia
	Unknown
Uncommon	Coagulopathy
	Congestive heart failure
	Pulmonary embolism
	Tuberculosis
	Wegener's
	Goodpasture's
Rare	Systemic HTN, pulmonary HTN, trauma, vasculitis, foreign body, collagen vascular disease, pulmonary arteriovenous malformation

Treatment

- Supplemental oxygen
- Place patient with bleeding side down.
- Suppress cough reflex (i.e., codeine).

Patients with massive hemoptysis usually require surgical involvement. Initial therapy includes:
- Intubation of the good lung
- Endobronchial cold saline or epinephrine
- Bronchial artery embolization

Typical scenario:
A patient with dyspnea, hemoptysis, and acute renal failure. *Think: Goodpasture's syndrome.*

MEDIASTINUM

Masses

Anterior
- Thymoma
- Teratoma
- Thyroid
- T-cell lymphoma

Middle
- Vascular lesions
- Lymph nodes

Posterior
- Neurogenic tumor

Inhalation **anthrax** is considered to be a likely agent to be used in the event of biological warfare. Nonmilitary persons are not immunized, and the disease is nearly 100% fatal once severe symptoms occur.

Mediastinitis

Causes of Mediastinitis
- Esophageal perforation
- Post-median sternotomy
- Inhalation anthrax (hemorrhagic mediastinitis)
- Tuberculosis, histoplasmosis (chronic)

Symptoms
- Initial symptoms similar to viral syndrome
- After 1 to 3 days, fever, dyspnea, hypoxia, hemorrhagic mediastinitis, and death occur.

Treatment
- High-dose penicillin, ciprofloxacin, or doxycycline is recommended.

Physical findings in pneumomediastinum. **Hamman's sign:** A crunching sound occurring with the heartbeat.

Pneumomediastinum

Causes
- Rupture of alveolus, bronchus, or trachea
- Esophageal rupture
- Dissection of cervical (neck) or abdominal free air into mediastinum

Treat underlying cause.

Small cell lung cancer has a rapid mitotic rate and therefore is sensitive to chemotherapy. Surgery is not indicated.

Two types of cancer share a "s"entral location:
- **Small cell**
- **Squamous cell**

Bronchoalveolar cancer, a type of adenocarcinoma, is not linked to smoking and is more common in women.

Chronic cough is the most common symptom of lung cancer.

Types

Small Cell Lung Cancer
- Central location
- Sensitive to chemotherapy
- Surgery is not indicated.
- Poor prognosis (2 to 4 months from diagnosis to death)

Non–Small Cell Lung Cancer
- Includes squamous, large cell, and adenocarcinoma
- Poor response to chemotherapy
- Treated with surgery (debulking)
- Prognosis varies with stage.

Epidemiology

- Leading cause of cancer death in both men and women in the United States
- Cases have been decreasing in men, but increasing in women.
- Smoking is by far the most important causative factor in the development of lung cancer.

Etiology

- Smoking
- Passive smoke exposure
- Radon gas exposure
- Asbestos
- Arsenic
- Nickel

Signs and Symptoms

- Cough
- Hemoptysis
- Stridor
- Dyspnea
- Hoarseness (recurrent laryngeal nerve paralysis)
- Postobstructive pneumonia
- Dysphagia
- Associated (paraneoplastic) syndromes (see Table 3-6)

Treatment

The two main types of lung cancer, small cell and non–small cell cancer, have different responses to radiotherapy, chemotherapy, and surgery (see Table 3-7).

HIGH-YIELD FACTS

Pulmonology

TABLE 3-6. Syndromes Associated with Lung Cancer

Horner's syndrome	Sympathetic nerve paralysis produces enophthalmos, ptosis, miosis, amd ipsilateral anhidrosis.
Pancoast's syndrome	Superior sulcus tumor injuring the 8th cervical nerve and the 1st and 2nd thoracic nerves and ribs, causing shoulder pain radiating to arm
Superior vena cava syndrome	Tumor causing obstruction of the superior vena cava and subsequent venous return, producing facial swelling, dyspnea, cough, headaches, epistaxis, syncope. Symptoms worsened with bending forward and on awakening in the morning.
Syndrome of inappropriate antidiuretic hormone (SIADH)	Ectopic antidiuretic hormone (ADH) release in the setting of plasma hyposmolarity, producing hyponatremia without edema. Also caused by other lung diseases, CNS trauma or infection, and certain medications.
Eaton–Lambert syndrome	Presynaptic nerve terminals attacked by antibodies, decreasing acetylcholine release. Treated by plasmapheresis and immunosuppression, 40% associated with small cell lung CA, 20% have other CA, 40% have no CA.
Trousseau's syndrome	Venous thrombosis associated with metastatic cancer

PLEURAL EFFUSION

Definition

Pleural effusion is classified as a transudate or exudate depending on origin.

Transudative pleural effusions are due to:
- Increased hydrostatic pressure
- Decreased oncotic pressure

Exudative pleural effusions are due to:
- Increased capillary permeability

Diagnosis

Thoracentesis: The effusion is an *exudate* if:
- Ratio of pleural to serum protein > 0.5

Transudates:
- CHF
- Cirrhosis
- Nephrosis

Exudates:
- Tumor
- Trauma
- Infection

TABLE 3-7. Distinction Between Small and Non–Small Cell Lung Cancer

Characteristic	Small Cell Lung Cancer	Non–Small Cell Lung Cancer
Histology	Small dark nuclei scant cytoplasm	Copious cytoplasm, pleomorphic nuclei
Ectopic peptide production	Gastrin, ACTH, ADH, calcitonin, ANF	PTH
Response to radiotherapy	80–90% will shrink	30–50% will shrink
Response to chemotherapy	Complete regression in 50%	Complete regression in 5%
Surgical resection for	Not indicated	Stages I, II, IIIA
Included subtypes	Small cell only	Adenocarcinoma, squamous cell, large cell, bronchoalveolar
5-year survival rate all stages	5%	11–83%

ACTH, adrenocorticotropic hormone; ADH, antidiuretic hormone; ANF, atrial natriuretic factor; PTH, parathyroid hormone.
Note: ADH is also known as arginine vasopressin (AVP).

- Ratio of pleural to serum lactic dehydrogenase (LDH) > 0.6
- Pleural fluid LDH > ⅔ upper normal limit

The effusion is *parapneumonic* if:
- Pleural fluid leukocyte count > 10,000/mm³ with high PMNs
- Parapneumonic effusions are always exudates.

Gross blood in pleural fluid is associated with:
- Tumor
- Trauma
- Pulmonary infarction
- Aortic dissection

Low glucose in pleural fluid is associated with:
- Empyema
- Rheumatoid arthritis
- Tumor
- Tuberculosis

High amylase in pleural fluid is associated with:
- Pancreatitis
- Renal failure
- Tumor
- Esophageal rupture

PULMONARY EMBOLISM

Definition

Pulmonary thromboembolism results from disruption of a deep venous thrombosis or local stasis, causing blockage of pulmonary blood flow beyond the embolus. Very large PEs that impede blood flow in both the right and left pulmonary arteries are called saddle emboli.

Risk Factors

- Immobilization
- Recent surgery
- Hypercoagulable state (malignancy, pregnancy, genetic)
- Proximal leg deep venous thrombosis
- Stroke

Diagnosis of PE is difficult, and a high clinical suspicion should be maintained.

Symptoms

- Dyspnea
- Tachypnea
- Pleuritic chest pain
- Cough
- Hemoptysis
- Syncope
- Anxiety
- Posterior leg pain or swelling

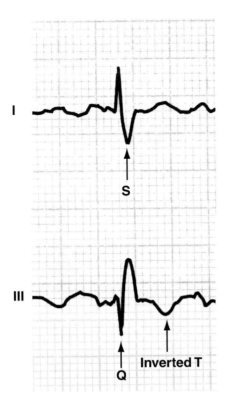

FIGURE 3-1. Pulmonary embolism. S_1-Q_3-T_3 pattern.

Diagnosis

- ECG: S in lead I, Q and inverted T waves in lead III, or may show diffuse ST changes, and tachycardia
- Chest film: May show an infiltrate or may be normal
- ABGs: Usually reveal hypoxemia, hypocapnia, and respiratory alkalosis
- D-dimer: Measures products of fibrin degradation
- Leg ultrasonography (venous duplex): To detect DVT
- Ventilation, perfusion scan (V/Q scan): To look for perfusion defects at site of PE
- Helical (spiral) CT: To look for embolus in the pulmonary vasculature. Does not detect small emboli.
- Pulmonary angiogram: The gold standard for detection of PE. Invasive test.

How to Use Tests to Diagnose PE

Multiple algorithms have been constructed, but most share the following principles:

1. Determine your level of clinical suspicion based on history, physical exam, EKG, and chest film as high, intermediate, or low risk.
2. Patients with a low risk of PE can be ruled out with a negative D-dimer test.
3. Patients can be ruled in and treated after a positive leg sonogram to look for DVT or a high-probability V/Q scan.
4. Low- and intermediate-risk patients with a normal V/Q scan are ruled out.
5. Intermediate-probability V/Q scans are not helpful and require further testing, either spiral CT or angiogram.

S_1-Q_3-T_3 on ECG is the classic ECG finding for PE, but the most frequent rhythm is sinus tachycardia (see Figure 3-1).

Angiography is the gold standard in the diagnosis of:
- Deep venous thrombosis
- Dissecting aortic aneurysm
- Ischemic bowel syndrome
- Pulmonary embolism

A V/Q result of "intermediate probability" is useless.

Treatment

Acute treatment of PE includes:

1. Anticoagulation with heparin or low-molecular-weight heparin
2. Thrombolysis
3. Interventional pulmonary angiography: Mechanical disintegration or local thrombolysis
4. Surgery: Embolectomy

Prolonged treatment:

1. Patients with DVTs are orally anticoagulated for 6 months.
2. Patients with PEs are orally anticoagulated for 1 year.

TUBERCULOSIS

Definition

Tuberculosis is a leading cause of death worldwide. In the United States, the incidence of tuberculosis decreased every year until 1984, but then rose again until 1993.

Pathophysiology

Transmission occurs by inhalation of droplet nuclei produced by the cough or sneeze of a patient with pulmonary TB disease. Particles may remain suspended in air for several hours:
- 5% of those infected will develop TB disease in 2 years.
- 5% more will develop TB disease in their lifetime.
- 90% will remain infected but disease free.

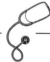

Sites of TB disease:
- Lungs (85% of all cases)
- Central nervous system (TB meningitis)
- Lymphatics
- Genitourinary system
- Bones (Pott's disease)
- Disseminated TB (miliary)

Epidemiology

High-Prevalence Groups
HIV-infected persons
Close contacts of persons with TB disease
IV drug users
Immunocompromised persons (non-HIV)
Foreign-born persons
Residents of medically underserved communities
Prisoners
Homeless

High Risk for TB Once Infected
HIV-infected persons
IV drug users
Immunocompromised persons (non-HIV)
Abnormal chest film

Symptoms

- Productive cough
- **Night sweats**
- **Hemoptysis**
- Anorexia
- Weight loss
- Fever
- Chills
- Chest pain
- Fatigue

Diagnosis

Findings
- Positive PPD
- Infiltrate or granuloma in upper lobes of lungs
- Acid-fast bacilli (AFB) on sputum microscopy
- Positive culture

Types of Stains for AFB
- Ziehl–Neelsen
- Kinyoun
- Auramine

How to Use the TB Skin Test

1. Screen patients in high-prevalence groups.
2. Gives a positive reaction 2 to 10 weeks after infection
3. Plant 0.1 mL of PPD intradermally on volar aspect of the forearm.
4. Read 48 to 72 hours after placement.
5. Measure induration, not erythema (see Table 3-8).

False Positives
- Bacillus Calmette–Guérin (BCG) vaccinated
- Nontuberculous mycobacterial infection

False Negatives
- Ten to 25% of patients with TB infection have negative skin tests.
- The two-step TB skin test is used in high-prevalence patients who have a negative first test: The first test boosts the immune response to a second skin test, which will turn positive in infected patients.

Patients who are anergic (do not mount response) can be screened by planting the common antigens *mumps* and *Candida.*

TABLE 3-8. Interpretation of PPD Skin Test

	Measured Induration	
15 mm or Greater	**10 mm or Greater**	**5 mm or Greater**
All patients are considered infected.	Considered infected if: Immunocompromised IV drug user Foreign born Medically underserved Nursing home resident Prisoner Child under age 4	Considered infected if: HIV Close contact Abnormal chest film

TABLE 3-9. Preventive Therapy for Patients with Positive TB Skin Test

INH 300 mg PO QD for 12 months reduces the risk of TB disease by 90%. Directly observed therapy (DOT) improves compliance.

Adult under 35	Over 35
Recent conversion (10 mm)	Conversion (15 mm) within 2 years of a previously negative PPD
No risk factors (15 mm) High prevalence (10 mm)	

- High-risk TB disease group always treated
- Close contacts with negative tests should be retested in 10 weeks
- Pregnant patients should be treated after delivery unless they are in a high-risk group (e.g., HIV)

Prevention

See Table 3-9. Preventive treatment is withheld for:
- Patients with liver disease
- Patients over age 35 unless high-risk group or recent conversion due to increased risk of isoniazid (INH)-related hepatitis

Treatment

Standard Regimen
- *6 months of:* INH, rifampin, and pyrazinamide *plus* ethambutol or streptomycin

Patients Unable to Take Pyrazinamide
- *9 months of:* INH, rifampin *plus* ethambutol or streptomycin

Pregnant with TB Disease
- *9 months of:* INH, rifampin, *plus* ethambutol

Negative-pressure rooms are used to prevent droplet nuclei from being transported into hospital hallways by air currents. Patient is no longer infectious after:
- Therapy for 10 days
- Three consecutive sputum smears negative for AFB

Toxicity of TB Medication

INH
- Bactericidal
- Peripheral neuropathy (can be prevented with administration of pyridoxine)
- Seizures in overdose: These can be very difficult to break with standard measures—remember to give pyridoxine!
- Hepatitis (check liver function tests each month)

Rifampin
- Bactericidal
- Induces hepatic microsomal enzymes
- Is excreted as a red-orange compound in urine, stool, sweat, and tears; will discolor contact lenses

Typical scenario:
A patient is brought in by ambulance in status epilepticus. The patient's family member says he has no medical history except tuberculosis. *Think: INH toxicity.* Treat with pyridoxine.

Ethambutol

- Bactericidal/bacteristatic at usual doses
- Optic neuritis and impaired color vision are related to cumulative dose.

Definition

Air in the pleural space

Epidemiology

- Spontaneous pneumothorax affects approximately 20,000 persons per year, usually from rupture of a subpleural bleb or pleural necrosis due to lung disease.
- Primary spontaneous pneumothorax occurs in an otherwise healthy person, while secondary spontaneous pneumothorax occurs in patients who have underlying lung disease.

Etiology

Primary Spontaneous Pneumothorax

- Male smokers
- Patients tall for weight

Secondary Spontaneous Pneumothorax

- COPD
- Cystic fibrosis
- Pneumonia
- HIV
- Cancer
- Substance abuse

Signs and Symptoms

- Chest pain
- Dyspnea
- Hyperresonance of affected side
- Decreased breath sounds of affected side
- Tracheal deviation *away* from affected side (in tension pneumothorax)

Diagnosis

- ECG: ST segment changes possible
- Upright chest x-ray is ~83% sensitive, demonstrates an absence of lung markings where the lung has collapsed.

Treatment

- Oxygen
- For pneumothoraces > 20%: Tube thoracostomy to remove air

Typical scenario:
A 20-year-old tall man arrives complaining of sudden onset of severe shortness of breath and pleuritic chest pain. *Think: Primary spontaneous pneumothorax.*

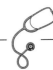

Expiratory chest film is more sensitive for pneumothorax than inspiratory chest film.

HIGH-YIELD FACTS

Pulmonology

79

- Pleurodesis to adhere the visceral and parietal pleura
- Treat underlying disorder in secondary pneumothorax.

TENSION PNEUMOTHORAX

Definition

Tension pneumothorax is created when air trapped in the pleural space exerts pressure on the lung and mediastinum, reducing both oxygenation and venous return.

Signs and Symptoms

- Severe dyspnea
- Tachycardia
- Hypotension
- Tracheal deviation away from side of pneumothorax
- Hemopneumothorax often associated with trauma

Treatment

Tension pneumothorax is an emergency and, if suspected on clinical grounds, should be treated prior to films with needle decompression followed by tube thoracostomy.

ENVIRONMENTAL LUNG DISEASE

Typical scenario:
A farmer presents with fever, cough, and difficulty breathing after several days of filling his silo with grain. *Think: Hypersensitivity pneumonitis.*

Definitions

Chronic exposure to particulate matter and dusts formed in industry causes disease:

Asbestosis: A diffuse interstitial lung disease caused by dusts of mineral silicates. Asbestos exposure is associated with an increased risk of squamous cell CA, adenocarcinoma, and mesotheliomas.

Silicosis: Nodular fibrosis of the lung caused by exposure to silica flour, sand blasting, or the manufacture of abrasive soaps. These patients are at a greater risk of developing pulmonary TB disease.

Coal workers' pneumoconiosis: An occupational hazard of ~50% of all coal miners; they develop progressive massive fibrosis.

Byssinosis (cotton dust exposure): Patients experience "chest tightness" with an associated decrease in FEV_1 with exposure to cotton dust. Treatment is to wear protective equipment and to use bronchodilators.

Farmer's lung: A *hypersensitivity pneumonitis* caused by exposure to spores of thermophilic actinomycetes. Thought to be associated with a suppressor T-cell defect, is IgG mediated. Symptoms include fever, chills, cough, and dyspnea, and episodes occur more frequently during wet weather. Treat with steroids, and avoid exposure. Long-term complications include pulmonary fibrosis and weight loss.

Neurology

R. Anand Narasimhan

CEREBROVASCULAR ACCIDENTS (CVAS)

Definitions

Abrupt onset of new neurologic deficits (see Table 4-1) caused by cerebrovascular disease.

Types of CVAs
- *Stroke:* CVA resulting in infarcted cerebral tissue, regardless of the presence or absence of neurologic deficits
- *Stroke in evolution:* Neurologic deficits continue to fluctuate or increase over time.
- *Completed stroke:* Neurologic deficits have remained stable for 24 to 72 hours.
- *Transient ischemic attack (TIA):* Neurologic deficit resolving completely in 24 hours (usually within 30 minutes) and resulting in no apparent infarcted tissue on magnetic resonance imaging (MRI)
- *Crescendo TIAs:* Two or more TIAs within 24 hours—highly predictive of impending stroke, constitutes a medical emergency
- *Reversible ischemic neurologic deficit (RIND):* Neurologic deficit lasting more than 24 hours but less than 3 weeks, improving progressively to complete or almost complete resolution

Some Jargon for CVA Sequelae
Anosognosia: The inability to identify body dysfunction—patients are unaware of their neurological deficits.
Aphasia: A defect in comprehension or expression of spoken or written language
Broca's aphasia: A deficit in speech and written expression
Wernicke's aphasia: Patients tend to articulate a fluent nonsense with natural rhythm, and comprehension is impaired.
Apraxia: Disturbance in the ability to perform learned motor tasks
Dysarthria: Disturbance in the articulation of speech
Dysphagia: Difficulty swallowing

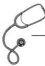

Ischemic penumbra: The tissue surrounding an infarcted zone that is dysfunctional but not infarcted and that may recover full functionality if the hypoxic state resolves. The volume of the ischemic penumbra is often greater than that of the infarcted core, and thus its salvage can dramatically reduce the degree of permanent deficit.

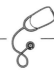

TIAs used to be defined as any CVA whose symptoms resolved completely within 24 hours. With the advent of MRI and the ability to detect "silent" infarctions, the definition has narrowed toward including only those cases with no detectable infarcts. *A word of caution:* You will find many physicians using the dated definition.

TABLE 4-1. Neurological Deficits in Stroke

Artery Occlusion	Deficit	Other
Middle cerebral	<ul><li>Contralateral hemiparesis (face and hand more affected)</li><li>Contralateral hemisensory deficit</li><li>Homonymous hemianopsia (blindness affecting the right or the left half of the visual fields of both eyes) opposite to occluded artery</li><li>If dominant MCA affected (left side in right-handed person), patient will be aphasic</li><li>If nondominant MCA affected, confusion, constructional apraxia, contralateral body neglect</li></ul>	
Anterior cerebral (see Figure 4-1)	<ul><li>Contralateral weakness of leg or foot</li><li>Broca's aphasia</li><li>Incontinence</li></ul>	
Internal carotid	<ul><li>Presentation similar to MCA occlusion</li></ul>	
Posterior cerebral (see Figure 4-2)	<ul><li>Homonymous hemianopsia of contralateral visual field</li><li>Other visual field defects including vertical gaze and oculomotor nerve palsy</li><li>If dominant sphere affected, anomic aphasia (difficulty naming objects) or alexia (inability to read) may occur</li></ul>	Pupillary reflexes spared
Posterior inferior cerebellar	Clinical: Sudden onset of:<ul><li>Nausea/vomiting</li><li>Vertigo</li><li>Hoarseness</li><li>Ataxia</li><li>Ipsilateral palate and tongue weakness</li><li>Contralateral disturbance of pain and temperature sensation</li><li>Dysphagia, dysarthria, and hiccup</li><li>Ipsilateral Horner's syndrome (ptosis, miosis, hemianhidrosis, and apparent enophthalmos)</li></ul>	1. Motor system typically spared 2. Lateral medullary (Wallenberg's) syndrome Horner's syndrome: **HORNE** **H**—hemianhidrosis (loss of sweating) **O**—one eye (usually unilateral) **R**—relaxed eyelid (ptosis) **N**—narrow pupil (miosis) **E**—enophthalmos (sunken eyes)
Anterior inferior cerebellar	Definition: Infarction of lateral portion of pons Clinical:<ul><li>Ipsilateral facial weakness</li><li>Gaze palsy</li><li>Deafness</li><li>Tinnitus</li></ul>	* No Horner's syndrome, dysphagia, or dysarthria
Lacunar	Lenticulostriate branches of the middle cerebral artery (midbrain) become occluded as a result of chronic hypertension.<ul><li>Symptoms may present gradually over several days.</li><li>CT or MRI may not detect stroke.</li></ul>Presentations:<ul><li>Pure motor hemiparesis: Affecting face, arm, leg without other disturbances</li><li>Pure sensory stroke: Hemisensory loss</li><li>Ataxic hemiparesis: Pure motor hemiparesis combined with ataxia</li><li>Dysarthria—clumsy hand syndrome: Dysarthria, dysphagia, facial weakness, and weakness/clumsiness of hand</li></ul>	

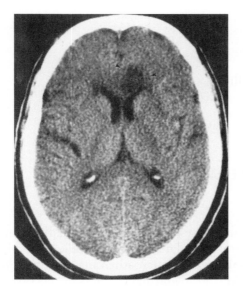

FIGURE 4-1. CT of ischemic stroke of the anterior cerebral artery (ACA). Note the lesion is hypodense.
(Reproduced, with permission, from Johnson MH. CT evaluation of the earliest signs of stroke. *The Radiologist* 1(4): 189–199, 1994.)

Epidemiology

- Third major cause of death and disability
- 500,000 strokes per year
- One third are fatal

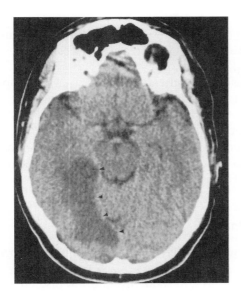

FIGURE 4-2. CT of ischemic stroke of the posterior cerebral artery (PCA). Note the lesion is hypodense.
(Reproduced, with permission, from Johnson MH. CT evaluation of the earliest signs of stroke. *The Radiologist* 1(4): 189–199, 1994.)

Risk Factors

- Hypertension
- Smoking
- Diabetes mellitus
- Coronary artery disease
- Atrial fibrillation
- Left ventricular hypertrophy

Classification and Etiology

Ischemic
- **Thrombotic:**
    - Large-vessel disease—atherosclerosis usually located at bifurcation of carotid, vertebrobasilar system, or middle cerebral artery
    - Small-vessel disease—microatheroma or lipohyalinosis usually due to HTN or DM, causing lacunar infarcts in subcortical tissues
- **Embolic:** Usually of cardiac origin (60%), source often unknown, sometimes carotid (artery-to-artery embolus)

Hemorrhagic
- **Subarachnoid:** Head trauma most common, aneurysms, AV malformations
- **Intracerebral:** Hypertension, amyloid, bleeding disorders

Hypoperfusion
- Shock, etc.; most affect *watershed* areas (most commonly parasagittal strips of cortex)

Pathophysiology

Ischemic Stroke
- Occlusion of artery feeding brain causes oxygen depletion and damage to neurons.
- The ensuing ischemia results in release of inflammatory cytokines, which decreases flow by increasing viscosity. These cytokines further damage neuronal function.
- With reperfusion of ischemic area, oxygen free radicals are produced, which also damage neurons.

Hemorrhagic Stroke (see Figure 4-3)
- Blood is extremely neurotoxic, hence the blood–brain barrier (BBB)
- Bleeding into or around the central nervous system (CNS) also compresses brain tissue and vascular structures.

Signs and Symptoms

- Thrombotic strokes often show relatively slow progressive onset, often during sleep.
- Embolic strokes present suddenly, often in discrete steps ("stuttering onset"), most often during waking hours.

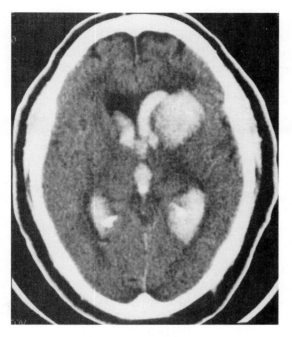

FIGURE 4-3. CT of hemorrhagic stroke due to hypertension. Note the lesion is hyperdense. Note bleeding into the ventricles. Effacement of sulci suggests edema. Mild mass effect is also present.

(Reproduced, with permission, from Lee, Rao, and Zimmerman. *Cranial MRI and CT.* New York: McGraw-Hill, 1999: 581.)

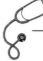

The initial CT should be done *without* contrast as fresh blood is radiolucent relative to old blood and normal cerebral tissue. Contrast-enhanced CT or MRI is useful subsequently to reveal regions of infarct.

- Hemorrhagic strokes evolve over minutes, invariably during waking hours.
- Twenty percent of stroke patients have a history of at least one TIA.

Diagnosis

- CT scan is useful for quick diagnosis and localization. It can also be helpful to exclude hemorrhagic infarcts.
- MRI for further study and follow-up
- Carotid ultrasound to screen for carotid stenosis
- Cardiac echocardiography may be used to screen for embolic source. Transesophageal echo (TEE) is most sensitive.

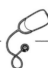

TIAs preceding thrombotic strokes tend to present with similar symptoms because the transient ischemia is locked to the distribution of the stenotic artery. Conversely, TIAs preceding embolic strokes tend to have more variable presentation.

Treatment

1. TIAs:
   - Antiplatelet therapy (aspirin, clopidogrel)
   - Anticoagulation for embolic causes (heparin, warfarin)
   - Carotid endarterectomy for anterior circulation TIAs with moderate- to high-grade carotid stenosis
2. Stroke in evolution:
   - Anticoagulation with heparin
   - Thrombolytic therapies are being studied.
3. Stroke:
   - Thrombolytic agents (ischemic strokes):
     - Lyses fibrin containing clots
     - Should be administered within 3 hours of onset

Thrombolytic therapy is not indicated for extremely mild or severe strokes. Other contraindications are the same as for MI.

- Major risk is hemorrhage
- Antiplatelet therapy (all)
- Anticoagulation in cases of cardiac embolus (heparin)
- Hemorrhagic stroke requires neurosurgical consult.

RABIES

Definition

A rapidly progressing viral infection affecting the human nervous system

Epidemiology

- Fewer than 10 cases per year in United States
- 50% of cases from raccoon bites
- Other cases transmitted by dogs, skunks, foxes, coyotes, bats, and bobcats
- Rare cases from tissue transplantation (cornea)

Pathophysiology

- After bite or scratch from animal, virus replicates in local sensory nerve fibers.
- It then ascends through unmyelinated nerve fibers to CNS.
- The virus finally progresses to the salivary glands and peripheral nerves.

Signs and Symptoms

- Two phases:
  - *Prodromal phase:* Pain, paresthesias, GI/respiratory symptoms, irritability, apprehension, **hydrophobia** (aversion to swallowing water because of pain), aerophobia (fear of fresh air)
  - *Excitation phase:* Hyperventilation, hyperactivity, disorientation, and seizures
- Patient becomes increasingly lethargic. Further involvement of cardiac and respiratory nerves leads to death.

Diagnosis

- Fluorescent antibody staining, polymerase chain reaction
- Presence of Negri bodies (postmortem)

Treatment

- Wash affected area thoroughly with soap and water.
- No antiviral therapy available
- Supportive treatment:
  - Rabies immunoglobulin (passive immunization)
  - Human diploid cell rabies vaccine (active immunization: Because of long incubation period, early injections provide sufficient time for protective immunity.

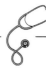

A patient with encephalitis, hydrophobia, and aerophobia should have rabies virus workup.
RABIES
R — Respiratory failure
A — Aerophobia, apprehension, aversion to water
B — Bad pains
I — Irritability
E — Excitation
S — Seizures

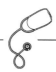

Rabies is universally fatal unless vaccine is given prior to the onset of symptoms. Immunize for:
- Raccoon bites
- Skunk bites
- Bat exposure (bite may be too small to see)
- Fox bites
- Bite from feral dog or cat

- Active and passive immunization are administered in different parts of body so that immunoglobulin (passive) does not neutralize the vaccine (active).
- Isolation
- Preexposure prevention with vaccine should be used for high-risk individuals like zookeepers and veterinarians.

Definition

Infection of the pia and arachnoid meninges (the leptomeninges)

Causes
- *Streptococcus pneumoniae* (40 to 60%)
- *Neisseria meningitidis* (young adults)
- *Listeria monocytogenes* (immunocompromised hosts)
- Gram-negative bacilli
- *Hemophilus influenzae* (unimmunized adults)
- Group B strep (neonates)

Pathophysiology

- Infection may be acquired by:
  - Septic patients through bloodstream
  - Direct invasion through trauma
- Indirectly through sinusitis or otitis

Signs and Symptoms

- Headache, stiff neck, fever (95%), and photophobia
- Mental changes like confusion, lethargy, or coma in 80%
- Seizures occur in 10 to 30%.

Diagnosis

- Leukocytosis
- Blood culture positive in 50 to 60%
- Lumbar puncture:
  - Neutrophil count, protein, and opening pressure increased
  - Monocytes may predominate in cases of *Listeria*.
  - Glucose decreased
  - Check Gram stain for presence of microorganisms.
  - Cerebrospinal fluid (CSF) culture positive in 80%
- See Table 4-2 for CSF findings.
- X-rays may reveal a primary infection site.

Kernig's sign: Extending the knee with the thigh at right angles causes pain in back and hamstring.
Brudzinski's sign: Forced neck flexion results in flexion at the knee and hip.

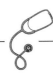

Herniation from LP occurs 1% of time and is more likely to occur in those with focal neurological findings.

Low glucose is caused by bacterial inhibition of glucose tra. :p: t into the CSF, not bacterial consumption. The value should be compared to a concurrently determined blood glucose level.

HIGH-YIELD FACTS

Neurology

TABLE 4-2. CSF Findings in Meningitis and Abscess

	WBCs	Diff.	Protein	Glucose	Opening Pressure
Bacterial meningitis	Very high	Polys	High	Low	High
Viral meningitis	High	Lymphs	Norm	Norm	Norm/high
TB/fungal meningitis	High	Lymphs	High	Low	High
Brain abscess	Norm/high	Polys	High	Low	Very high

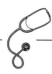

When meningitis is suspected on clinical grounds, do not wait for results of lab tests or imaging studies: Treat empirically!

Treatment

- Empiric treatment with antibiotics based on age. This is adjusted once when the Gram stain or sensitivity results are completed.
- *Streptococcus pneumoniae:* Vancomycin + cefotaxime or ceftriaxone
- *N. meningitidis:* Penicillin G or ceftriaxone
- *L. monocytogenes:* Ampicillin + gentamicin

VIRAL MENINGITIS

- Also called aseptic meningitis
- More common than bacterial
- Course is more benign.
- Signs and symptoms are similar to bacterial, but less pronounced (patient does not appear toxic).
- CSF shows normal to low protein, normal to high glucose, and lymphocytosis.
- Treatment is supportive.

BRAIN NEOPLASMS

See Table 4-3 for individual types.

Etiology

- Exposure to ionizing radiation
- Hereditary syndromes
- HIV

Astrocytomas are the most common primary intracranial neoplasms.

Epidemiology

- Kills > 13,000 per year
- Most common solid tumor of childhood
- Originates from brain, spinal cord, or meninges
- Most common:
  - Glial origin (50 to 60%)
  - Meningiomas (25%)
  - Schwannomas (8%)

TABLE 4-3. CNS Tumors

Tumor	Description
Astrocytoma	■ Most common neuroectodermal tumor ■ Those occurring in adults are usually high grade—poor prognosis. ■ *Glioblastoma multiforme* (GBM) is an aggressive anaplastic type.
Central nervous system lymphomas	■ Originate from B cells that have entered the CNS ■ Commonly affects eyes, spinal cord, or leptomeninges ■ Presents with headache, vision problems, and behavioral/personality changes ■ Diagnose by identifying malignant lymphocytes. ■ Treatment with chemotherapy and radiation
Oligodendrogliomas	■ Tend to calcify ■ More benign and better prognosis than astrocytoma
Ependymoma	■ In adults, characteristically found in spinal canal ■ In children, most common location in 4th ventricle ■ With excision, 5-year survival rate is 80%.
Meningiomas	■ Most common mesodermal tumor ■ Usually benign and slow growing, but usually discovered at large size ■ Clinically, may present as a cranial nerve palsy
Schwannomas	■ Most common cranial nerve tumor ■ Vestibular (acoustic) neuromas are 8th cranial nerve tumors. Anyone with unilateral deafness should have this ruled out.
Pituitary tumors	See endocrinology section.
Metastatic tumors to CNS	■ 80,000 per year ■ More common than primary tumors ■ Metastases common from lung, breast, and malignant melanoma

Signs and Symptoms

- Headache (40%):
    - Present upon awakening and disappears within 1 hour
    - Can wake patient from sleep
    - Worse while lying supine
    - New headache in middle-aged or older person
    - Change in headache character in person with chronic headaches
- Nausea or vomiting especially on awakening
- Irritability
- Apathy
- Sometimes vision loss, weakness of extremities
- Seizures
- Focal neurologic deficits

In migraines, prolonged headache may be followed several hours later by vomiting. In brain tumors, acute headache is followed immediately by vomiting.

Diagnosis

- MRI for detection of mass and preliminary diagnosis
- Biopsy for histology and definitive diagnosis

Treatment

- Corticosteroids to decrease edema and intracranial pressure
- Surgical resection, if possible
- Radiation and perhaps chemotherapy for high-grade tumors

EPILEPSY

Definition

- Seizure: Abnormal neuronal discharge causing a transient disturbance of cerebral function
- Epilepsy: Recurrent seizures
- 1 to 2% of population has disease

Classification

- Partial: Focal, only part of cortex involved:
  - Simple: No loss of consciousness (LOC), no postictal state
  - Complex: Postictal state present, LOC may or may not be present
- Generalized: Always associated with LOC, whole cortex is involved:
  - Absence (petit mal): Brief episode of nonresponsiveness to external or internal stimuli; motor tone is preserved
  - Tonic–clonic (grand mal): Generalized convulsion

Etiology

Status epilepticus is a long continuous seizure lasting 30 minutes or two or more seizures in a row without a lucid interval.

- Fever
- Idiopathic
- Head trauma
- Stroke
- Mass lesions
- Meningitis/encephalitis (infectious)
- Metabolic: Hypoglycemia, hyponatremia, hyperosmolarity, hypocalcemia, uremia, hepatic encephalopathy, porphyria, drugs, eclampsia, hyperthermia

Diagnosis

3-Hz spike and wave is the pathognomonic EEG pattern of absence seizures.

- Electroencephalogram (EEG)
- CT or MRI to rule out any lesions

Treatment

INH causes seizures refractory to anticonvulsant therapy. They are treated with pyridoxine (B$_6$).

- Address underlying cause if appropriate.
- Anticonvulsant therapy:
  - Benzodiazepines to break on-going seizure
  - Phenytoin, carbamazepine, and valproic acid are common preventive medications for seizure.

Definition

A toxin formed by *Clostridium botulinum* that produces paralysis

Etiology

- Ingestion of improperly prepared home processed foods, canned foods
- Wound contamination

Pathophysiology

- Toxin blocks the release of acetylcholine at the peripheral nerve endings.
- Usual incubation period is 18 to 36 hours.

Botulinum spores in honey can replicate in the gut of a newborn (who does not have normal bacterial flora yet) and cause botulism.

Signs and Symptoms

- *Neurologic:* Dry mouth, diplopia, dysphagia, dysarthria, descending weakness of the extremities and muscles of ventilation
- *GI:* Nausea, vomiting, diarrhea, abdominal cramps

Signs of botulism
"5 Ds"
- **D**ry mouth
- **D**iplopia
- **D**ysphagia
- **D**ysarthria
- **D**escending weakness

Diagnosis

- Detection of neurotoxin by serology

Treatment

Ingestion
- Antitoxin
- Vomiting and cathartics can be used to decrease absorption.

Wound Contamination
- Drainage of lesion, antitoxin, and penicillin

For Both
- Intubation with ventilatory support

Prevention

The toxin can be inactivated after 10 minutes in boiling water. The spores, however, can withstand boiling temperatures for several hours.

Pathophysiology

Autoimmune disease in which antibodies against the postsynaptic nicotinic acetylcholine receptor prevent acetylcholine from binding. Therefore, an end plate potential cannot be generated at the neuromuscular junction.

Epidemiology

- Two peaks of incidence:
  - Women in 2nd to 3rd decade
  - Men older than 60
- 20% have thyroid disease.

Signs and Symptoms

- Muscular weakness and fatigue
- Ptosis and diplopia (by affecting muscles of eye)
- Proximal muscle weakness
- Intact reflexes

Diagnosis

Edrophonium (Tensilon™) test: Edrophonium inhibits acetylcholinesterase (enzyme which breaks down acetylcholine). Therefore, more acetylcholine is available to stimulate the receptors at the postsynaptic junction. The patient's muscle strength improves during administration of the drug.

Labs and Tests

- Antibody presence against acetylcholine receptor (AChR)
- Chest MRI to evaluate any thymus abnormalities

Treatment

- If mild, anticholinesterase drug
- Thymectomy when indicated
- Prednisone as first line therapy
- Cyclosporine or azathioprine if prednisone not effective

GUILLAIN–BARRÉ SYNDROME

Definition

Syndrome of transient immune-mediated ascending paralysis usually following a viral upper respiratory tract infection

Forty to 50% of patients with ocular myasthenia gravis go on to develop generalized myasthenia gravis.

Symptoms worsen as day progresses. (This is the opposite of rheumatoid arthritis.)

In myasthenia gravis, repetitive muscle use quickly induces fatigue, whereas in Eaton–Lambert syndrome, repetitive muscle use improves muscle strength.

Aminoglycosides can precipitate myasthenic crisis.

Pathophysiology

Removal of myelin from axons of nerves by macrophages

Signs and Symptoms

- Prodrome 1 to 3 weeks: Initial symptoms are paresthesias beginning in the feet and spreading symmetrically and proximally (ascending paralysis).
- Distal muscle weakness is common soon afterward—may last a few weeks.
- Deep aching pain in back and legs
- Areflexia
- Tachypnea
- Quadriparesis and respiratory muscle paralysis occur in 30% of patients.
- Respiratory muscle paralysis can be fatal.

Follow peak flows for a measure of declining respiratory muscle function.

Diagnosis

- CSF shows increased protein, but no WBCs.
- EMG shows signs of demyelination with marked decrease in action potential conduction velocities.

Treatment

- Mechanical ventilation for respiratory muscle paralysis
- Plasma exchange and IV immunoglobulin in selected patients
- Reassurance
- Most cases resolve spontaneously over the course of a few weeks.

HEADACHE

Top 10 Causes of Headache
- Chronic headache syndromes (migraine, cluster, tension headaches)
- Subarachnoid hemorrhage
- Meningitis
- Hypertension
- Mass lesion
- Temporal arteritis
- Trigeminal neuralgia
- Brain abscess
- Pseudotumor cerebri
- Subdural hematoma

MIGRAINE HEADACHE

Pathophysiology

According to the vasogenic theory, cerebral vasoconstriction is followed by vasodilation.

Epidemiology

- 60% have family history.
- 12% in United States affected
- Females > males

Signs and Symptoms

1. *Migraine with aura (classic):* Patient suffers from aura approximately 1 hour before onset. The focal neurological dysfunction can include photophobia, sonophobia, nausea, vomiting, vertigo, dysarthria, tinnitus, diploplia, weakness, and ataxia. Patient may also complain of scintillating scotoma or homonymous hemianopsia.
2. *Migraine without aura (common):* Photophobia and sonophobia are again noted, along with anorexia, nausea, vomiting, and general malaise. Specific visual findings are usually not involved.

Both types have prodromal symptoms 1 to 2 days before attack. These include lethargy, craving of food, depression, and fluid retention.

Headache phase of migraine may last several hours. It is characterized by a unilateral, throbbing head pain.

Treatment

- Nonpharmacologic: Avoidance of triggers, stress reduction, dark quiet environment
- Acute treatment:
  - Nonsteroidal anti-inflammatory drugs (NSAIDs)
  - Ergotamine derivatives
  - 5-HT receptor agonists (sumatriptan)
  - Antiemetics (metoclopramide IV)

Prophylaxis: Calcium channel blockers, beta blockers, tricyclics, and serotonergic drugs

Abdominal pain regularly accompanying migraine headaches is called *abdominal migraine.*

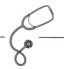

5-HT receptor agonists can cause coronary vasospasm.

TENSION HEADACHE

Signs and Symptoms

- Muscular contractions causing bandlike pain located in head and neck
- Neck stiffness
- Usually bilateral
- No prodrome
- Worsens as the day progresses

Treatment

- Aspirin or acetaminophen
- Narcotics if severe
- Prophylaxis with tricyclics like amitriptyline

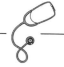

Tension headache may benefit from head and neck massage.

Epidemiology

- Increased incidence in males than females
- Increased incidence after alcohol, nitrates, or stress

Signs and Symptoms

- Unrelenting unilateral facial pain, which tends to occur in clusters
- Pain so severe it can lead to suicide
- Headaches are often seasonal.
- Accompanied by ipsilateral autonomic signs, including conjunctival injection, lacrimation, rhinorrhea, nasal congestion, ptosis, miosis, eyelid edema, and facial sweating

Treatment

Acute Episodes
- High-flow oxygen
- Intranasal lidocaine
- Ergotamine, sumatriptan, and antiemetics if the above fail

Prophylaxis
- Verapamil, methysergide, high-dose prednisone followed by rapid taper, or indomethacin

Definition

Idiopathic inflammation of temporal artery histologically characterized by giant multinucleated cells

Etiology

Idiopathic

Epidemiology

More common in women and persons older than 60

Signs and Symptoms

- Unilateral headache in distribution of temporal artery
- Thickened, tender temporal arteries
- Ipsilateral visual loss (late finding)
- Claudication of the masseter, temporalis, and tongue muscles
- Scalp tenderness
- Pulsating temporal artery

More than 50% of patients with temporal arteritis have polymyalgia rheumatica.

Typical scenario:
A 62-year-old woman presents with headache, pain when she chews, and scalp tenderness.
Think: Temporal arteritis. Treat with steriods.

Diagnosis

- High erythrocyte sedimentation rate (ESR), C-reactive protein
- Definitive diagnosis by temporal artery biopsy

Treatment

- Corticosteroids as soon as suspected; can lead to blindness if treatment is delayed
- NSAIDs for pain relief

Involve ophthalmology early when suspecting temporal arteritis to aid in prevention of vision loss.

The most common cause of blindness in the United States is macular degeneration.

ACUTE VISION LOSS

See Table 4-4 for differential diagnosis.

TABLE 4-4. Differential Diagnosis for Acute Vision Loss

Differential Diagnosis	Description	Treatment
Central retinal artery occlusion	<ul><li>Typically painless loss of vision</li><li>Causes ischemic stroke of retina</li><li>Cherry red spot on fovea</li></ul>	Dissolve or dislodge embolus.
Retinal detachment	<ul><li>Symptoms include flashes of light.</li><li>Floaters</li><li>Vision loss</li></ul>	Surgery or laser treatment.
Vitreous hemorrhage	<ul><li>Caused by bleeding into vitreous humor</li><li>Common causes are diabetic retinopathy and retinal tears.</li><li>Symptoms initially include floaters, which progress to vision loss.</li></ul>	Photocoagulation or vitrectomy
Optic neuritis	<ul><li>Painful, unilateral vision loss with partial resolution</li><li>Inflammation of optic nerve</li><li>Caused by demyelination</li><li>Visual acuity at its worst in 1 week</li><li>Other symptoms include headache and eye pain with movement.</li><li>Many patients have progression to multiple sclerosis.</li></ul>	Steroids quicken recovery.
Temporal (giant cell) arteritis	<ul><li>See description under Headaches</li></ul>	

DEMENTIA

Definition

Loss of cognitive function with normal sensorium

Etiology

- CVAs
- Infection (particularly syphilis, AIDS, Creutzfeldt–Jakob)
- Epilepsy
- Vitamin deficiency (folate, B$_{12}$, thiamin, niacin)
- Normal pressure hydrocephalus (NPH)
- Neurodegenerative disorders (Alzheimer's, Parkinson's, Huntington's, amyotrophic lateral sclerosis)
- Trauma
- Toxins
- Tumors

Causes of dementia:
Vincent **V**an **G**ogh **w**as demented.
Vitamin deficiency
Infection
NPH
CVA
Epilepsy
Neurodegeneration
Trauma, tumors, toxins

Diagnosis

Dementia workup should include CBC, electrolyte panel, B$_{12}$, folate, rapid plasma reagin (RPR), and head CT.

Treatment

- Treat underlying disorder.
- Optimize sensory function (vision aids, hearing aids).
- Simplify activities of daily living (simplify floor plans, stairs).
- Ensure physical safety (bedrails, companions).

NORMAL PRESSURE HYDROCEPHALUS (NPH)

Definition

Increased CSF without increased intracranial pressure

Etiology

Usually sequela of some other CNS event (Subarachnoid hemorrhage, meningitis, trauma, tumor)

Signs and Symptoms

Classic Triad
- Gait disorder (most responsive to treatment)
- Urinary incontinence
- Dementia (most refractory to treatment)

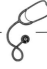

NPH is one of the few reversible causes of dementia.

Diagnosis

- Normal pressure on lumbar puncture (LP)
- Enlarged ventricles on CT or MRI
- Clinical improvement after LP and removal of a volume of CSF

Treatment

- CSF ventricular shunt
- Choroid plexectomy in some cases

ALZHEIMER'S DISEASE

Alzheimer's is the most common cause of dementia.

Definition

- Slowly progressive dementia characterized by amyloid plaques and neurofibrillary tangles in the neurons of the cerebral cortex (mostly temporal lobe)

Epidemiology

- Older people
- Family history (apolipoprotein E genotype)
- Higher incidence in patients with Down's syndrome

Alzheimer's disease is definitively diagnosed by tissue examination on autopsy.

Signs and Symptoms

- Usually present with memory deficits (key feature)
- Aphasia, apraxia, agnosia

Diagnosis

- Diagnosis is mainly clinical.
- Cortical atrophy on CT or MRI (see Figure 4-4)
- EEG slowing

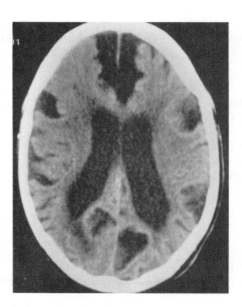

FIGURE 4-4. Alzheimer's disease. Note the severe frontal atrophy.

(Reproduced, with permission, from Lee, Rao, and Zimmerman. *Cranial MRI and CT*. New York: McGraw-Hill, 1999: 194.)

Treatment

- Donepezil, tacrine, and selegiline may slow cognitive decline.
- Gingko biloba and vitamin E may be protective.
- Behavioral symptoms can be treated with neuroleptics, anxiolytics, and antidepressants.

PARKINSON'S DISEASE

Definition

Complex progressive disorder involving movement and higher cognitive function

Etiology

- Degeneration of neurons in the substantia nigra
- May be secondary to toxins (manganese, carbon monoxide, designer drugs) and encephalitis

Epidemiology

Mean age is 55—more common in men (3:2).

Signs and Symptoms

Signs and symptoms fluctuate:
- **Pill-rolling resting tremor**
- **Cogwheel rigidity**
- **Bradykinesia**
- Shuffling gait
- Mask facies
- Depression
- Hallucinations

Cognitive decline is a late feature of Parkinson's.

Diagnosis

- Clinical presentation
- Response to levodopa–carbidopa

Treatment

- Amantadine may improve tremor and bradykinesia in early disease by blocking reuptake of dopamine into presynaptic neurons.
- Levodopa: Converted to dopamine in substantia nigra; co-administer with carbidopa (does not cross BBB) to block metabolism of levodopa in peripheral tissues.
- Anticholinergics: Block cholinergic inhibition of dopaminergic neurons in substantia nigra; commonly trihexyphenidyl, benztropine mesylate

The pathophysiologic opposite of Parkinson's disease (dopamine paucity) is schizophrenia (dopamine excess).

- Selegiline: Selective MAO-B inhibitor, blocks central metabolism of dopamine
- Dopamine receptor agonists such as bromocriptine, pergolide

FEATURES OF BRAIN DEATH

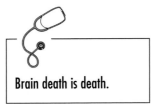

Brain death is death.

- Preserved cardiac function
- No spontaneous respiratory function
- No cranial nerve reflexes (especially pupils)
- No posturing (decerebrate or decorticate)
- No evidence of hypothermia
- No known reversibility of state

Gastroenterology

Eric Michael Fields and Barbara G. Lock

GASTROINTESTINAL DISORDERS

ABDOMINAL PAIN

Types of Pain

Visceral Pain
- Vague, dull, and poorly localized pain
- Midline location due to bilateral innervation of organs based on their embryological origin
- Associated with stretching, inflammation, or ischemia, involving bowel walls or organ capsules

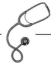

V is for Vague. **Example:** Early appendicitis; initially dull, periumbilical pain.

Parietal Pain
- Sharp, well-localized pain; peritonitis associated with rebound and involuntary guarding
- Pain location correlates with associated dermatomes.
- Occurs commonly with inflammation, frank pus, blood, or bile in or adjacent to the peritoneum

Peritonitis is associated with rebound tenderness and involuntary guarding.

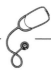

P is for Pinpoint. **Example:** Late appendicitis; local inflammation leads to tenderness in the right lower quadrant.

Referred Pain
- Pain stimuli generated at an afflicted location are perceived as originating from a site in which there is no current pathology.
- These sites are usually related by a common embryological origin.
- The pain can sometimes be perceived in both locations.

Example: Ureteral obstruction can produce pain in the ipsilateral testicle.

Typical scenario:
A 45-year-old obese woman complains of fever, RUQ pain, and nausea that is worse when she eats. *Think: Cholecystitis.*

Typical scenario:
A 26-year-old woman complains of severe left lower quadrant pain, vaginal bleeding, weakness, and light-headedness. Last menstrual period was 6 weeks ago. *Think: Ectopic pregnancy.*

Typical scenario:
A 28-year-old woman presents with diffuse abdominal pain, nausea, and confusion. She is not pregnant. She currently takes a stained-glass class. *Think: Lead poisoning.*

Causes of Abdominal Pain

Right Upper Quadrant
Gastric ulcer
Peptic ulcer
Biliary disease
Hepatitis
Pancreatitis
Retrocecal appendicitis
Renal stone
Pyelonephritis
Myocardial infarction
Pulmonary embolus
Pneumonia

Left Upper Quadrant
Gastric ulcer
Gastritis
Pancreatitis
Splenic injury
Renal stone
Pyelonephritis
Myocardial infarction
Pulmonary embolus
Pneumonia

Right Lower Quadrant
Appendicitis
Ovarian cyst
Mittelschmerz
Pregnancy (ectopic or normal)
Tubo-ovarian abscess
Pelvic inflammatory disease
Ovarian torsion
Cystitis
Prostatitis
Ureteral stone
Testicular torsion
Epididymitis
Diverticulitis/perforation
Abdominal aortic aneurysm

Left Lower Quadrant
Diverticulitis
Ovarian cyst
Mittelschmerz
Pregnancy (ectopic or normal)
Tubo-ovarian abscess
Pelvic inflammatory disease
Ovarian torsion
Cystitis
Prostatitis
Ureteral stone
Testicular torsion
Epididymitis
Diverticular perforation
Abdominal aortic aneurysm

Note: All premenopausal women with abdominal pain must have a pregnancy test, even if they say they are not sexually active.

Other Causes of Abdominal Pain

Abdominal Wall
- Hernia
- Rectus sheath hematoma

Metabolic
- Diabetic ketoacidosis
- Acute intermittent porphyria
- Hypercalcemia

Infectious
- Herpes zoster
- Mononucleosis
- HIV

Drugs/Toxins
- Heavy metal poisoning
- Black widow spider envenomation

Other

- Sickle cell anemia
- Mesenteric ischemia

Abdominal Pain in the Elderly

Elderly patients who present with abdominal pain must be treated with particular caution. Common problems include:

- Difficulty communicating
- Comorbid disease
- Inability to tolerate intravascular volume loss
- Unusual presentation of common disease
- May not mount a white blood cell count or a fever
- Complaint often incommensurate with severity of disease

Note: Up to 2% of elderly patients with an MI will present with abdominal pain.

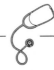

In elderly patients with abdominal pain, always consider vascular causes, including:
- AAA
- Mesenteric ischemia
- Myocardial infarction

ABDOMINAL AORTIC ANEURYSM

Definition

Abdominal aortic aneurysms are associated with atherosclerosis. Acute expansion or leak of an AAA causes pain and may precede rupture, a life-threatening emergency.

Risk Factors

- Atherosclerosis
- Aneurysms > 5 cm associated with 20 to 40% 5-year risk of rupture

Signs and Symptoms

- Syncope or light-headedness
- Abdominal or back pain
- Pulsatile mass in abdomen
- Hypotension
- History of vascular disease or atherosclerosis

Typical scenario:
A 63-year-old obese man complains of pain in his "kidney" for 3 days. He has a history of MI × 2. He has no back tenderness. *Think: Abdominal aortic aneurysm.*

Diagnosis

Ultrasound: Can detect aneurysm's dimensions. Not currently helpful in demonstrating leak or thrombus. Operator and patient dependent.
MRI or CT scan with IV contrast: Can demonstrate size of aneurysm and location of leak or rupture. May replace angiogram as gold standard.
Angiogram: Can demonstrate size of aneurysm and location of leak or rupture. Can underestimate size of aneurysm with mural thrombus.

Treatment

All patients should have good IV access and a type and cross. Patients with a suspected rupture in progress require emergent surgical repair.

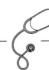

For suspected AAA rupture in progress, diagnostic tests may be eliminated and the patient may be taken directly to the OR.

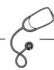
MESENTERIC ISCHEMIA

Definition

Ischemia of the small bowel due to compromised mesenteric blood supply

Causes

- Atherosclerosis causing obstruction of SMA, IMA, or celiac artery
- Atrial fibrillation: Embolus
- Low-flow state: Hypotension, poor cardiac output
- Mesenteric venous thrombosis
- Hypercoagulability

Signs and Symptoms

- Severe abdominal pain out of proportion to exam
- History of similar abdominal pain after eating
- Late: Metabolic acidosis, increased lactic acid, bloody stools

Diagnosis

- Gold standard is angiography.
- Spiral CT scan with PO and IV contrast is often useful.

Treatment

- Maintain tissue perfusion.
- Early surgical involvement

DISORDERS OF THE ESOPHAGUS AND STOMACH

INFECTIOUS ESOPHAGITIS

Etiology

Viral Esophagitis
- Herpes simplex virus
- Varicella-zoster virus
- Cytomegalovirus

Bacterial Esophagitis
- *Lactobacillus*
- *Streptococcus*
- *Cryptosporidium*
- *Pneumocystis carinii*
- *Mycobacterium tuberculosis*

Other Causes
- *Candida*
- Radiation exposure or therapy
- Corrosive exposure

Signs and Symptoms
- Odynophagia
- Dysphagia
- Esophageal bleeding
- Nausea/vomiting
- Chest pain
- May be asymptomatic

Diagnosis

Candida: Nodular filling defects on barium esophagogram
HSV, VZV: Vesicles and discrete erosions on endoscopy
CMV: Intranuclear inclusions on biopsy via endoscopy

Treatment

Candida: Fluconazole PO
HSV: Acyclovir IV
CMV: Ganciclovir IV

Differential: A patient with HIV and odynophagia (pain on swallowing) has esophagitis most likely due to:
- Candida
- CMV
- Herpes

ESOPHAGEAL PERFORATION OR RUPTURE

Definition

Iatrogenic or pathologic trauma to the esophagus, which may result in leakage of air and esophageal contents into the mediastinum. Carries a 50% mortality.

Etiology

Iatrogenic: This often occurs in an already diseased esophagus. Comprises 50 to 75% of cases of esophageal rupture:
- Endoscopy
- Dilation
- Blakemore tubes
- Intubation of the esophagus
- Nasogastric tube placement

Typical scenario:
An alcoholic man presents after severe retching, complaining of retrosternal and upper abdominal pain. *Think: Boerhaave's syndrome (full thickness) or Mallory–Weiss syndrome (partial thickness).*

Boerhaave's syndrome: A *full-thickness* tear. Generally occurs in the relatively weak left posterolateral wall of distal esophagus. Due to:
- Forceful vomiting
- Cough
- Labor
- Lifting
- Trauma

Mallory–Weiss syndrome: A *partial-thickness* tear. Usually occurs in the right posterolateral wall of the distal esophagus and results in bleeding that generally resolves spontaneously. Due to:
- Forceful vomiting

Foreign body ingestion: Objects usually lodge near anatomic narrowings:
- Distal to the upper esophageal sphincter
- Near the aortic arch
- At lower esophageal sphincter

Subcutaneous and mediastinal emphysema are due to a full-thickness tear.

Signs and Symptoms

- Severe, constant pain in chest, abdomen, and back
- Dysphagia
- Dyspnea
- Subcutaneous emphysema
- Mediastinal emphysema heard as a "crunching sound" with heartbeat (Hammon's crunch)

Diagnosis

- **Chest x-ray:** Left-sided pleural effusion, mediastinal or subcutaneous emphysema
- **Esophagogram with *water-soluble* contrast:** Shows extravasation of contrast
- **Other studies:** Endoscopy, CT, and pleurocentesis (check fluid for low pH and high amylase)

Treatment

Surgical repair of full-thickness tears. Partial-thickness tears may resolve spontaneously.

ZENKER'S DIVERTICULUM

Zenker's is a pulsion diverticulum: arises from pressure of swallowing.

Definition

Pharyngeal or esophageal pouch due to a defect in the muscular wall of the posterior hypopharynx

Signs and Symptoms

- Halitosis
- Frequent aspiration
- Esophageal obstruction

Diagnosis

- Barium swallow
- Endoscopy

Treatment

Surgical removal or cricopharyngeal myotomy

ESOPHAGEAL SPASM

See Table 5-1.

Etiology

- Achalasia is thought to arise from scarring in Auerbach's plexus.
- DES shows no physical abnormality in Auerbach's plexus but is thought to arise from hypoactive inhibitory interneurons within it.

Epidemiology

Achalasia has equal incidence in males and females. Ratio not known for diffuse esophageal spasm (DES).

Diagnosis

- Barium swallow (see Figures 5-1 and 5-2)
- Manometry: Achalasia will show normal to increased pressure at LES with no relaxation upon swallowing; DES will show high amplitude contractions, possibly including proximal esophagus.

Barium swallow:
- Bird's beak or steeple sign: Achalasia
- Corkscrew-shaped: DES

TABLE 5-1. Comparison of Achalasia and Diffuse Esophageal Spasm

	Achalasia	Diffuse Esophageal Spasm
Signs and symptoms	Weight loss, cough, diffuse chest pain	Dysphagia, diffuse chest pain
Pattern of contraction	Failure of LES to relax on swallowing Classic: Simultaneous small wave Vigorous: Simultaneous large wave	Swallow-induced large wave
Relieved by	Nitroglycerin	Nitroglycerin
X-ray findings	Absence of gastric bubble, narrowing of terminal esophagus that looks like a beak	Corkscrew appearance
Treatment	Nitroglycerin, local botulinum toxin, balloon dilatation, sphincter myotomy	Nitroglycerin, anticholinergics

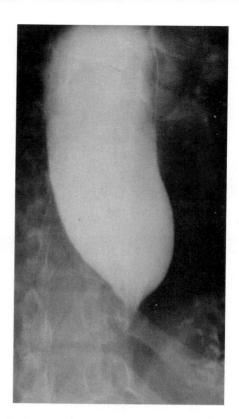

FIGURE 5-1. Achalasia. Barium esophagogram in a patient with achalasia demonstrates a dilated esophagus with a sharply tapered "bird's beak" narrowing.

(Reproduced, with permission, from Waters PF, DeMeester TR. Foregut motor disorders and their surgical management. *Med Clin North Am* 65:1244, 1981.)

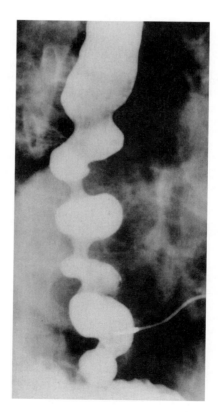

FIGURE 5-2. Diffuse esophageal spasm. Barium esophagogram in a patient with diffuse esophageal spasm demonstrates the characteristic "corkscrew" pattern.

(Reproduced, with permission, from *Schwartz's Principles of Surgery*, 7th ed. New York, NY: McGraw-Hill, 2000: 1129.)

Plummer–Vinson Syndrome

Hypopharyngeal webs associated with iron deficiency anemia

Schatzki Ring

A narrow lower esophageal ring associated with dysphagia (see Figure 5-3)

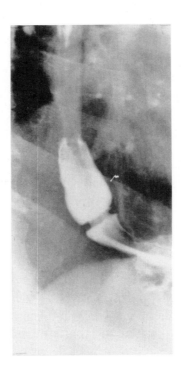

FIGURE 5-3. Schatzki's ring. Barium esophagogram in a patient with Schatzki's ring demonstrates a distal esophageal ring at the gastroesophageal junction.
(Reproduced, with permission, from *Schwartz's Principles of Surgery,* 7th ed. New York, NY: McGraw-Hill, 2000: 1168.)

GASTROESOPHAGEAL REFLUX DISEASE

Definition

GERD: Reflux of acidic gastric contents into the esophagus

Causes of GERD

- Relaxed or incompetent lower esophageal sphincter (LES)
- Hiatal hernia
- Delayed gastric emptying
- Decreased esophageal motility

Causes of delayed gastric emptying:
- Diabetes mellitus
- Gastroparesis
- Gastric outlet obstruction
- Anticholinergic use
- Fatty foods

Causes of Lowered LES Tone

- Coffee
- Cigarettes
- Alcohol
- Chocolate
- Peppermint
- Anticholinergics
- Progesterone
- Estrogen
- Nitrates
- Calcium channel blockers

Signs and Symptoms

- Substernal burning pain
- Dysphagia
- Hypersalivation (water brash)
- Cough

Diagnosis

Barium swallow, esophagoscopy, mucosal biopsy

Treatment

- Elevate head of bed.
- Discontinue foods which decrease LES tone
- Oral antacids
- H$_2$ blocker or proton pump inhibitor
- Patients with hiatal hernia may be candidates for Nissen fundoplication (the stomach is wrapped around the distal esophagus to create a "new sphincter").

Complications of GERD

- **Esophagitis:** Esophageal damage, bleeding, and friability due to prolonged exposure to gastric contents
- **Peptic stricture:** Occurs in about 10% of patients with GERD
- **Barrett's esophagus:** Transformation of normal squamous epithelium to columnar epithelium, sometimes accompanied by an ulcer or stricture
- **Esophageal cancer:** Upper ⅔ squamous, lower ⅓ adenocarcinoma

PEPTIC ULCER DISEASE (PUD)

PUD consists of duodenal ulcers (DU) and gastric ulcers (GU).

Epidemiology

- Two times more common in men
- Incidence increases with age.
- Smoking and EtOH increase risk.

Pathophysiology

Key Concepts
- Parietal cells secrete HCl into the gastric lumen and bicarbonate into the gastric venous circulation (alkaline tide) and into the protective gastric mucous gel.
- A proton pump exchanges potassium in the gastric lumen for protons.
- The parietal cells are stimulated by gastrin and the vagus nerve.
- Gastrin release is stimulated by gastrin-releasing peptide and is inhibited by somatostatin.
- Histamine receptors on parietal cells also stimulate HCl secretion.
- Gastric bicarbonate secretion into the mucous gel is inhibited by non-steroidal anti-inflammatory drugs (NSAIDs), acetazolamide, alpha blockers, and alcohol.
- Gel thickness is increased by prostaglandin E (PGE) and reduced by steroids and NSAIDs.

Typical scenario:
A patient with known PUD presents with sudden onset of severe epigastric pain. Physical exam reveals guarding and rebound tenderness.
Think: Perforation.

Complications

- **Bleeding:** 20% incidence
- **Perforation:**
    - 7% incidence
    - Posterior perforation of a duodenal ulcer will cause pain that radiates to the back and can cause pancreatitis. A chest or abdominal film will not show free air because the posterior duodenum is retroperitoneal.
    - Anterior perforation will show free air under the diaphragm in 70% of cases (see Figure 5-4).
- **Gastric outlet obstruction,** due to scarring and edema

Typical scenario:
A 52-year-old woman presents due to 3 months of early satiety, weight loss, and vomiting.
Think: Gastric outlet obstruction.

DUODENAL ULCER (DU)

Pathophysiology

Increased acid production

Etiology

H. pylori
- A bacterium that produces urease, which breaks down the protective mucous lining of the stomach. Ten to 20% of persons with *H. pylori* develop PUD.

NSAIDs/Steroids
- Inhibit production of PGE thereby inhibiting mucosal barrier production

Zollinger–Ellison Syndrome
- A gastrin-secreting tumor in or near the pancreas. ZE can be part of multiple endocrine neoplasia type I (MEN I). Diarrhea is common.

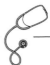

Over 90% of patients with ZE have peptic ulcer disease.

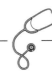

H. pylori may colonize 90% of the population — infection does not necessitate disease.

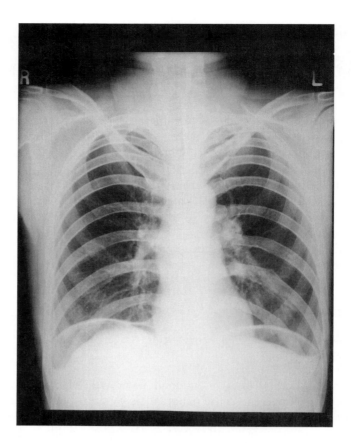

FIGURE 5-4. Free air. Upright chest film in a patient with perforated duodenal ulcer demonstrates free air underneath both right and left hemidiaphragms.
(Reproduced, with permission, from *Schwartz's Principles of Surgery*, 7th ed. New York, NY: McGraw-Hill, 2000: 1195.)

Typical scenario:
A 33-year-old female smoker presents with burning epigastric pain that is improved after eating a meal.
Think: Duodenal ulcer.

Clinical Features

- Burning gnawing epigastric pain that occurs with an empty stomach: Pain is relieved within 30 minutes by food.
- Nighttime awakening (when stomach empties)
- Nausea, vomiting
- Associated with blood type O

Diagnosis

DU

- Via endoscopy; however, most symptomatic cases of DU are easily diagnosed clinically. If patient responds to DU therapy, there is no need to do the biopsy.

H. pylori

- Endoscopy with biopsy—allows culture and sensitivity for *H. pylori* (organism is notoriously hard to culture—multiple specimens required during biopsy)
- Serology: Anti–*H. pylori* IgG indicates current or prior infection.
- *Urease breath test:* $C^{13/14}$ labeled urea is ingested. If gastric urease is present, the carbon isotope can be detected as CO_2 isotopes in the breath.

ZE

- Secretin stimulation test: Secretin, a gastrin inhibitor, is delivered parenterally (usually with Ca^{2+}), and its effect on gastrin secretion is measured. In ZE syndrome, there is a paradoxical astronomic rise in serum gastrin.

Treatment

- Discontinue NSAIDs, steroids, and smoking.
- Triple therapy for *H. pylori* (e.g., proton pump inhibitor, amoxicillin, and clarithromycin)
- Antacids
- H_2 blockers
- Prostaglandin analogs (misoprostol)
- Mucosal barrier enhancers (sucralfate)
- Proton pump inhibitors
- Surgery is indicated when ulcer is refractory to 12 weeks of medical treatment, or if hemorrhage, obstruction, or perforation is present.

GASTRIC ULCER (GU)

Pathophysiology

Decreased protection against acid: *normal or low acid production*

Etiology

- *H. pylori* (less than for duodenal)
- NSAIDs/steroids

Clinical Features

- Burning gnawing epigastric pain that occurs with anything in the stomach: Pain is **worst 30 minutes after food.**
- Anorexia/weight loss
- Vomiting
- Associated with blood type A

Diagnosis

Via endoscopy; 3% of GUs are associated with gastric cancer, so all GUs are biopsied.

Treatment

Same as for DU

- NSAIDs and steroids inhibit production of PGE.
- PGE stimulates production of the gastric mucosal barrier.
- *H. pylori* produces urease, which breaks down the gastric mucosal barrier.

Gastric ulcers can even occur with achlorhydria.

Smoking is a risk factor for GU.

Typical scenario:
A 45-year-old Japanese male smoker presents with epigastric pain, exacerbated by eating, and weight loss. *Think: Gastric ulcer.*

- Burnt paper CURLS
- CrUSHING'S ulcer

SPECIAL GASTRIC ULCERS

- Curling's ulcers: Gastric stress ulcers in patients with severe burns
- Cushing's ulcers: Gastric stress ulcer related to severe CNS damage

GASTRITIS

Definition

- Acute or chronic inflammation of the stomach lining

Etiologies of gastritis:
"GNASHING"
- **G**astric reflux (bile or pancreatic secretions)
- **N**icotine
- **A**lcohol
- **S**tress
- **H**elicobacter pylori and other infections
- **I**schemia
- **N**SAIDs
- **G**lucocorticoids (long term use)

Etiology

- Increased acid: Smoking, alcohol, stress
- Decreased mucosal barrier: NSAIDs, steroids
- Direct irritant: Pancreatic and biliary reflux, infection

Signs and Symptoms

- Burning or gnawing pain
- Pain *usually worsened with food* and relieved by antacids
- Vomiting may relieve the pain after eating.

Diagnosis

Diagnosis is made by endoscopy.

Treatment

- Dicontinue NSAIDs.
- Triple therapy to eradicate *H. pylori* if present
- Abstain from cigarettes and alcohol.
- H₂ blockers (e.g., cimetidine, ranitidine), sucralfate, or misoprostol
- Over-the-counter antacids

Cimetidine is a p450 inhibitor and, therefore, prolongs the action of drugs cleared in the liver by this system.

Complications of Gastritis

Chronic gastritis leads to:
- Gastric atrophy
- Gastric metaplasia
- Pernicious anemia (decreased production of intrinsic factor from gastric parietal cells due to **idiopathic** atrophy of the gastric mucosa and subsequent malabsorption of vitamin B_{12})

Gastrointestinal Bleeds

Etiology

- Mallory–Weiss tear
- Varices
- Gastritis
- Arteriovenous malformation
- Ulcer (peptic)

Signs and Symptoms

- Hematemesis (bright red or coffee grounds)
- Hypotension
- Tachycardia
- Bleeding that produces 60 cc of blood or more will produce black, tarry stool.
- Very brisk upper GI bleeds can be associated with bright red blood per rectum.

Diagnosis

- Gastric lavage with normal saline or free water to assess severity of bleeding (old versus new blood)
- Rectal exam
- CBC
- Endoscopy
- Bleeding scan
- Arteriography

Treatment

- Depends on etiology and severity
- Bleeding varices are ligated, tamponaded, or sclerosed via endoscopy.
- Most Mallory–Weiss tears resolve spontaneously.
- For severe bleeds:
  - Intravenous fluids and blood products as needed
  - Somatostatin (inhibits gastric, intestinal, and biliary motility, decreases visceral blood flow)
  - Consider balloon tamponade.

Etiology of UGI bleeds:
Mallory's **V**ices **G**ave (her) **A**n **U**lcer.

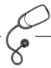

Coffee grounds is the term used to describe old, brown, digested blood found on gastric lavage. It usually indicates a source of bleeding proximal to the ligament of Treitz.

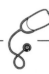

A bleeding scan detects *active* bleeding by infusing a radioactive colloid or radiolabeled autologous RBCs and watching for their collection in the GI tract.

HIGH-YIELD FACTS

Gastroenterology

Etiology of UGI bleeds: **Can U Cure Aunt Di's Hemorrhoids.**

CBC in hemorrhage will not reflect the true severity of the bleed for 4 to 6 hours, as it takes time for the concentration to change.

Patients with GI bleeds should have two large-bore IVs and a type and cross. These patients can bleed rapidly.

Etiology

- Cancer or polyps
- Upper GI bleed
- Colitis (infectious, inflammatory bowel disease, ischemic, etc.)
- Angiodysplasia
- Diverticulosis
- Hemorrhoids

Signs and Symptoms

- Bright red blood per rectum
- Melena (black or maroon tarry stool)
- Hypotension
- Tachycardia

Diagnosis

- Gastric lavage to rule out upper GI source
- Rectal exam
- CBC
- Colonoscopy
- Bleeding scan
- Arteriography

Treatment

- Fluids, blood products as needed
- Surgical involvement
- Bowel prep
- Very severe cases may require colectomy.

MAJOR TYPES OF MALABSORPTION

MALABSORPTION

Definition

Disruption in absorption of food, water, or vitamins due to alterations in intestinal function. For sites of absorption of specific nutrients, see Table 5-2.

TABLE 5-2. GI Absorption

Nutrient	Site	Comments
Monosaccharides	Whole small bowel	■ Only monosaccharides are absorbed. ■ Complex carbohydrate (starch) is degraded by salivary and pancreatic amylase to disaccharides (mostly maltose), which cannot be absorbed. ■ Brush border enzymes cleave disaccharides to monosaccharides. ■ Glucose and galactose are cotransported with Na^+, energy derived from Na^+ gradient maintained by Na^+-K^+ ATPase. Low Na^+ meals reduce the gradient, retarding absorption. ■ Fructose uses facilitated diffusion independent of Na^+ and does not require energy. However, the fructose carrier proteins are relatively sparse and can be overwhelmed, resulting in an osmotic diarrhea following a high-fructose meal. ■ Pentoses cross by passive diffusion.
Lipids and lipid-soluble vitamins (A, D, E, and K)	Duodenum > jejunum	■ Pancreatic lipase hydrolyzes triglycerides to fatty acids and monoglycerides. ■ Bile salts combine with fatty acids, cholesterol, and monoglycerides to form micelles, which allow passive diffusion of the lipids into the brush border cells. ■ Bile salts are not absorbed here but are recycled until they reach the ileum. ■ Lipid-soluble vitamins absorbed into micelles—low-fat meals inhibit absorption of these nutrients.
Amino acids	Jejunum > duodenum	■ Protein digestion begins in the stomach, with pepsins yielding small polypeptides. ■ In the duodenum, pancreatic enzymes (trypsin, chymotrypsin, elastase) and brush border enzymes digest the gastric polypeptides to amino acids, dipeptides, and tripeptides. ■ Most amino acids cotransported with Na^+ similar to glucose ■ Many different Na^+-independent transporters for specific amino acids, dipeptides, and tripeptides
Nucleic acids	Whole small bowel	■ Split into pentoses and bases by pancreatic nucleases. ■ Pentoses diffuse freely throughout small bowel. ■ Bases absorbed by active transport in duodenum and jejunum
Water	Jejunum > ileum > colon	■ Average intake of 2 L/day, endogenous secretions amount to an additional 7 L/day, all but ~200 mL is reabsorbed. ■ Most water reabsorbed in small bowel, most colonic water reabsorbed in cecum ■ Water moves freely in response to osmotic gradients.
Water-soluble vitamins	Duodenum > jejunum	■ Most cross by passive diffusion.
Vitamin B_{12}	Ileum	■ Bound to intrinsic factor from gastric parietal cells ■ Unknown mechanism of absorption by ileal mucosa
Bile salts	Ileum	■ Active transport in ileum
Na^+	Whole small bowel	■ Active and passive absorption thoughout ■ Secretion throughout by Na^+-K^+ ATPase
K^+	Whole small bowel	■ *Secreted* in colon

(*continues*)

HIGH-YIELD FACTS

Gastroenterology

TABLE 5-2. GI Absorption (continued)

Nutrient	Site	Comments
Cl⁻	Duodenum > jejunum	• Some secretion, but net absorption • Slow absorption in ileum and colon, HCO_3^- is secreted in exchange, creating basic milieu in the lumen
Ca^{2+}	Duodenum > jejunum	• Active transport facilitated by 1,25-dihydroxycholecalciferol, a vitamin D metabolite • Absorption facilitated by protein • Absorption inhibited by phosphates and oxalates, which form insoluble Ca^{2+} salts
Fe^{2+}	Duodenum > jejunum	• Poorly absorbed—only about 3 to 6% of amount ingested • Ferric form (Fe^{3+}) constitutes most dietary iron but is not absorbed. • The acidic environment of stomach allows reduction of Fe^{3+} to Fe^{2+}. • Postgastrectomy patients often suffer from Fe deficiency anemia. • The ferrous form (Fe^{2+}) freely diffuses into mucosal cells and binds to apoferritin, a storage molecule. • Most Fe^{2+} enters the blood by moving from apoferritin to transferrin in a concentration-dependent manner—decreased transferrin saturation increases the release of iron from intestinal mucosal cells.

Etiology

- Incomplete digestion
- Impaired intestinal bile salt distribution
- Surgical alteration of the bowel
- Lymphatic obstruction
- Deficiency of mucosal absorption
- Endocrine derangements
- Infection (tapeworm, bacterial overgrowth)

Signs and Symptoms

- Weight loss
- Diarrhea
- Flatus
- Abdominal pain
- Amenorrhea
- Anemia
- Easy bruising
- Neuropathy

CELIAC SPRUE

Definition

A gluten-induced enteropathy in susceptible persons diffusely affecting the entire small bowel (also called celiac disease, nontropical sprue, gluten-induced enteropathy). Glutens are a class of high-molecular-weight proteins found in wheat, rye, and barley.

Epidemiology

- More common in women (3:2)
- Associated with HLA DR3 and HLA DQw2

Signs and Symptoms

- Diarrhea
- Bloating/abdominal distention
- Steatorrhea
- Weight loss
- Cerebellar ataxia
- Seizures

Pathology

- Infiltration of **lymphocytes**
- Hyperplasia and lengthening of intestinal crypts
- Very flattened intestinal villi

Diagnosis

- 7% fat in 72-hour fecal fat collection
- Antigliadal IgG and IgA antibodies
- Antiendomysial antibody
- Antireticulin antibody

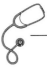

Except for the CNS manifestations, these are symptoms of any malabsorptive syndrome.

Dermatitis herpetiformis is a pruritic rash associated with celiac sprue, responds to treatment of topical sulfone, resolves with regression of disease.

Definitive diagnosis of celiac sprue requires a normal biopsy following a trial of a gluten-free diet.

Treatment of celiac sprue: All grains are to be eliminated from diet, except rice and corn.

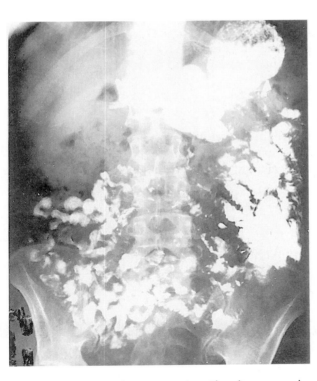

FIGURE 5-5. Celiac sprue. Barium study in a patient with celiac sprue showing dilation of small bowel, lack of mucosal markings, and segmentation and clumping of barium.

(Reproduced, with permission, from Fauci et al. *Harrison's Principles of Internal Medicine,* 14th ed. New York, NY: McGraw-Hill, 1998: 1622.)

- Decreased prothrombin time (PT)
- Decreased total protein, calcium iron, folic acid, vitamins A, B_{12}, C
- Anemia
- Barium swallow shows clumping of barium and loss of mucosal folds (see Figure 5-5).

Treatment

- Avoid gluten-containing foods.
- Consider course of glucocorticoids for severe cases.

TROPICAL SPRUE

Definition

- Malabsorption disease of unknown etiology affecting the jejunum
- Occurs in inhabitants and visitors of the tropics
- Can be seen several years after exposure
- Characterized by protein malnutrition and folic acid deficiency

Signs and Symptoms

Symptoms of malabsorption plus those seen due to folic acid deficiency (cheilosis, glossitis, stomatitis)

Pathology

- Jejunal infiltration of **monocytes**
- Mildly flattened intestinal villi

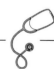

The presence of a normal jejunal biopsy practically excludes the diagnosis of tropical sprue.

Diagnosis

- Requires malabsorption of at least two nutrients
- Megaloblastic anemia
- Decreased calcium, B_{12}, iron, folic acid, cholesterol, albumin, magnesium

Treatment

- Vitamin B_{12} and folate supplementation
- Tetracycline for a few months

LACTASE DEFICIENCY

- Lactase is required to digest lactose, a carbohydrate found in dairy products.
- Congenital deficiency is rare; a milder late-onset form is found in a majority of adult African Americans, Asians, and in 5 to 15% of adult whites.

Signs and Symptoms

- Abdominal cramps
- Flatus
- Diarrhea

Treatment

- Lactase supplementation
- Avoidance of dairy products

WHIPPLE'S DISEASE

Definition

- Devastating illness beginning in the GI tract, but spreading systemically
- Profound malabsorption syndrome due to destruction of intestinal lamina propria
- Causative organism is *Trophermyma whippleii*, a gram-negative rod of the Actinomycetes genus.

Whipple's is a rare disease that is fatal if untreated, but otherwise completely curable. It is also a favorite on exams.

Epidemiology

- More common in males (8:1)
- More common in Caucasians
- Peak incidence in 4th to 6th decades

Signs and Symptoms

- Arthralgia
- Abdominal pain
- Malabsorption: Diarrhea, weight loss, steatorrhea, hypoproteinemia, anemia, etc.
- Bacteremia—present but not detectable
- Frequently:
  - Low-grade fever
  - Increased skin pigmentation
  - Uveitis
  - Cardiac involvement: Heart failure, endocarditis
  - CNS involvement: Confusion, memory deficits, CN palsies, nystagmus, ophthalmoplegia

Typical scenario:
A 54-year-old farmer who has been suffering with diarrhea, weight loss, and arthralgias for the past few months is brought in by his wife for memory deficits that have been occurring for the past 3 weeks.
Think: Whipple's disease.

Diagnosis

- Demonstration of replacement of intestinal lamina propria by PAS-positive macrophages
- PCR of peripheral blood since *T. whippleii* cannot be cultured

Treatment

- Long-term antibiotic therapy (e.g., TMP-SMX for 1 year)
- Clinical remission in almost all cases if treated
- Complete histologic reversal has been observed in some cases.

PROTEIN-LOSING ENTEROPATHY

- The GI tract is the primary site for endogenous protein turnover (proteolysis) in the body. During this process, 10 to 20% of the protein is normally lost to the GI lumen.
- Protein-losing enteropathy occurs when plasma proteins (principally albumin) are lost to the GI lumen in excess.

Causes

Myriad causes, most relating to disorders affecting GI mucosa or heart failure

Signs and Symptoms

- Diarrhea
- Edema
- Steatorrhea

Diagnosis

- Alpha-1-antitrypsin is resistant to proteolysis in the gut and, thus, is used to measure protein loss by comparing levels in the serum and stool.
- Lab abnormalities may include low calcium and low B_{12}, in addition to low protein.

Treatment

- Low-fat diet
- Treat underlying cause

MÉNÉTRIER'S DISEASE

Definition

- Protein-losing enteropathy
- Enlarged, tortuous gastric rugae
- Mucosal thickening due to hyperplasia of glandular cells replacing chief and parietal cells
- Low-grade inflammatory infiltrate—*not* a form of gastritis

Signs and Symptoms

- Epigastric pain
- Symptoms of protein-losing enteropathy
- Decreased gastric acid secretion
- Less commonly:
  - Nausea, vomiting
  - Anorexia, weight loss
  - Occult GI bleed

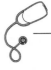

Ménétrier's can look like gastric cancer on barium study.

Diagnosis

- Endoscopy with deep mucosal biopsy is definitive.
- Barium swallow will reveal large gastric folds.

Complications

- Gastric ulcer
- Gastric cancer

Treatment

- Anticholinergics, H_2 blockers to reduce protein loss
- High-protein diet
- Treatment of ulcers/CA if present
- Severe disease may require gastrectomy

Anticholinergics are thought to reduce the width of tight junctions between gastric mucosal cells.

DIARRHEA

Definition

- > 200 g daily stool weight
- Often with increased stool frequency and liquidity

Signs and Symptoms

- Fever
- May note signs of dehydration

Diarrhea Onset
- Shigella: Longest delay (7 hours to 5 days)
- S. aureus toxin: Shortest delay (< 5 hours)
- Others: 5 to 24 hours

Opiate antidiarrheal agents such as loperamide are *contraindicated* in diarrhea due to infectious agents; they promote longer contact time between bacteria and intestinal mucosa.

Diagnosis

- Stool for fecal leukocytes
- Stool for ova and parasites
- Metabolic alkalosis
- Hypokalemia

Bloody diarrhea: **"CASES"**
- **C**ampylobacter
- **A**moeba (E. histolytica)
- **S**higella
- **E.** coli
- **S**almonella

Etiology

Partial List
- Infection:
  - Enterotoxigenic *E. coli*
  - *Vibrio cholera*
  - *E. coli* 0157:H7 (undercooked beef)
  - *Giardia lamblia* (contaminated water, camping)
  - Rotavirus, Norwalk virus
  - *Salmonella* (undercooked poultry)
  - *Clostridium difficile* (pseudomembranous colitis)
- Medications
- Osmotic diarrhea (celiac sprue, lactase deficiency)
- Secretory diarrhea (carcinoid syndrome, ZE)
- Altered intestinal motility (irritable bowel syndrome)
- Inflammatory (UC, Crohn's, infections associated with AIDS)

CONSTIPATION

Definition

Stool frequency < 3 times per week

Etiology

- Low fiber, low fluid intake
- Obstruction
- Disturbed colonic motility
- Medications
- Hypothyroidism
- Diabetes mellitus

Treatment

- Increase fiber to 30 g/day.
- Increase fluid intake.
- Bulk-forming and emollient laxatives

PANCREAS

ACUTE PANCREATITIS

Definition

- Inflammation of the pancreas due to parenchymal autodigestion by proteolytic enzymes
- In severe cases, it can be associated with a *systemic inflammatory response syndrome* (SIRS), which can progress to multi-organ system failure and ARDS.

Normal Function of the Pancreas

Exocrine: Bicarbonate, amylase, lipase, tyrosine, and other digestive enzymes
Endocrine: Insulin, glucagon, somatostatin

Etiologies

Posterior perforation of peptic ulcer
Alcohol
Neoplasm
Cholelithiasis (biliary disease)
Renal disease (end stage)
ERCP
Anorexia (malnutrition)
Trauma
Infections
Toxins (drugs)
Incineration (burns)
Surgery, scorpion bite

Hypercalcemia can cause pancreatitis, and pancreatitis can cause hypocalcemia.

Signs and Symptoms

- Severe, constant midepigastric or LUQ pain, *radiates to the back*
- Pain sometimes improved when patient sits up and leans forward
- Nausea, vomiting
- Low-grade fever
- Tachypnea
- Abdomen is usually tender with guarding, but no rebound.

Diagnostic Markers

Amylase
- Secreted by the pancreas to break down carbohydrates
- Also found in salivary glands, small bowel, ovaries, testes, skeletal muscle
- May be persistently elevated in renal insufficiency
- A level three times the upper limit of normal is 75% specific and 80 to 90% sensitive for pancreatitis.

Lipase
- Secreted by the pancreas to break down triglycerides
- Also found in gastric and intestinal mucosa, and liver
- A level two times the upper limit of normal is 90% specific and 80 to 90% sensitive.

Typical scenario:
A 50-year-old male alcoholic presents with midepigastric pain radiating to the back. He is leaning forward on his stretcher and vomiting. *Think: Pancreatitis.*

Typical scenario:
A 66-year-old female with HTN and seizures for which she is on furosemide and valproic acid, presents with abdominal pain, back pain, and fever. Her nonfasting glucose is noted to be 300. *Think: Pancreatitis.*

Imaging Pancreatitis

- Chest film: May see pleural effusion, elevated hemidiaphragm.
- Abdominal film: May see calcification of pancreas, which is indicative of chronic pancreatitis or the "sentinel loop" of a localized small bowel ileus.

- Ultrasound: May identify gallstones as the cause
- ERCP: Allows direct visualization and sphincterotomy of Ampulla of Vater for relief of biliary obstruction
- Contrast-enhanced dynamic CT (CECT): May show degree of pancreatic necrosis

Prognosis

Ranson's criteria (see Table 5-3)

TABLE 5-3. Ranson's Criteria (Predicts Risk of Mortality in Pancreatitis)

On Admission	After 48 hours
Age > 55	Drop in hematocrit > 10%
Blood sugar > 200	Increase in BUN > 5
WBC > 16,000	Calcium < 8
SGOT > 250	PO_2 < 60 mm Hg
LDH > 700	Base deficit > 4
	Fluid deficit > 6 L

Number of Risk Factors	Mortality
< 3	1%
3 or 4	16%
5 or 6	40%
> 6	Approaches 100%

Treatment

- Bowel rest, NG tube for vomiting or associated ileus
- Hydrate to normal urine output (1 to 2 cc/kg/hr).
- Analgesics and antiemetics as needed
- Treat underlying cause.

CHRONIC PANCREATITIS

Definition

Recurrent episodes of acute pancreatitis, usually from alcohol abuse (70 to 80%), which leads to inflammation, scarring, and duct obstruction

Signs and Symptoms

- Pain similar to acute pancreatitis
- Malabsorption
- Steatorrhea

- Elevated blood sugars
- Polyuria
- Associated with chronic liver disease

Treatment

Same as for acute pancreatitis, with emphasis on pain control and abstinence from alcohol

BILE STORAGE AND RELEASE

Bile is produced in the liver and stored in the gallbladder where it is acidified and concentrated. The presence of fat and amino acids in the proximal duodenum causes release of cholecystokinin, which stimulates gallbladder contraction.

CHOLELITHIASIS

Definition

Gallstones

Mechanisms of Gallstone Formation

- Increased secretion of cholesterol in bile
- Decreased hepatic secretion of bile
- Increased formation of solid cholesterol nuclei
- Formation of biliary sludge
- Also associated with pregnancy, and a very low calorie diet

Signs and Symptoms

- RUQ pain that lasts between 2 and 6 hours. About two thirds of patients will have pain after meals—often worse with fatty foods.
- Nausea and vomiting are common.
- On exam, the patient will be mildly tender in the RUQ *without* guarding or rebound.

Diagnosis

- AST/ALT to evaluate for hepatitis
- Alkaline phosphatase and bilirubin (direct fraction more elevated than indirect) to evaluate for common duct stones
- Amylase/lipase for concomitant pancreatitis
- RUQ ultrasound to detect gallstones

Risk factors for cholelithiasis: **(8 Fs)**
Female
Fat
Fertile
Forty
Fibrosis, cystic
Familial
Fasting
F-Hgb (sickle cell disease)
Also:
Diabetes
Oral contraceptives

Gallstone composition:
- Cholesterol (70%): Radiolucent
- Pigment (20%): Radiodense
- Mixed (10%)

Treatment

- Chenodeoxycholate to dissolve stones (not very effective)
- Lithotripsy (extracorporeal shock wave treatment; breaks up stones)
- Analgesia and antiemetics as needed
- Low-fat diet
- Cholecystectomy

CHOLECYSTITIS

Definition

Gallbladder inflammation, ischemia, or infection usually due to an obstructing stone

Note: Infection *is not necessary* to make the diagnosis of acute cholecystitis but may complicate up to 75% of the cases.

Etiology

- Tumor
- Abscess
- Infection:
  - *E. coli*
  - *Klebsiella*
  - *Enterococcus*
  - *Bacteroides*

Signs and Symptoms

- RUQ pain often longer than the 6 hours duration
- Guarding and rebound may occur
- Fever
- Tachycardia
- Murphy's sign

Murphy's sign: The arrest of inspiration while palpating the RUQ. This test is > 95% sensitive for acute cholecystitis, but less sensitive in the elderly.

Diagnosis

- Elevated white cell count with increased PMNs
- Ultrasound findings: Presence of gallstones, thickened gallbladder wall, pericholecystic fluid (presence of all three has a positive predictive value of > 90%)
- **HIDA** *(the study of choice):* For this test, technetium 99m-labeled iminodiacetic acid is injected IV and is taken up by hepatocytes. In normals, the gallbladder is outlined within 1 hour.

Gold standard test for cholecystitis is HIDA scan.

Treatment

- Pain control
- Administration of second- or third-generation cephalosporin
- The definitive treatment is cholecystectomy.

Complications

Fistula, gallstone ileus, perforation, pancreatitis, gangrene

ACALCULOUS CHOLECYSTITIS

- 5 to 10% of cases of cholecystitis
- More rapid downhill clinical course
- Increased morbidity and mortality

Risk factors include increased age, DM, multiple trauma, HIV, extensive burn, major surgery, prolonged labor, systemic vasculitides, gallbladder torsion, and infections of the biliary tract.

ASCENDING CHOLANGITIS

Definition

Complete obstruction of the biliary outflow tract due to a stone obstructing the common bile duct (choledocholelithiasis), a stricture or tumor.

This is a life-threatening emergency.

Signs and Symptoms

- *Charcot's triad* occurs in only about 25% of patients and lacks specificity.
- Patients may also develop shock and altered mental status, (Reynold's pented)which carries a worse prognosis.

Charcot's triad:
- RUQ pain
- Jaundice
- Fever

Reynold's pentad:
- Shock (hypotension)
- Altered mental status

Diagnosis

Ultrasound may show stones in the common bile duct.

Treatment

- Fluid resuscitation, vasopressors as needed
- Antibiotics to cover *E. coli*, *Klebsiella*, *Enterococcus*, and *Bacteroides*
- ERCP may allow removal of obstruction (associated with 5 to 10% morbidity and 1% mortality)
- Early surgical decompression of obstructed biliary tract

PRIMARY SCLEROSING CHOLANGITIS

Definition

Chronic progressive disorder of unknown etiology characterized by inflammation, fibrosis, and strictures of the medium- and large-diameter intrahepatic and extrahepatic biliary tree

Most patients with primary sclerosing cholangitis also have ulcerative colitis.

Treatment

Balloon dilatation of obstructed biliary tree or surgical intervention

EMPHYSEMATOUS CHOLECYSTITIS

Definition

- A rare variant (1%) caused by gas-forming bacteria in the wall of the gallbladder, particularly *Clostridium*
- Greater than 25% are acalculous, and there is a higher incidence of gangrene and perforation.

Treatment

Antibiotics and surgical intervention

LIVER

NORMAL FUNCTION OF THE LIVER

- Carbohydrate metabolism (glucose homeostasis)
- Plasma protein synthesis
- Bile acid synthesis
- Coagulation factor synthesis
- Lipid synthesis
- Vitamin storage
- Detoxification of many endogenous and exogenous substances
- Hormone metabolism
- Nitrogenous waste processing (urea cycle)

See Table 5-4 for explanation of liver function tests.

TABLE 5-4. A Comparison of Lab Findings in Obstructive and Parenchymal Liver Disease

Test	Obstructive	Parenchymal
AST/ALT	Slight elevation	Very high
Alkaline phosphatase	Very high	Slight elevation
Albumin	Normal	Decreased
PT	Normal—slight elevation	Very high
Bilirubin: Direct (conjugated)	Normal—very high	Normal—very high
Bilirubin: Indirect (unconjugated)	Normal—slight elevation	Normal—very high
GGT	Very high	Normal—very high

PT and albumin are the only true tests of liver function; they are both synthesized by the liver.

Definition

Chronic hepatic injury associated with hepatocellular necrosis, fibrosis, and nodular regeneration

ALCOHOLIC CIRRHOSIS

Most common cause of cirrhosis in North America

Etiology

Caused by chronic alcoholism. *Alcoholic fatty liver*, a mostly asymptomatic, reversible form of liver injury, often precedes cirrhosis. *Alcoholic hepatitis* initiates the necrosis.

Signs and Symptoms

- Loss of appetite
- Nausea, vomiting
- Jaundice
- Tender hepatomegaly
- Spider angiomata (superficial venous radial branching on belly)
- Ascites
- Edema
- Bleeding
- Encephalopathy
- Palmar erythema
- Dupuytren's contractures (contractures of palmar fascia resulting in flexion of 4th digit)

Diagnosis

Common Laboratory Abnormalities
- Anemia
- Elevated bilirubin (direct and indirect)
- AST/ALT ratio > 2
- Elevated GGT
- In severe disease: Prolonged PT and low albumin

Treatment

- Cease alcohol consumption.
- High-protein diet (1 g/kg body weight) and multivitamins
- Avoid hepatotoxins (e.g., acetaminophen, INH).
- Consider glucocorticoids and colchicine to decrease inflammation.
- Spironolactone (potassium-sparing diuretic) for ascites

Non-alchoholic causes of cirrhosis:
- Postviral
- Primary biliary cirrhosis
- Secondary biliary cirrhosis
- Cardiac cirrhosis
- Wilson's disease
- Alpha-1-antitrypsin deficiency
- Hemochromatosis

HIGH-YIELD FACTS

Gastroenterology

GGT is the most sensitive serum marker for recent alcohol binging.

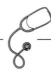

Cirrhotic patients should receive extra protein (on top of high-protein diet) during times of stress (alcohol binge, infection, surgery, trauma).

PRIMARY BILIARY CIRRHOSIS

Definition

Autoimmune disease causing destruction of *intrahepatic* bile ducts

Etiology

Unknown, but *antimitochondrial antibodies* are the serologic hallmark and the pathology results from an autoimmune response to the biliary epithelium.

Epidemiology

More common in women

Signs and Symptoms

- Pruritus
- Fatigue
- Jaundice
- Xanthelasmas, xanthomas
- Presence of an additional (extrahepatic) autoimmune disorder (e.g., RA or Sjögren's)

Do not mix up *primary biliary cirrhosis* with *primary sclerosing cholangitis.*

Diagnosis

- Presence of antimitochondrial antibodies
- Hyperlipidemia
- Increased alkaline phosphatase

Treatment

- Liver transplant
- Medical therapy is largely unsuccessful.

PORTAL HYPERTENSION

Schistosomiasis is the most common cause of portal hypertension worldwide.

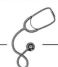

Medusa was a Greek goddess with a head of blue snakes.

Definition

Increased portal vascular resistance caused by cirrhosis, portal vein obstruction, or hepatic vein thrombosis

Complications of Portal Hypertension

- Esophageal varices
- Splenomegaly
- Ascites
- Hemorrhoids
- Caput medusae (periumbilical collaterals visible on abdomen)

Treatment

- Portasystemic shunt surgery
- TIPS (transjugular intrahepatic portacaval shunt) between hepatic and portal veins
- Propranolol reduces portal pressure and prevents variceal bleeds.
- Liver transplant

VARICEAL BLEEDING

Definition

Variceal bleeding presents as hematemesis or postural hypotension in a patient with known or suspected portal hypertension.

Treatment

- Maintain perfusion pressure with normal saline and blood as needed.
- Replace clotting factors with FFP.
- Vasopressin or somatostatin
- Beta blockade
- Endoscopic sclerotherapy or banding
- Balloon tamponade

GI functions of somatostatin:
- Inhibit visceral blood flow
- Inhibit gastric acid secretion
- Inhibit gastric motility
- Inhibit gallbladder emptying
- Inhibit pancreatic enzyme and bicarbonate secretion
- Inhibit intestinal absorption of glucose, water, amino acids, and triglycerides

HEPATIC ENCEPHALOPATHY

Definition

Neurobehavioral changes associated with hepatocellular dysfunction

Etiology

- Increased CNS GABA due to high circulating precursor amino acids
- Increased endogenous benzodiazepines
- Cerebral edema
- The direct role of ammonia is questioned.

Hepatic encephalopathy precipitated by:
- Gastrointestinal bleed
- Increased dietary protein
- Infection

Signs and Symptoms

- Mental status progression from mild to moderate to marked confusion, to coma
- Asterixis (unless patient is in coma)
- Fetor hepaticus (peculiar breath smell) may be present.

Diagnosis

- Exclude acute alcohol intoxication, delirium tremens, infection, trauma, and metabolic disorders.

Asterixis is nonrhythmic downward flapping motion of hands held in dorsiflexion ("liver flap" or "bye-bye sign").

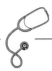

In early liver disease, patients are placed on a high-protein diet because the general state of protein malnutrition puts the body at a disadvantage to fight other stresses such as infection. In end-stage liver disease, the liver cannot break down protein, and the excess accumulation can cause encephalopathy. At this stage, the patient is protein restricted.

Most common organism in SBP: *E. coli*

Treatment

- Protein restriction
- Lactulose (is metabolized by gut bacteria to small acids. The acidification of the stool favors conversion of ammonia to ammonium ion, which gets trapped in the colonic lumen)
- Neomycin (kills urease-producing bacteria in the gut, so that urea can be excreted, rather than ammonia reabsorbed)
- Look for source of infection and consider empiric antibiotics.
- Consider flumazenil cautiously to reverse effects of endogenous benzodiazepines. *Note:* Overreversal may precipitate seizures.

SPONTANEOUS BACTERIAL PERITONITIS

Definition

An acute bacterial peritonitis in patients with ascites

Signs and Symptoms

- Presence of ascites
- Fever, chills
- Generalized abdominal pain with rebound
- May progress to sepsis with change in level of consciousness

Diagnosis

Via Paracentesis (Abdominal Tap)
- > 250 polymorphonuclear cells/µL considered diagnostic
- Gram stain
- Culture and sensitivity

Treatment

- Cover enteric gram negatives (e.g., cefuroxime).
- Monitor electrolytes carefully (hypokalemia and hypernatremia common)

HEPATORENAL SYNDROME

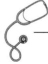

Hepatorenal syndrome can be precipitated by aggressive diuresis, paracentesis, contrast dye, aminoglycosides, or GI bleeding.

Definition

The development of acute renal failure in patients with advanced hepatic disease, characterized by azotemia, sodium retention, and oliguria

Signs and Symptoms

- Worsening azotemia
- Oliguria
- Hypotension

Diagnosis

- Urine sodium < 10 meq/L
- Hyponatremia

Treatment

- None proven effective
- Restoring plasma volume if low is occasionally successful.

HEPATITIS

Definition

Systemic infection or inflammation of the liver due to viral agents, toxins, or alcohol

Etiology

- Viral hepatitis A, B, C, D ("delta"), E, or G
- Alcohol
- Toxins: Acetaminophen, aflatoxin (found in peanuts)

Signs and Symptoms

- Right upper quadrant pain
- Fatigue
- Anorexia
- Nausea, vomiting
- Arthralgias, malaise, headache
- Low-grade fever (100 to 102°F)
- Dark urine
- Jaundice

HEPATITIS A VIRUS

Definition

- RNA virus
- Spread by fecal–oral route
- 15- to 50-day incubation
- No chronic carrier or infection state

Etiology of viral hepatitis:
- Vowels from the bowels (A and E, fecal–oral route)
- Consonants from "consumance" (B, C, D, G from sex and blood)

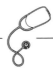

Hepatotoxicity due to acetaminophen (APAP) can be *prevented* by early determination of APAP levels and administration of N-acetylcysteine.

Gastroenterology

Diagnosis

- Anti-HAV IgM = acute infection
- Anti-HAV IgG = immunity from prior infection

Treatment

- Treatment is symptomatic.
- Self-limited, no progression to chronic liver disease
- Prevention:
  - A vaccine is available if traveling to developing nations; it becomes effective 3 weeks after administration.
  - Anti-HAV immunoglobulin is 90% effective if given within 2 weeks of exposure.

HEPATITIS B VIRUS

HBV is the *only* DNA hepatic virus.

Definition

- DNA virus
- Spread by percutaneous or mucous membrane exposure to blood, semen, and saliva
- 45- to 160-day incubation

Diagnosis

- HbsAg positive = infection is present
- IgM anti-HBc = the infection is acute (window period)

For explanation of more Hep B markers, see Table 5-5.

TABLE 5-5. Hepatitis B Markers

Disease State	Marker	Approximate Time from Exposure to Detection in Serum	Explanation
Early infection	HBcAg (hepatitis B core antigen)	Never detectable	Intracellular antigen expressed in infected hepatocytes; not detectable in the serum
Acute infection	Anti-HBc IgM	1.5–6 months	Window period (there can be a several week gap between the disappearance of HBsAg and the appearance of anti-HBs in the serum, during this time infection can be detected with anti-HBc IgM)
Active hepatitis or carrier	HBsAg	1–6 months	Viral protein coat
High infectivity, chronic hepatitis	HBeAg	1–4 months	Indicates ongoing viral replication
Low infectivity	Anti-HBe	4 months–years	Present in acute phase
Immunity	Anti-HBs	6 months–years	In serum after disappearance of HBsAg
Remote infection	Anti-HBc IgG	6 months–years	Remains detectable longest

Treatment

- Hep B immune globulin (HBIG)
- Interferon
- Prevention: Vaccination (series of three), standard blood and body fluid precautions.

HBIG is most effective if given within 7 days of exposure.

Complications

- 1% will develop fulminant hepatic necrosis.
- 10% of adults (90% neonates) will develop chronic carrier state or chronic hepatitis with an increased hepatocellular cancer risk.

HEPATITIS C VIRUS

Definition

- RNA virus
- Spread by blood and body fluid contact
- Incubation 15 to 160 days

Hep C is the most common cause of viral hepatitis in the United States.

Diagnosis

Anti-HCV presents 1 to 6 months after infectivity and indicates chronic infection.

Treatment

- Interferon—remission in 50% of cases, with sustained response in only 10%. May be used in conjunction with ribavirin.
- Amantadine or rimantadine for nonresponders
- Prevention: Standard blood and body fluid precautions

Donor blood is currently not screened for HCV.

Complications

Fifty to 80% develop chronic hepatitis and may develop cirrhosis and/or hepatocellular carcinoma.

Note: Hepatitis G virus is very similar to HCV.

HEPATITIS D VIRUS OR "DELTA" AGENT

Definition

- "Defective" RNA virus; *requires HBV for replication and expression*
- Spread by blood or body fluid exposure as a *co-infection* (simultaneously with HBV) or a *super-infection* (patient already infected with HBV)
- Increased incidence of chronic hepatitis and cirrhosis

HEPATITIS E VIRUS

Definition

- RNA virus
- Incubation 15 to 60 days
- Fecal–oral transmission
- Occurs in India, Asia, Africa, and Central America
- High rate of fulminant liver failure
- No chronic carrier or infection state

Diagnosis

No marker

Treatment

- Supportive care
- Prevention: Hand washing, sanitation

LIVER TRANSPLANTATION

Definition

- Used in selected cases of severe, irreversible liver disease
- Currently has a 5-year survival rate of better than 80%

Indications for liver transplant:
- Cirrhosis (biliary, alcoholic.)
- 1° sclerosing cholangitis
- Hepatitis (chronic, fulminant)
- Hepatocellular carcinoma
- Hepatic vein thrombosis

Immunosuppression

- Cyclophosphamide
- Tacrolimus
- OKT3

Acute Rejection

Suspect in transplant recipients with:
- Fever
- RUQ pain
- Increased serum bilirubin
- Increased aminotransferases

Treatment of Rejection

- Methylprednisolone (first line)
- Lymphocyte antibodies

Donor Liver

- Needs to be size and ABO matched
- Does not require Rh or HLA matching

Liver Dialysis

A new technology similar to renal hemodialysis that functions as surrogate liver until donor liver becomes available. Presently used for cases of fulminant hepatitis. Still considered experimental.

COLON

CARCINOID TUMOR

Definition

- Neuroendocrine tumor arising from ectodermal stem cells in the gut
- Generally slow growing
- 90% in ileum—most in appendix
- Secretes neurotransmitters and hormones, commonly:
  - Serotonin (5-HT)
  - Bradykinin
  - ACTH
  - Histamine
  - Dopamine
- Metastases (in order of frequency):
  - Regional lymph nodes
  - Liver (graver prognosis)
  - Lung

Etiology

- Most idiopathic
- No familial tendencies
- Part of MEN type I
- Increased incidence in Gardner syndrome and Crohn's disease

Signs and Symptoms

- Many are asymptomatic—radiographic incidentalomas.
- Appendicitis
- Small bowel obstruction
- Weight loss
- Liver metastases: RUQ pain, elevated LFTs
- Lung metastases: Pneumonia, obstructed bronchus
- Carcinoid syndrome:
  - Occurs in only 5 to 10% of carcinoid tumors
  - Classic triad:
    1. Flushing—bradykinin
    2. Diarrhea—serotonin
    3. Right-sided valvular heart disease—serotonin
  - Wheezing is also common.

Carcinoid constitutes one third of all primary gut neoplasms.

Types of GI cancer differ based on region:
- Esophagus: Squamous and adenocarcinoma
- Duodenum and jejunum: Adenocarcinoma
- Ileum: Carcinoid, lipoma, and lymphoma

HIGH-YIELD FACTS

Gastroenterology

Diagnosis

- \> 10 mg/24 hr urine 5-HIAA is 75% sensitive and 100% specific.
- Elevated serum and urinary 5-HT
- Chest x-ray or CT for lung metastases
- Abdominal CT for primary tumors, lymph nodes, and liver metastases
- Barium study with small bowel follow-through

Treatment

- Surgical excision
- Radiation therapy
- Antihormonal therapy as needed
- For liver metastases: Resection, embolization, alpha interferon

Prognosis

- With carcinoid syndrome, median survival is 3 years.
- Appendiceal primaries have 99% 5-year survival.
- Extra-appendiceal primaries have 50% 5-year survival.

DIVERTICULOSIS

Definition

- An *acquired* condition of the colon in which saclike protrusions of colonic mucosa herniate through a defect in the muscle layer (where nutrient arteries insert) (see Figure 5-6)
- Diverticulae are most common in the sigmoid colon, probably because this is the narrowest area of the colon and therefore subject to the highest pressures.

Etiology

- Low-fiber diet, less bulk in the stool
- Frequency increases directly with age—50% affected by age 65 in the United States.

Diverticulosis is the most common cause of massive lower GI bleeding in patients over age 60.

Signs and Symptoms

- Usually asymptomatic
- Can cause painless rectal bleeding

Pathophysiology of Diverticular Bleeding

- An inflamed diverticulum erodes through a colonic artery causing sudden, profuse, painless bleeding, usually from right-sided diverticula.
- Seventy-five to 95% of the cases stop bleeding spontaneously.

Treatment of Diverticular Bleeding

Same as for any lower GI bleed

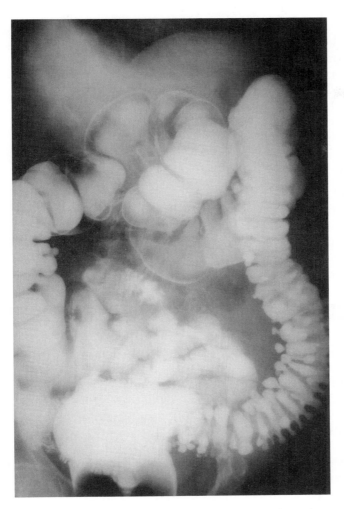

FIGURE 5-6. Diverticulosis. Barium study in a patient with diverticulosis demonstrates many small contrast-filled outpouchings in the sigmoid colon.

(Reproduced, with permission, from *Schwartz's Principles of Surgery,* 7th ed. New York, NY: McGraw-Hill, 2000: 1277.)

DIVERTICULITIS

Definition

Inflammation and or infection of a diverticulum due to impaction of fecal material in the diverticular neck

Signs and Symptoms

- LLQ pain
- Fever
- Constipation more than diarrhea
- Increased flatus
- Urinary symptoms secondary to irritation from protruding diverticulae
- Recurrent infections can occur secondary to fistula formation.
- Peritonitis is seen with perforation.

Diagnosis

Abdominal CT may help define the extent of disease:

- Inflammation of pericolic fat
- Diverticula
- Bowel-wall thickening
- Possible abscess
- Elevated WBC

Treatment

- NPO, IV fluids, pain control
- Antibiotics to cover gram-negative anaerobes, particularly *E. coli*, *Klebsiella*, *Enterobacter*, *Bacteroides*, and *Enterococcus*
- Patients under 40 have a 25% risk of recurrence and may benefit from sigmoid resection.

PSEUDOMEMBRANOUS COLITIS

C. difficile is the most common cause of nosocomial enteric infection.

Definition

Colonic infection caused by *Clostridium difficile*, a spore-forming anaerobe found normally in GI tract. When *C. difficile* overgrows, due to eradication of competing gut flora by antibiotics, it may release a toxin, which damages colon mucosa.

Classically caused by clindamycin, but many antibiotics can do it—even metronidazole and vancomycin, which are used to treat it.

Typical scenario:
A 68-year-old man in the hospital for 3 weeks for pneumonia returns with new-onset diarrhea. *Think: C. difficile.*

Signs and Symptoms

- Crampy, diffuse abdominal pain
- Fever
- Watery (occasionally bloody) diarrhea

Diagnosis

- *C. difficile* toxin in stool
- Fecal leukocytes
- Sigmoidoscopy: Yellowish membranous plaques (pseudomembranes) adherent to colonic mucosa are pathognomonic.

Vancomycin is almost never given PO, except in the case of pseudomembranous colitis. The reason is because it has such poor GI absorption.

Treatment

- Stop the offending antibiotic if possible.
- Metronidazole PO or vancomycin PO

Complications

Toxic megacolon can occur when inflammation and infection spread through all layers of the colon wall. Severe diarrhea and toxicity develop. Plain radiography may show a long, colon loop with diameter > 6 cm and "thumbprinting" (bowel-wall edema)—these patients will likely need a colectomy.

IRRITABLE BOWEL SYNDROME

Definition

An alteration of intestinal motility that leads to changes in bowel habits. The "resting pressures" in patients with IBS may fluctuate between spasm (constipation) and laxity (diarrhea). Patients are particularly sensitive to cholecystokinin, cholinergics, and distension from gas.

There is a strong relationship between symptoms and psychosocial stress in irritable bowel syndrome.

Epidemiology

- 20 to 40 years old
- Female (2:1)

Signs and Symptoms

- Fluctuating constipation and diarrhea
- Increased with stress
- Lack of systemic symptoms

Giardia infection and lactose intolerance may present similarly.

Treatment

- Reassurance
- High-fiber and low-fat diet
- Anxiolytic, antispasmodic, or antidiarrheal may help with more severe cases.

INFLAMMATORY BOWEL DISEASE

Definition

A chronic, inflammatory disease affecting GI tract. Two major types are Crohn's disease (CD) and ulcerative colitis (UC).

Epidemiology

- More common in people of Caucasian and Jewish background
- Peak incidence in ages 15 to 35
- Occurs with familial clustering
- Incidence: UC = 2–10/100,000; CD = 1–6/100,000
- UC more common in women
- CD more common in men
- Associated risk of colon cancer is 10 to 30 times for UC and 3 times for CD.

Crohn's: Lower incidence, lower risk of cancer, more common in men than UC.

143

Symptoms improve with nicotine. Patients can wear dermal patches.

Signs and Symptoms

UC
- Bloody diarrhea (more prominent than in CD)
- Rectal pain

CD
- Fever
- Malaise
- Weight loss
- Crampy abdominal pain
- Tender RLQ mass

Extraintestinal manifestations affect 20% of patients with IBD (see Table 5-6).

Pathology

UC
- Inflammation of the **mucosa only** (exudate of pus, blood, and mucous from the *crypt abscess*)
- Always **starts in rectum** (up to ⅓ don't progress).

CD
- Inflammation involves **all bowel-wall layers,** which is what may lead to fistulas and abscess.
- Rectal sparing in 50%

Diagnosis (Colonoscopy Findings)

UC
- **Continuous lesions**
- **Apthous ulcers rare**
- **Lead pipe colon** appearance due to chronic scarring and subsequent retraction and loss of haustra

CD
- **Skip lesions:** Interspersed normal and diseased bowel
- **Aphthous ulcers common**
- **Cobblestone** appearance (from submucosal thickening interspersed with mucosal ulceration)

Complications

UC
- Perforation
- Stricture
- Megacolon

CD
- Abscess
- Fistulas
- Obstruction
- Perianal disease

Treatment

Supportive Care

Antidiarrheals:
- Decrease frequency of stool.
- Loperamide and diphenoxylate are used for patients with fatty acid–induced diarrhea.
- Cholestyramine is used for patients without FA-induced diarrhea.
- Contraindicated in severe colitis due to risk of toxic megacolon

Anticholinergics:
- Reduce abdominal cramping, pain, and urgency.
- Opium–belladonna combination works well to control diarrhea and pain.

TABLE 5-6. Extraintestinal Manifestations of Inflammatory Bowel Disease

Eye involvement	■ Uveitis	CD > UC
	■ Episcleritis	Uveitis, erythema nodosum, and colitic arthritis are commonly seen together.
Dermatologic	■ Erythema nodosum	CD, especially in children > UC Parallels disease course (gets better as IBD improves)
	■ Pyoderma gangrenosum	UC > CD May or may not follow disease course
	■ Aphthous ulcers	CD
Arthritis	■ Colitic arthritis	CD > UC Parallels disease course
	■ Ankylosing spondylitis	30 times more common in UC Unrelated to disease course
Hematologic	■ Anemia ■ Thromboembolism	
Hepatobiliary	■ Fatty liver ■ Hepatitis ■ Cholelithiasis ■ Primary sclerosing cholangitis	 UC > CD
Renal	■ Secondary amyloidosis leading to renal failure	CD Unrelated to disease course

Specific Therapy

Sulfasalazine:
- Consists of 5-ASA (active component) and sulfapyridine (toxic effects are due to this moiety)
- How it works in IBD is unknown (because other NSAIDs do not work), but its mechanisms of action include:
    - Altering action of microbial agents
    - Inhibition of leukocyte motility
    - Free radical scavenger
    - Inhibition of prostaglandin and leukotriene synthesis
- Side effects include gastric distress in one third of patients (give enteric-coated preparation), decreases folic acid absorption, and causes male infertility (reversible).
- Drug appears safe in children and pregnant women.

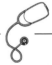

Sulfasalazine is also used to treat rheumatoid arthritis, but in RA, it is the sulfapyridine component that is the active one.

Corticosteroids:
- Early phase of action blocks vascular permeability, vasodilation, and infiltration of neutrophils.
- Late phase of action blocks vascular proliferation, fibroblast activation, and collagen deposition.
- May be given as enemas (decreases systemic absorption)

Drugs with only the 5-ASA component are not effective.

Antibiotics (used for CD):
- 3 week courses of metronidazole and ciprofloxacin have been used to induce disease remission with some success.
- Mechanism of action unknown, because other antibiotics with similar antimicrobial spectrum have not been shown to be effective.

Immunomodulators:
- Used in refractory cases, especially in CD
- Include azathioprine, 6-mercaptopurine, and methotrexate

Experimental therapy:
- Includes anti-TNF antibodies, recombinant anti-TNF cytokines

COLORECTAL CANCER

Villous polyps are the villain in colorectal cancer.

Definition

Colorectal cancer is the second most common cause of cancer death in the United States. Most cases are thought to arise from adenomatous polyps, usually sessile, villous polyps.

Fifty percent of colorectal cancer is within reach of the examiner's finger on rectal exam.

Signs and Symptoms

Constitutional Symptoms
- Weight loss
- Anorexia
- Malaise

Right Colon
- Signs of anemia: Pallor, weakness
- Dull abdominal pain may or may not be present.

Left Colon
- Pencil-thin stools
- Rectal bleeding
- Signs of obstruction (constipation, vomiting)
- Mass on rectal exam

Signs Related to Metastases
- Hepatomegaly
- Palpable abdominal masses

Typical scenario:
A 70-year-old woman presents with a few months of hard stools, weight loss, and a vague abdominal pain that is not related to food or time of day.
Think: Colorectal cancer.

Screening

American Cancer Society recommendations for screening:
- Annual digital rectal exam beginning at age 40
- Annual fecal occult blood test (FOBT) screening beginning at age 50
- Flexible sigmoidoscopy—every 3 to 5 years beginning at age 50, if asymptomatic with no risk factors
- Colonoscopy is recommended for abnormal FOBT or sigmoidoscopy and for patients with inflammatory bowel disease or hereditary colorectal cancer syndromes

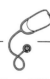

Up to 50% of patients with colorectal cancer can have a negative FOBT.

Diagnosis

Imaging (see Figure 5-7)
- Barium enema
- CT scan with PO contrast
- Consider CXR to look for metastases.

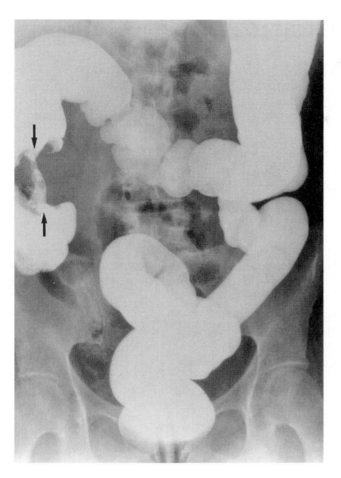

FIGURE 5-7. Colon cancer. Barium study in a patient with colon cancer demonstrates an "apple core"–shaped filling defect at the site of a circumferential neoplasm.
(Reproduced, with permission, from *Schwartz's Principles of Surgery,* 7th ed. New York, NY: McGraw-Hill, 2000: 1347.)

Laboratory
- Anemia
- Elevated CEA (carcinoembryonic antigen)
- Check LFTs (elevations may indicate metastases).

Duke's Classification for Staging and Prognosis

Staging		5-Year Survival
A	Confined to mucosa and submucosa	> 80%
B	Invasion of muscularis propria	60%
C	Local node involvement	20%
D	Distant metastases	3%

Treatment

- Surgical resection: Cures about 50% of cases
- Radiation therapy: Useful for stages B and C
- Chemotherapy: 5-Fluorouracil (FU) and levimasole for stages B at high risk and all C.

Familial polyposis coli (high risk for colorectal cancer):
- Autosomal dominant condition in which thousands of adenomatous polyps appear throughout the colon by age 25
- Most untreated patients develop colon cancer by age 40.

Hereditary nonpolyposis colon cancer (HNPCC) (high risk):
- Autosomal dominant condition in which three or more relatives of a patient, and at least one first-degree relative, develop colon cancer at an early age
- Often multiple other primary cancers in family

Gardner's syndrome (high risk):
- Autosomal dominant disorder characterized by polyposis coli, supernumerary teeth, osteomas, and fibrous dysplasia of the skull

Peutz–Jegher's (low to moderate risk):
- Multiple polyposis of small intestine with multiple pigmented melanin macules in oral mucosa
- Associated with gynecological cancers

HIGH-YIELD FACTS

Gastroenterology

Hematology—Oncology

R. Anand Narasimhan

IRON DEFICIENCY ANEMIA

Definition

Anemia due to decreased iron stores

Pathophysiology

Defect in hemoglobin synthesis due to decreased iron

Etiology

Blood loss (chronic GI bleed or menorrhagia most common)
Malnutrition
Pregnancy

Epidemiology

Most common cause of anemia in the world

Signs and Symptoms

- Fatigue
- Decreased exercise tolerance
- Headaches
- Irritability
- Paresthesias
- Glossitis
- Angular cheilosis (cracking at the corners of mouth)
- Pallor
- Koilonychia (spoon nails)
- Pica (ingestion of clay, ice)

Features of iron deficiency anemia: Fe KAP
"Fe (Iron) Kap"
Fatigue
Exercise tolerance ↓
Koilonychia
Angular cheilosis
Pica, Pallor

Diagnosis

- Low hemoglobin/hematocrit
- Low MCV (microcytic)
- Low TIBC, ferritin
- Low reticulocyte count

Treatment

Oral iron replacement and investigation into underlying cause.

CAUSES OF MACROCYTOSIS (MCV > 100)

- Folate deficiency
- Vitamin B_{12} deficiency
- Alcohol abuse
- Liver disease
- Hypothyroidism
- Myelodysplasia

FOLATE DEFICIENCY ANEMIA

Definition

Decreased hemoglobin content of red blood cells due to impaired production

Pathophysiology

Defect in pathway of DNA synthesis (transfer of one-carbon units)

Risk Factors

- Alcoholism
- Homelessness
- Diet low in folic acid
- Pregnancy
- Tropical sprue

Signs and Symptoms

- Diarrhea
- Cheilosis
- Glossitis

Diagnosis

Blood smear: macrocytosis (high mean corpuscular volume [MCV]), basophilic stippling, hypersegmented neutrophils, low reticulocyte count

Folate deficiency can be differentiated from vitamin B_{12} deficiency by the lack of neurologic abnormalities.

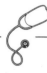

Glossitis is a chronic appearance of the tongue characterized by redness (beefy red), swelling, and loss of papillae.

Treatment

Folic acid replacement: 1 mg/day orally

VITAMIN B₁₂ (Cobalamin) Deficiency

Definition

Anemia due to lack of available vitamin B_{12}

Etiology

- Pernicious anemia
- Vegan diet (excludes meat, eggs, milk products)
- Gastric surgery or ileal resection
- GI bacterial overgrowth (B_{12} consumed before absorbed)
- Fish tapeworm (*Diphyllobothrium latum*)
- Any disorder which decreases absorptive capacity of terminal ileum (regional enteritis, Whipple's disease, tropical sprue)
- Low pancreatic lipase, by any number of conditions (lipase cleaves R moiety from B_{12}—necessary for absorption)

Pathophysiology

Defect in pathway of DNA synthesis (essential cofactor for enzymes producing DNA)

Signs and Symptoms

- Symptoms of anemia
- Neurologic symptoms from subacute combined degeneration of the dorsal columns causing paresthesias, positive Romberg, slowed reflexes, impaired touch and temperature sensitivity, ataxia
- Dementia
- Atrophy of lingual papillae and glossitis

Diagnosis

- Blood smear shows macrocytosis, basophilic stippling, hypersegmented neutrophils, low reticulocyte count
- Decreased plasma cobalamin levels

Treatment

- Vitamin B_{12} replacement (usually IM) and specific therapy related to underlying disorder

Causes of vitamin B_{12} deficiency "VITAMIN B"
Vegan
Ileal resection
Tapeworm
Autoimmune (pernicious anemia)
Megaloblastic anemia
Inflammation of terminal ileum
Nitrous oxide
Bacterial overgrowth

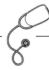

Anemia precedes neurologic symptoms in vitamin B_{12} deficiency.

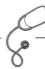

B_{12} replacement can cause hypokalemia. Should see reticulocytes in peripheral smear by 4th day.

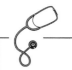

Pernicious anemia is associated with an increased risk of gastric cancer.

HIGH-YIELD FACTS

Hematology—Oncology

Pathophysiology

- Absence of intrinsic factor (IF) causing vitamin B_{12} deficiency.
- Normally, IF and hydrogen ions are both produced by parietal cells of stomach.
- IF binds to vitamin B_{12} and is absorbed in the terminal ileum.
- An autoimmune mechanism is thought to produce antibodies against parietal cells, which destroys them.

Etiology

- Antiparietal cell autoantibodies
- Gastrectomy

Signs and Symptoms

- Same as vitamin B_{12} deficiency; insidious onset
- Associated with vitiligo
- Associated with chronic gastritis

Diagnosis

Schilling Test, anti-IF antibody levels

Schilling Test

Purpose: To assess endogenous presence of IF

Steps:
1. Unlabeled vitamin B_{12} is given parenterally (preloading)—this saturates the cobalamin receptors such that a significant proportion of the radioactive vitamin B_{12} is absorbed in intestine and excreted in the urine.
2. Radioactively labeled vitamin B_{12} is administered orally.
3. If the amount of labeled cobalamin measured in an accurately collected 24-hour urine sample is less than 10% of the amount that was administered orally, there is poor absorption of cobalamin in the intestine.

Interpretation:
One may repeat the Schilling test adding intrinsic factor. In cases of pernicious anemia, IF will correct the cobalamin absorption.

Treatment

Because a small amount of cobalamin is absorbed even in the absence of IF, oral cobalamin dosages of 300 to 1,000 μg/day have proved adequate.

Biochemistry

- Glucose-6-phosphate dehydrogenase (G6PD) is the first enzyme in the hexose monophosphate (HMP) shunt and the *only entry point into this pathway* from glycolysis.
- HMP shunt produces the reducing agent, reduced glutathione (GSH), which is used to protect the RBC against oxidative insults.
- Glutathione cycles between its reduced form (monomer—GSH) and its oxidized form (dimer—GSSG).

Metabolism

- The HMP shunt metabolizes ~10% of glucose used by red blood cells.
- Accumulated oxidants react with hemoglobin and structural proteins → loss of function and lysis.
- Normally, GSH (in conjunction with the enzyme glutathione peroxidase) reduces oxidants before they can cause damage.
- Activity of G6PD decreases with normal RBC age, half-life of single molecule is 62 days, in G6PD deficient cell half-life may be as low as 13 days.

G6PD deficiency is the most common metabolic disorder of red blood cells.

Genetics

- Gene on X chromosome, sex-linked trait
- Heterozygous females fare better than males: Only 50% RBCs affected due to lyonization of erythroid precursors.
- Homozygous females and males are affected in equal severity.

Complete absence of G6PD is incompatible with life.

Pathology

- Not a total absence of enzyme: reduced half-life or catalytic activity
- Most patients have no anemia in the steady state:
  - Normal reticulocyte counts
  - Mildly reduced RBC lifespan
  - Minority of cases suffer chronic hemolysis
- Most hemolysis is extravascular (liver and spleen), but some occurs intravascularly causing hemoglobinemia and hemoglobinuria.

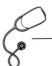

Precipitates of oxidized Hgb bound to cell membranes are called **Heinz** bodies.

Epidemiology

- Worldwide prevalence:
  - African-Americans:
    Usually Gd^{A-} variant (milder)
    12% of men
    20% of women heterozygous, 1% homozygous
  - Mediterraneans (Greeks, Italians, Arabs):
    Usually Gd^{Med} variant (more severe)
    20 to 30% of men
  - Kurdish and Sephardic Jews: 60 to 70% of men

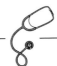

G6PD
Think: Africa, Mediterranean, Middle East, Asia — all fairly contiguous land masses with warm climates

HIGH-YIELD FACTS

Hematology—Oncology

153

- Cambodian: 14% of men
- Chinese: 6% of men
- Asian Indian: 3% of men
- Correlated with incidence of *Plasmodium falciparum* malaria, which confers selective advantage in endemic areas.

Signs and Symptoms

Acute Hemolysis
- Jaundice, dark urine, acute tubular necrosis due to hemoglobinemia
- Anemia: Pallor, tachycardia, systolic ejection murmur
- Mesenteric and renal ischemia: Abdominal and back pain
- Sudden drop of 3 to 4 g/dL in RBC Hgb

Chronic Hemolysis
- Hepatosplenomegaly

Triggers

G6PD crisis is triggered by anything that causes release of oxidants by macrophages.

- Infection (most common)
- Drugs
  - Antimalarials, quinolones, sulfa drugs, NSAIDs, nitrofurantoin, fava beans, vitamin C (acids), naphthalene (in moth balls)
- Diabetic ketoacidosis (DKA)
- Low pH is oxidative stress.

Diagnosis

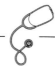

Typical scenario:
A 35-year-old Italian male presents complaining of weakness, back pain, and jaundice. He reports being started on ciprofloxacin 2 days ago for a pneumonia. *Think: G6PD deficiency.*

- Hemolysis:
  - Peripheral smear: *Microcytosis, schistocytosis, Heinz bodies*
  - CBC/reticulocyte count: *Anemia, reticulocytosis*
  - Haptoglobin: *Low*
  - Direct and indirect Coombs': *Negative*
  - Fractionated bilirubin: *Elevated direct and indirect*
  - Membrane osmotic fragility: *Normal*
  - U/A: *Hemoglobinuria, elevated urobilinogen, acute tubular necrosis*
- G6PD assay: Requires 3-week wait after acute hemolytic episode to avoid false-negative result from preponderance of younger cells

Treatment

- Volume loading—renal protection
- Removal of oxidative stressor if possible (discontinue drug, treat infection)
- RBC replacement as necessary; severe cases may require exchange transfusion
- Acute crises will resolve spontaneously after ~1 week due to new erythrocytes with more G6PD activity replacing lysed RBCs, and frequently the source of oxidative stress has been removed.
- Education most effective therapeutic measure

Definition

Marrow failure resulting in severe pancytopenia

Pathophysiology

Two mechanisms for are postulated:
- Stem cell defect
- Immune-mediated destruction

Etiology

- Viral hepatitis
- Chloramphenicol (idiosyncratic)
- Parvovirus B19 with sickle cell anemia
- Benzene (dose related), lindane, DDT
- Others

Signs and Symptoms

- Insidious onset
- Weakness
- Fatigue
- Mucosal bleeding
- Pallor

Diagnosis

- Normochromic, normocytic pancytopenia
- Low reticulocyte count
- Normal peripheral smear
- Thrombocytopenia with normal-sized platelets

Treatment

- Bone marrow transplant is treatment of choice, prior blood transfusions can impair success due to sensitization to minor HLA antigens.
- Immunosuppression (steroids, cyclophosphamide)

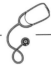

Patients with erythema infectiosum (causative agent: parvovirus B19) should avoid contact with patients with sickle cell anemia due to the risk of aplastic anemia.

ANEMIA OF CHRONIC INFLAMMATION

Definition

Anemia observed in patients with infectious, inflammatory, or neoplastic diseases

Etiology

- Tuberculosis
- Malignancies
- Rheumatologic disorders that put body in a state of prolonged inflammation

Pathophysiology

Iron deficiency in the presence of ample iron stores

Signs and Symptoms

Signs and symptoms of the underlying disorder

Diagnosis

- Ferritin is normal to increased; serum iron, total iron-binding capacity (TIBC), and transferrin all decreased.
- Erythropoietin appropriately elevated
- Normocytic, normochromic anemia

Treatment

Identification and treatment of underlying disease

TYPES OF HEMOGLOBIN

- Hemoglobin A: α_2/β_2 globin chains (normal hemoglobin)
- Hemoglobin F: α_2/γ_2 globin chains (fetal hemoglobin)
- Hemoglobin A_2: α_2/δ_2
- Normal distribution of Hb in adults is:
  - 96% Hb A
  - 3% Hb F
  - 1% Hb A_2
- There are 2-α and 1-β genes on each chromosome, making a total of 4-α genes and 2-β genes in each chromosome pair.

ALPHA-THALASSEMIA

Definition

Genetic defects causing gene deletions of α chains

Epidemiology

$\alpha\alpha$/—thalassemia trait is most common in Asians.
α–/α–thalassemia trait is most common in Africans.

Pathophysiology

- Ineffective production of alpha globin chains causes β globin chains to accumulate.

Signs and Symptoms

Depends on how many of the four foci are deleted or mutated:
  1/4 foci involved = silent thalassemia
  - Asymptomatic
  2/4 foci involved = thalassemia trait
  - Mild anemia
  3/4 foci involved = Hemoglobin H disease
  - Microcytic, hypochromic, hemolytic anemia with marked splenomegaly. Patient may need occasional transfusions.
  4/4 foci involved = Hemoglobin Barts, hydrops fetalis
  - Incompatible with life

Diagnosis

- Blood smear: Microcytic anemia, hypochromia, target cells, Heinz bodies
- HbH precipitates on staining with brilliant cresyl blue

β-THALASSEMIA

Definition

Gene defects including deletions, abnormalities of transcription and translation, and instability of mRNA in β globin hemoglobin

Pathophysiology

- Ineffective production of β globin chains causes α globin chains to accumulate in the cell.
- The accumulation of α chains form insoluble aggregates that damage cell membranes.
- A partial compensatory increase of the δ and γ chains yields elevated levels of Hb A_2 ($\alpha_2\delta_2$) or Hb F ($\alpha_2\gamma_2$).

Signs and Symptoms

β-Thalassemia major (Cooley's anemia): Associated with jaundice, hepatosplenomegaly, and jaundice
β-Thalassemia minor: Mild or no anemia

Diagnosis

Elevated Hb F and Hb A_2 measurements

Treatment

β-Thalassemia major: Aggressive transfusions, splenectomy to enhance survival of RBCs, bone marrow transplant
β-Thalassemia minor: No treatment indicated.

SICKLE CELL ANEMIA (SCA)

Pathophysiology

- Genetic disease characterized by the presence of hemoglobin S in RBCs.
- Hemoglobin S is formed by substitution of valine for glutamine in the sixth position of the β-hemoglobin chain.
- During periods of high oxygen consumption, this abnormal hemoglobin distorts and causes red blood cell to sickle.
- Sickle cell trait: Heterozygous for sickle gene
- Sickle cell disease: Homozygous for sickle gene

Epidemiology

- More common in blacks than whites.
- Increased incidence in populations from Africa, the Mediterranean, Middle East, and India.

Signs and Symptoms

Acute Crisis
- Symptoms include arthralgias and pain
- Caused by vascular sludging and thrombosis. These vaso-occlusive crises may cause organ failure (secondary to infarction), dehydration, fever, and leukocytosis.

Chronic
- Skeletal: Aseptic necrosis of femoral head
- Biliary disease: Pigmented gallstones (increased bilirubin)
- Renal: Chronic hematuria, renal papillary necrosis
- Liver disease: Congestion (heart failure) and viral hepatitis (transfusions)
- Pulmonary: Local infection and vascular occlusions (acute chest syndrome)
- Heart: Enlarged, flow murmur
- Immune: Increased susceptibility to infections, functional asplenism (due to repeated infarction)
- Eye: Ischemic retinopathy
- GU: Priapism

Diagnosis

- Blood smear: Howell–Jolly bodies (cytoplasmic remnants of nuclear chromatin that are normally removed by the spleen), sickled cells

---

Signs of SCA: "SICKLE"
Splenomegaly, sludging
Infection
Cholelithiasis
Kidney — hematuria
Liver congestion, leg ulcers
Eye changes

Renal papillary necrosis occurs in SCA because of the very high osmolalities in renal medulla needed to pull the water from the collecting ducts causing the RBCs to sickle.

Patients with SCA are prone to infection with encapsulated organisms. *Salmonella* osteomyelitis is most common among patients with SCA.

- Blood tests show anemia, increased reticulocyte count, increased indirect bilirubin.
- Hemoglobin electrophoresis will show Hb S.

Treatment

- Acute crisis: Analgesia and hydration
- Hydroxyurea acts by increasing amount of fetal hemoglobin.
- *Hemophilus influenza* and pneumococcal vaccines for prophylaxis
- Acute chest syndrome: Respiratory support and exchange transfusion

Best treatment for SCA patients is education about their disease, specifically, how to avoid vaso-occlusive crises.

IMMUNE-MEDIATED HEMOLYTIC ANEMIA

Presence of autoantibodies to one's RBCs, resulting in hemolysis and splenomegaly

WARM HEMOLYTIC ANEMIA

- Most common form of immune-mediated hemolytic anemia
- IgG antibodies to Rh factor
- Do not usually fix complement
- Active at body temperature
- Treated with steroids
- Seen with lymphomas, leukemias, systemic lupus erythematosus (SLE), and other autoimmune diseases, and drugs. Sixty percent of cases are idiopathic.

COLD HEMOLYTIC ANEMIA

- IgM antibodies
- Active at cool temperatures (dissociate at 30°C) such as in distal body parts
- Fixes complement
- Seen acutely with mycoplasma and infectious mononucleosis (resolve spontaneously) and chronically with myeloproliferative disorders
- Degree of hemolysis is variable.
- Treatment includes keeping warm and corticosteroids.

PAROXYSMAL COLD HEMOGLOBINURIA

- Also called cold hemolysis
- IgG antibodies against P group antigen (Donath–Landsteiner Ab)
- Active at cool temperatures, dissociate at 30°C to cause hemolysis
- Fix complement
- Clinically characterized by acute intermittent massive hemolysis and hemoglobinuria following exposure to cold

Ab Against Foreign RBC Ag

ABO Incompatibility
- Most common transfusion reaction
- Almost invariably due to **human error**
- Patients are immunized against A/B Ag without prior exposure because endogenous bacteria produce glycoproteins with structures similar to the A/B Ag.

Excluding ABO Incompatibility
- Uncommon, occurring mostly in multitransfused patients
- 1 to 1.5% risk of red cell alloimmunization per unit transfused
- 15 to 20% incidence in multitransfused patients
- Most commonly Ab to Rh and Kell (K) Ag, less frequently Duffy (Fy) and Kidd (Jk) Ag
- Rh⁻ mothers who give birth to Rh⁺ children have a 15 to 20% chance of developing anti-Rh Ab due to fetal–maternal blood mixing.
- Anti-Rh IgG (RhoGAM) is routinely given to Rh⁻ mothers pre- and perinatally to prevent Rh immunization.
- The most common reasons for Rh immunizations are:
  - Childbirth in developing countries
  - Older (parous) women
  - Lack of prenatal/perinatal care
  - Human error

Ab Against Foreign WBC Ag

- Usually against HLA group Ag
- Risk groups:
  - Multiparous women
  - Multitransfused patients
  - Cardiac surgery
  - Transfusions for aplastic anemia or acute leukemia (up to 70% incidence)
  - Prior platelet transfusions (anti-HLA Ab)

Ab Against Foreign Platelet Ag

- Foreign platelets commonly stimulate Ab against HLA Ag.
- Ab against platelet-specific antigens cause posttransfusion purpura.
- Ab due to fetal–maternal blood mixing cause neonatal thrombocytopenia.
- Most common platelet-specific antigen is HPA-1a.

Ab Against Foreign Plasma Proteins

- Rare cause of transfusion reactions
- Ab against lipoproteins and Gm and Inv determinants on IgG are often found in multitransfused patients.
- Anaphylactic reactions are most often due to anti-IgA Ab.

Hemolytic Transfusion Reactions

- Destruction of donor, not recipient RBCs (with rare exceptions)
- Clinical significance ranges from trivial to life threatening.
- Hemolysis may occur immediately within the circulation, or more slowly within the reticuloendothelial system.
- Most common in females due to prior RBC immunization during childbirth
- ~85% of fatal hemolytic transfusion reactions are due to ABO incompatibility, and of these ~90% are due to human error.

Immediate Hemolytic Transfusion Reactions

- Occur intravascularly
- Usually due to ABO incompatibility
- Anti-A/B Ab are predominantly IgM, and thus can bind complement causing immediate destruction of RBCs.
- Immediate hemolysis due to other RBC Ag such as Duffy (Fy) and Kidd (Jk), Kell (K) and Rh occur less frequently.

SIGNS AND SYMPTOMS

- Begins soon after the transfusion
- Usually sudden clinical deterioration:
  - Fever +/– chills
  - Dyspnea
  - Tachycardia
  - Anxiety
  - Back pain
  - Chest pain
  - Flushing
  - Hypotension
  - Rarely subtle or mild
- Sequelae:
  - Death (40%)
  - Acute renal failure
  - Shock
  - Disseminated intravascular coagulation (DIC)

PATHOPHYSIOLOGY

- Interaction between Ab and the RBC generating immune complexes
- Activation of the complement cascade → release of C3a and C5a with anaphylatoxic activity
- Activation of the coagulation mechanism via cytokines and factor XII → consumption coagulopathy and generation of bradykinin
- Vasomotor mediators (histamine, serotonin, cytokines) cause widespread vasodilation resulting in shock.
- Renal failure primarily due to ischemia, caused by a combination of hypotension, vasoconstriction, and intravascular coagulation.

General anesthesia is a frequent setting for blood transfusion. In this setting, immediate hemolytic transfusion reaction should be suspected with:
- Severe hypotension
- Coagulopathic oozing
- Hemoglobinuria

Precipitation of free hemoglobin in the renal tubules is *not* a major contributor to renal failure.

DIAGNOSIS

- Confirm patient's identity.
- Check donor blood and recipient's records for blood type mismatch.
- Check posttransfusion blood sample for hemolysis: Free plasma hemoglobin can be detected quickly by centrifuging a tube of blood anticoagulated with EDTA or heparin; pink plasma indicates intravascular hemolysis.
- Repeat ABO and Rh typing on all specimens.
- Assess for DIC:
  - Fibrin split products
  - Coagulation profile
  - d-Dimers
  - Platelet count
- Check and follow renal function:
  - Blood urea nitrogen/creatinine (BUN/Cr)
  - Urinary hemosiderin, hemoglobinuria, wine-colored urine
  - Urine output
- Reduced serum haptoglobin
- Hyperbilirubinemia

Heparinization of patients with disseminated intravascular coagulation is controversial.

TREATMENT

- Discontinue transfusion.
- Send new sample of patient's blood to blood bank along with the suspect donor blood.
- Severity of reaction related to the volume of RBCs transfused: As little as 30 cc of incompatible blood can be lethal, most severe reactions require > 200 cc.
- Hydrate to prevent renal failure and increase BP: Use normal saline (NS) to maintain intravascular volume.
- Increase renal perfusion: Dopamine, diuretics (furosemide)
- Dopamine also effective against hypotension (higher dose)
- Oliguric renal failure → fluid restriction, careful electrolyte management, and dialysis
- Coagulopathy may require management with platelets, cryoprecipitate, or fresh frozen plasma
- Exchange transfusion may be necessary; most reactions can be managed conservatively.

PREVENTION

- Most frequent cause is human error:
  - Patient sample mislabeled
  - Sample drawn from the wrong patient
  - Transcription errors
  - Improper identification of unit with the recipient
- With proper mechanisms in place, the frequency of serious transfusion reactions can be reduced dramatically.

Delayed Hemolytic Transfusion Reactions

PATHOPHYSIOLOGY

- Milder than immediate type
- Predominantly extravascular hemolysis
- Occur 2 to 10 days after transfusion
- Due to anamnestic antibody response
- Pretransfusion antibody level low → screening and cross-match tests usually negative
- Rarely 1° immunization from transfusion generates delayed type response, but time course usually too slow

SIGNS AND SYMPTOMS

Most Common
- Fever
- Recurrent anemia

Less Common
- Jaundice
- Hemoglobinemia/hemoglobinuria
- Renal failure → death

DIAGNOSIS

- Screen fresh blood sample for RBC Ab
- Direct antiglobulin test (DAT):
  - If positive, elute antibodies from RBCs and identify.
  - If transfused cells are already destroyed, DAT will be negative, but Ab should be detectable in patient's serum.
  - Patient should keep record of antibody identity on his person at all times.

TREATMENT

- Usually no treatment required
- More severe reactions may require hydration, transfusion of properly crossmatched RBCs.

Febrile Nonhemolytic Transfusion Reactions

- 0.5 to 3.0% of patients receiving transfusions
- More common in multitransfused patients
- Chill followed by fever within a few hours of transfusion
- Possibly headache, malaise
- Usually mild, but may be fatal
- Lasts only a few hours
- Most commonly due to preformed Ab against antigens on transfused leukocytes and platelets
- Bacterial contamination or endotoxin less likely but must be considered

The use of leukocyte-reduced blood products may reduce the incidence of febrile nonhemolytic transfusion reactions.

TREATMENT

- Discontinue transfusion.
- Rule out acute hemolysis (see *Immediate Hemolytic Transfusion Reactions* on page 161).

- Send donor unit to blood bank for culture and further investigation.
- Antipyretic (acetaminophen) for fever

Allergic Reactions to Plasma

- Incidence of 1 to 3%
- Large range of manifestations:
  - Urticarial lesions (hives) or other rashes
  - Bronchospasm
  - Angioedema
  - Anaphylaxis, shock
- Minor urticarial reactions do not necessitate immediate discontinuance of transfusion
- Incidence of anaphylactic reactions very low
- Causes of most reactions unknown
- Anaphylactic reactions often due to Ab against donor IgA

Posttransfusion Purpura

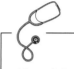

Additional platelet transfusions can worsen the thrombocytopenia in post-transfusion purpura.

- Rare, life-threatening thrombocytopenia
- Occurs 5 to 10 days after transfusion
- Caused by the development of Ab against platelet-specific Ag
- Anti-HPA-1a most common
- 2° immune response to platelet-specific Ag
- Most patients prior 1° immunization (usually pregnancy or transfusion)
- Donor *and* recipient's platelets are destroyed.
- Mechanism of destruction of the *recipient's* platelets is unknown.
- Limited form associated with the passive administration of a platelet-specific Ab
- Management includes high-dose IV Ig or plasma exchange; steroids may be useful adjunct.

Transfusion-Related Acute Lung Injury

- Sudden severe respiratory distress similar to adult respiratory distress syndrome (ARDS)
- Occurs within several hours of transfusion
- Incidence ~1 in 5,000 transfusions
- Caused by donor Ab against recipient granulocytes → agglutination of granulocytes and complement activation in the pulmonary vascular bed → capillary endothelial damage → fluid leak into the alveoli
- Resolves within 48 to 96 hours without residual effects (interim respiratory support often required)

SIGNS AND SYMPTOMS

- Chills/fever
- Chest pain
- Hypotension
- Cyanosis, dyspnea, crackles/rales
- Chest x-ray (CXR) shows diffuse pulmonary edema

TREATMENT

- Supportive measures for the pulmonary edema and hypoxia, including ventilatory support
- Steroids to block granulocyte aggregation and further vascular damage
- If fluid overload → diuretics

POLYCYTHEMIA VERA

Definition

A myeloproliferative disease that results in overproduction of all blood cell lines

Etiology

- Primary—idiopathic
- Secondary:
  - Hypoxia (high altitudes, lung disease)
  - Smoking (due to carboxyhemoglobin)
  - Renal cell carcinoma (decreased erythropoietin production)
  - Myelodysplasias
  - Dehydration

2° polycythemia is associated with hypernephroma, cerebellar hemangioma, hepatoma, and giant uterine myomas.

Epidemiology

- Males more commonly affected
- More common in people > 60
- Associated with increased incidence of cerebrovascular accidents (CVAs) and gastric ulcers

Signs and Symptoms

- General malaise
- Pruritus
- Plethora
- Splenomegaly
- Epistaxis

Diagnosis

- Low erythropoietin
- Low erythrocyte sedimentation rate (ESR)
- Pan elevation of all blood cell lines (WBCs, RBCs, platelets)

Treatment

- Serial phlebotomy to decrease blood volume
- Consider hydroxyurea for myelosuppression
- Aspirin to prevent thromboses

Bone marrow fibrosis is a late complication of polycythemia vera.

PORPHYRIA

Definition

- Group of disorders characterized by disturbances in porphyrin metabolism
- Porphyrins are pigments present in hemoglobin, myoglobin, and cytochromes.
- Major types:
  - Congenital erythropoietic porphyria
  - Erythrohepatic protoporphyria
  - Acute intermittent porphyria
  - Porphyria cutanea tarda
  - Mixed porphyria

ACUTE INTERMITTENT PORPHYRIA

Definition

Autosomal dominant disorder characterized by deficiency of porphobilinogen deaminase (hydroxymethylbilane [HMB] synthase)

Precipitating Factors

- Drugs (barbiturates, carbamazepine, valproic acid, sulfonamides)
- Steroid hormones (endogenous and exogenous)
- Low-calorie diet
- Alcohol
- Diet
- Infection
- Surgery

Signs and Symptoms

Asymptomatic unless exposed to stressor. Acute symptoms are due to neurologic dysfunction and include:
- Diffuse abdominal and pelvic pain (autonomic nervous system)
- Disturbances in temperature and blood pressure control (brainstem): Tachycardia, hypertension, diaphoresis
- Peripheral neuropathy, proximal muscle weakness
- Psychiatric symptoms: Convulsions, anxiety, paranoia, insomnia (cerebral cortex)

Diagnosis

Presence of δ-aminolevulinic acid and porphobilinogen in the urine

Treatment

- For acute attacks:
  - Intravenous heme as soon as possible
  - Analgesics for body pain
  - Phenothiazines for nausea, vomiting
  - Benzodiazepines for restlessness, tremors, and anxiety
- Education about disease, avoidance of stressors, maintain high-carbohydrate diet

COAGULATION CASCADE

Common pathway factors: I, II, V, X (see Figure 6-1)

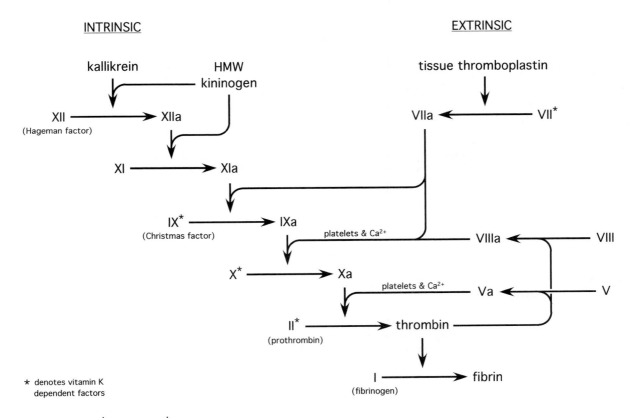

* denotes vitamin K dependent factors

FIGURE 6-1. Coagulation cascade.

HEPARIN

- Increases partial thromboplastin time (PTT)
- Affects intrinsic pathway
- Decreased fibrinogen levels
- Primarily affects factors VIII, IX, X, XI, XII

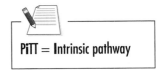

PiTT = Intrinsic pathway

Heparin goes with **Intrinsic** pathway because **H** comes right before **I.**

- Low-molecular-weight heparins have 10 times activity against factor Xa.
- Safe in pregnancy
- Adverse effects include bleeding, thrombocytopenia, and osteoporosis.

WARFARIN

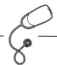

PeT = PT measures extrinsic pathway.

- Increases prothrombin time (PT)
- Affects extrinsic pathway
- Decreased vitamin K
- Primarily affects II, V, VII
- Teratogenic

ACTIVATED PARTIAL THROMBOPLASTIN TIME (aPTT)

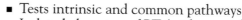

Leafy green vegetables are relatively contraindicated in patients on warfarin therapy due to their high vitamin K content.

- Tests extrinsic and common pathways
- Isolated elevation of PTT (with normal PT) seen in:
  - Heparin therapy
  - Deficiencies of factors VIII (hemophilia A), factor IX (hemophilia B), factor XI, and factor XII (asymptomatic)

PROTHROMBIN TIME (PT)

Warfarin has an initial *pro*coagulant effect, taking 48 to 72 hours to become anticoagulant. Concurrent coverage with heparin during this time is needed, and oral warfarin dose is titrated slowly.

- Tests intrinsic and common pathways
- Isolated elevation of PT (with normal PTT) seen in:
  - Vitamin K deficiency
  - Warfarin therapy
  - Liver disease (decreased factor production)
  - Congenital (rare)

THROMBIN TIME (TT)

- Measures the time it takes to convert fibrinogen into a fibrin clot
- Elevated in:
  - DIC (consumes fibrinogen)
  - Liver disease (decreased production of fibrinogen)
  - Heparin therapy (inhibits fibrinogen formation)
  - Hypofibrinogenemia (low fibrinogen to start)

BLEEDING TIME

- Measures time from start of skin incision to formation of clot (normal = 3 to 8 min)
- Independent of coagulation cascade
- Elevated in:
  - Thrombocytopenia
  - Qualitative platelet disorders
  - von Willebrand's disease

DIRECT COOMBS

- Ability of anti-IgG or anti-C3 to agglutinate patient's RBC
- Elevated in:
  - Drug therapy (α-methyldopa, penicillin, tetracyclines, quinidine, insulin)
  - SLE
  - Autoimmune hemolytic anemia
  - Transfusion reactions

INDIRECT COOMBS

- Detection of anti IgG antibody in sample of patient's blood incubated with normal antigen bearing red blood cells
- Elevated in:
  - Acquired hemolytic anemia
  - Incompatible crossmatched blood
  - Anti-Rh antibodies
  - Drug therapy (mefenamic acid, α-methyldopa)

IDIOPATHIC THROMBOCYTOPENIC PURPURA (ITP)

Definition

Immune-mediated thrombocytopenia of unknown etiology

Pathophysiology

Development of antibodies against a platelet surface antigen. The antibody–antigen complexes effectively decrease platelet count by being removed from circulation.

Causes of thrombocytopenia:
"PLATELETS"
Platelet disorders: TTP, ITP, DIC
Leukemia
Anemia
Trauma
Enlarged spleen
Liver disease
EtOH
Toxins (benzene, heparins, aspirin, chemotherapy agents, etc.)
Sepsis

HIGH-YIELD FACTS

Hematology—Oncology

Signs and Symptoms

- Petechiae and purpura over trunk and limbs
- Guaiac-positive stool
- Mucosal bleeding

Diagnosis

- Thrombocytopenia on CBC
- Absence of other factors to explain thrombocytopenia (diagnosis of exclusion)

Treatment

- Corticosteroids acutely
- May also consider intravenous immunoglobulin for severe cases
- Platelet transfusion if significant bleeding present
- Splenectomy electively to decrease recurrence
- Takes a few weeks to resolve; caution against strenuous activity during this time

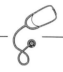

One unit of platelets increases platelet count by 10,000.

THROMBOTIC THROMBOCYTOPENIC PURPURA (TTP)

Definition

A hemolytic anemia that results from deposition of abnormal vWF multimers into microvasculature

Pathophysiology

- Normally, when endothelial cell damage occurs, vWF and platelets migrate to the site and form clot.
- In TTP, abnormal vWF, in the form of multimers, is present. The presence of such multimers are thought to be due to a defective or missing protease.
- These abnormal vWF multimers migrate to site of endothelial damage and attract platelets as usual, but due to their size, cause clumping of the platelets at the site of repair.
- The clumping of large numbers of platelets effectively decreases their number in circulation.
- This mechanical obstruction within microvasculature causes a shearing of the RBCs as they pass through, resulting in a hemolytic anemia.

Typical scenario:
A 27-year-old HIV+ female presents with fever, waxing and waning mental status, and hematuria. CBC shows pancytopenia.
Think: TTP.

Classic pentad of TTP:
- Hemolytic anemia
- Thrombocytopenia
- Neurologic changes
- Decreased renal function
- Fever

Epidemiology

- More common in women
- Peak age is age 12 to 45 years

Risk Factors

- Infection (especially HIV and *E. coli* 0157:H7)
- Malignancy
- Drugs (antiplatelet agents, chemotherapy agents, contraceptives)
- Autoimmune disorders
- Pregnancy

Signs and Symptoms

Diagnostic Pentad

- Fever
- Altered mental status (waxing and waning, depending on location and movement of clot)
- Renal dysfunction (hematuria, oliguria)
- Thrombocytopenia—can be mild to severe
- Microangiopathic hemolytic anemia

Others

- Petechiae, purpura
- Pallor, jaundice

Diagnosis

Clinical features of pentad:

- Evidence of hemolysis on peripheral smear: Schistocytes, helmet cells
- BUN and creatinine may be elevated
- CBC: Elevated reticulocyte count, anemia, thrombocytopenia
- Decreased haptoglobin level
- Increased lactic dehydrogenase (LDH)
- May note casts, or RBCs in urine

Treatment

- **Do Not Transfuse Platelets.**
- Plasmapheresis is mainstay of treatment (given daily, until platelet count rises to normal).
- May give FFP if plasmapheresis not available
- Transfuse PRBCs if anemia causes symptoms (tachycardia, orthostatic hypotension, hypoxia).
- Consider corticosteroids, vincristine, antiplatelet agents and splenectomy for refractory cases.
- Monitor for and treat acute bleeds (remember to look for intracranial bleed as well).
- Admit patients to the intensive care unit (ICU).

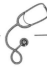

E. coli 0157:H7 is an invasive gastroenteritis resulting in hemolytic uremic syndrome (HUS). HUS differs from TTP in severity and lack of neurologic symptoms.

Diagnostic pentad for TTP:
FAT RN
Fever
Anemia
Thrombocytopenia
Renal dysfunction
Neurologic dysfunction

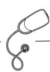

Transfusing platelets in TTP is thought to "fuel the fire" and exacerbate consumption of platelets and clotting factors, resulting in more thrombi in the microvasculature.

Definition

Acquired coagulation defect that results in consumption of coagulation factors I, V, VIII, and XIII, causing bleeding and thrombosis. Can be acute and life threatening or can be chronic, as seen with malignancies.

Risk Factors

- Obstetric problems (retained dead fetus, abruptio placentae, second-trimester abortion, amniotic fluid embolism)
- Sepsis (particularly with RMSF, HUS, Malaria, gram negatives)
- Local tissue damage: (snake bites, burns, frostbite)
- Trauma
- Malignancy
- Heatstroke
- Transfusion
- Liver disease

Typical scenario:
A 50-year-old female who is in the ICU for sepsis has purpura and gingival bleeding on day 2 of her hospital stay. All her coagulation factors are elevated. *Think: DIC.*

Signs and Symptoms

- Petechiae
- Purpura
- Mucosal bleeding
- Patients with chronic DIC may only have laboratory abnormalities.

Diagnosis

- Thrombocytopenia
- Elevated PT, aPTT, and TT
- Decreased fibrinogen
- Presence of fibrin split products
- Evidence of hemolysis on peripheral smear

PT, PTT are normal in TTP, whereas they are elevated in DIC.

Treatment

- Treat underlying cause
- Platelets, FFP, and cryoprecipitate to control bleeding
- Heparin with or without antithrombin III concentrate to control thrombosis (controversial)

VON WILLEBRAND'S DISEASE

Definition

Genetic disease, most commonly autosomal dominant, characterized by lack of a von Willebrand factor (vWF)

- *P. vivax* and *P. ovale* cause persistent infection in the liver.
- Symptoms of fever and chills occur about 1 to 4 weeks after infection.
- Others symptoms include headache, increased sweating, back pain, myalgias, diarrhea, nausea, vomiting, and cough.

Diagnosis

- Blood smear
- Should be considered in any person with febrile illness who immigrates or has traveled to malaria infested region
- WBC count usually normal
- Anemia, thrombocytopenia, and elevated liver enzymes may be present.

Treatment

- Chloroquine is effective only for erythrocytic stages. Therefore, in cases of *P. vivax* and *P. ovale*, primaquine is used for the hepatic phase.
- If chloroquine resistant, use mefloquine + proguanil or doxycycline

Patients with fever which follows a cyclical pattern every 48 or 72 hours should be considered for malaria.

ACUTE LEUKEMIA

Etiology

- Ionizing radiation
- Therapeutic external beam radiation
- Chemical carcinogens
- Genetic translocations
- Benzene exposure
- Genetic disorders such as Down's syndrome

Pathophysiology

- Hematopoietic disorder in which progenitor cells have transformed into malignant cells
- These leukemic cells accumulate in the bone marrow to disrupt the differentiation of normal cells.
- Clinical manifestations occur because of the loss of normal bone marrow elements and by infiltration of the body's tissues by malignant cells.

Signs and Symptoms

- Anemia: Weakness, fatigue, pallor, cardiopulmonary compromise
- Neutropenia: Infections, fever
- Thrombocytopenia: Purpura, hemorrhages
- Marrow infiltration: Bone pain
- Leukemic infiltration: Lymphadenopathy, splenomegaly, hepatomegaly

Signs of *"LEUKEMIA"*
Light skin (pallor)
Energy decreased
Underweight
Kidney failure
Excess heat (fever)
Mottled skin (hemorrhages)
Infections
Anemia

Diagnosis

- Blasts, anemia, thrombocytopenia on CBC
- Bone marrow biopsy showing > 30% immature cells confirms diagnosis.

Treatment

Three steps of chemotherapy:
- *Induction:* High doses of chemotherapy are used to reduce the number of malignant cells.
- *Consolidation:* Chemotherapy is then administered to eradicate residual, undetectable malignant cells.
- *Maintenance:* Chemotherapy

Complete remission is the goal in cancer patients. This is achieved if normal marrow elements are being produced and less than 5% residual blasts are present in the bone marrow.

ACUTE MYELOCYTIC LEUKEMIA (AML)

Epidemiology

More common in adults; association with benzene 8 subtypes M0–M7:
- M1–M3 have granulocytic differentiation.
- M4 and M5 are monocytic precursors.
- M6 have predominance of erythroblasts.
- M7 is mainly megakaryocytic.

Signs and Symptoms

- Fatigue, hemorrhage, or bruising (30%)
- Infection of lung, skin (25%)
- Splenomegaly, hepatomegaly, and lymphadenopathy (< 25%)

Diagnosis

- Elevated leukocyte count
- Blasts in peripheral blood
- Absolute neutrophil count, hematocrit, and platelet count decreased
- Auer rods, stains positively with Sudan black and myeloperoxidase (10% of patients)

$M_3 = DIC$

Subtypes based on morphology (FAB classification):
- M_3: DIC, t(15;17)
- M_5: Associated with gingival hyperplasia (50%)

Treatment

- Cytogenic analysis indicates prognosis.
- *Induction:* Cytarabine + an anthracycline (daunorubicin)—50 to 80% receive remission
- *Consolidation:* Same chemotherapy as induction
- *Maintenance:* Clinical trials determining best drugs
- Stem cell transplantation for those who do not achieve remission
- M_3 treated with *all*-trans-retinoic acid in addition to cytarabine and daunorubicin.

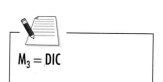

Adverse effects of chemotherapy agents:
Cisplatin = nephrotoxicity
Bleomycin = pulmonary fibrosis
Vincristine = neurotoxic, palsies
Doxorubicin = cardiotoxic
Tamoxifen = vaginal bleeding

Epidemiology

Primarily a disease of children, but accounts for 20% of adult leukemias:

- 3 subtypes L1–L3
- L1 occurs in 80% of ALL cases in children.
- Majority of adult cases are L2.
- L3 cell is identical morphologically to the neoplastic cells of Burkitt Lymphoma t(8;14).

Signs and Symptoms

- Symptoms acute at onset often beginning within a few weeks of diagnosis
- Malaise, fever, lethargy, weight loss, bone pain, infection, and hemorrhage
- Lymphadenopathy, splenomegaly, hepatomegaly in about 50%

Diagnosis

- Elevated leukocyte count
- Blasts in peripheral blood
- Absolute neutrophil count, hematocrit, and platelet count decreased
- 25 to 30%: Philadelphia chromosome (chromosome 22) arising from t(9;22)—poorer prognosis
- Periodic acid-Schiff (PAS) reaction will react positive in L1 and L2 subtypes
- TdT+ (terminal deoxyribonucleotidyl transferase)
- Since 80% from B-cell lineage, express CD10 (CALLA antigen), CD19, and/or CD20
- 15 to 20% of T-cell lineage and express CD2, CD5, and CD7

Treatment

- Patients with Philadelphia chromosome often need bone marrow transplantation.
- *Induction:* Four or five drugs such as vincristine, prednisone, daunorubicin, L-asparaginase, and cyclophosphamide are used.
- *Consolidation:* Cell-cycle phase-specific antimetabolites
- *Maintenance:* Low-dose chemotherapy is standard.

Pathophysiology

Clonal disorder in which the leukemic stem cell gives rise to red cells, neutrophils, eosinophils, basophils, monocyte–macrophages, platelets, T cells, and B cells

Signs and Symptoms

- *Chronic phase:* WBC counts increase, spleen and liver enlarge
- *Accelerated phase:* RBC, platelets decrease; symptoms include bone pain, fever, night sweats, and weight loss
- *Blastic phase:* Peripheral blood and marrow are filled with rapidly proliferating leukemic blast cells.

Diagnosis

- Examining the peripheral blood film shows increased myeloblasts and basophils, white blood cells
- Leukocyte alkaline phosphatase is low in CML cells.
- 90% have Philadelphia chromosome t(9;22).

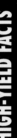

90% of patients with CML have the Philadelphia chromosome t(9;22).

Treatment

- Allogenic bone marrow transplant treatment of choice for younger patients
- Chemotherapy consists of busulfan and hydroxyurea for those that cannot have BMT (chronic phase) and vincristine and prednisone for those in the accelerated/blastic phase.

CHRONIC LYMPHOCYTIC LEUKEMIA (CLL)

Pathophysiology

- Malignant clonal disorder of mature lymphocytes which can disrupt normal marrow elements of production
- Since it predominantly affects the B cells, there is an impairment of the humoral immunity

Signs and Symptoms

- Lymphadenopathy and splenomegaly often present at discovery of disease
- Infections because of neutropenia, hypogammaglobulinemia
- At later stages of disease, patient may have symptoms of fever, night sweats, weight loss

Diagnosis

- Often suspected or found incidentally on routine CBC
- Lymph node biopsy
- Lymphocytosis
- Usually B cell origin

Treatment

- Alkylating agent like chlorambucil, steroids
- COP: Cyclophosphamide, vincristine, prednisone
- CHOP (COP plus doxorubicin)
- IgG for hypogammaglobulinemia

MULTIPLE MYELOMA

Pathophysiology

Malignant disease of plasma cells that is characterized by:
- Presence of monoclonal immunoglobulin or light chains in the serum and urine
- Bone destruction

Epidemiology

- Median age at diagnosis 68
- Twice as common in blacks than whites

Signs and Symptoms

- Hypercalcemia
- Pathologic fractures
- Lytic bone lesions
- Bone pain
- Renal failure
- Anemia

Diagnosis

- *Radiography:* Lytic lesions on x-ray
- *Electrophoresis:* Monoclonal elevation of one immunoglobulin
- *Urinalysis:* Free kappa and lambda light chains (Bence Jones proteins)
- *Bone marrow biopsy:* 10 to 20% plasma cells (normal is < 5%)

Treatment

- Chemotherapy:
  - Alkylating agent (melphalan or cyclophosphamide)
  - Prednisone
- Calcitonin
- Allopurinol
- Plasmapheresis for acute renal failure

Multiple myeloma: Common triad of back pain, anemia, and renal insufficiency.

Typical scenario:
A 60-year-old man with punched out lytic lesions in the skull and mild anemia. Think: *Multiple myeloma.*

Pathophysiology

- Follicular B cells undergo a transformation to malignant cells.

Four subtypes based on histology of lymph node and cell type:

1. *Lymphocyte predominant*
2. *Nodular sclerosing:* Most common type; typically presents as cervical lymph node enlargement or mediastinal mass
3. *Mixed cellularity*
4. *Lymphocyte depleted:* Rare, worst prognosis

Epidemiology

- Disease with bimodal distribution having peaks in 30s and 70s
- May have an association with Epstein–Barr virus (EBV)

Clinical

- Presents with asymptomatic lymph node enlargement or CXR showing mediastinal mass
- "B" symptoms may occur in patients with more widespread disease. These include fever, night sweats, weight loss, and shortness of breath.

Diagnosis

- Lymph node biopsy
- Presence of Reed–Sternberg cells confirms diagnosis.

Treatment

Based on staging and pathology, chemotherapy and radiotherapy are both utilized; prognosis dependent on extension of disease

Pathophysiology

Most originate from B cells. B cell lymphomas are further classified based on the tissue type origination from lymph node: Germinal center, mantle zone, or marginal zone:

- Working classification most widely used in the United States. Categorizes lymphoma by low, intermediate, and high grade based on median survival.

Signs and Symptoms/Treatment

- Fatigue, weight loss, fever, and night sweats are common symptoms.
- Involvement of mesenteric nodes and extranodal disease is more common.

Specific Types

Follicular Small Cleaved Cell

- A common presentation of the low-grade follicular lymphomas is asymptomatic, painless, diffuse, long-standing lymphadenopathy in a middle-aged individual.
- Bone marrow involvement is present in the majority of patients.
- t(14;18) translocation involving the bcl-2 gene
- Treatment includes alkylating agent (cyclophosphamide) and prednisone.

Diffuse Large Cell Lymphoma

- Most common intermediate-grade lymphoma
- Diffuse large cell lymphoma may present in a variety of extranodal sites, particularly the gastrointestinal tract and the head and neck.
- Patients treated with chemotherapy—CHOP (cyclophosphamide, doxorubicin [hydroxydaunomycin], vincristine [Oncovin], prednisone)

Lymphoblastic Lymphoma

- High grade lymphomas derived from thymic T-cells
- Often seen in children
- Associated with a large mediastinal mass and testicular, central nervous system (CNS), and marrow involvement

Burkitt Lymphoma

- High-grade lymphoma more common in children than adults
- High incidence of bone marrow involvement
- African type has higher association with EBV and jaw involvement than American type.
- Marrow with "starry-sky" appearance
- Treatment includes high-dose cyclophosphamide, methotrexate, and cytarabine and intensive CNS prophylaxis.

Diagnosis

- Pathologic subtype (tissue architecture, predominant cell), immunophenotypes, molecular analysis
- Unlike Hodgkin's disease, histology of the nodes is a major predictor of prognosis.

Prognosis

- Depends on histology of malignancy, not spread of disease.

Rheumatology

Jonathan Posner

RHEUMATOLOGIC AND MUSCULOSKELETAL DISORDERS

Rheumatology is a broad discipline covering diseases of the joints, connective tissue, and certain immunological disorders. Also covered in this chapter are conditions that are not typically classified as rheumatology but nonetheless affect the musculoskeletal system. Table 7-1 discusses laboratory data commonly used in rheumatology.

TABLE 7-1. Laboratory Data Commonly Used in Rheumatology

Finding	Significance
Erythrocyte sedimentation rate	Determined by filling a tube with whole blood and measuring the rate of sedimentation of red cells—changes in the rate are seen with increased plasma proteins. Certain proteins called *acute-phase reactants* (negatively charged proteins) and are produced at an increased rate during an inflammatory response. These proteins cause RBCs to adhere to one another like stacks of coins called **rouleaux,** which fall through the plasma faster than free RBCs. This is a very nonspecific test. An increased ESR is seen in infections, tissue infarctions, malignancies, collagen-vascular diseases, and states of increased physiologic stress (pregnancy, extreme exercise).
Antinuclear antibodies	Found in many rheumatologic disorders, such as: ■ SLE ■ Rheumatoid arthritis ■ Scleroderma ■ Polymyositis and dermatomyositis
Rheumatoid factor	This is an IgM antibody directed against the Fc portion of IgG. Found mainly in rheumatoid arthritis but also in vasculitides
Complement levels	Complement levels drop when there is decreased production in the liver or increased loss—either through the formation of immune complexes or from glomerular disease. Complement levels should be drawn with: ■ Liver disease (viral hepatitis) ■ SLE nephritis ■ Glomerulonephritis (C3 is the most reduced) ■ Bacterial endocarditis ■ Serum sickness ■ Rheumatoid arthritis with vasculitis

LEADING CAUSES OF LOWER BACK PAIN

Leading causes of low back pain: **ACTIONS**

- **A**rthritis (RA, OA)
- **C**ongenital Anomalies (not covered here)
- **T**rauma (strains, sprains, fractures, and lumbar disc herniation)
- **I**nfection
- **O**steoporosis
- **N**eoplasms
- **S**pinal Stenosis

Osteoarthritis can lead to osteophytes and hypertrophy of spinal facets, which can compress nerve roots.

LUMBAR DISC HERNIATION

Definition

- Disc herniation is a common cause of chronic lower back pain.
- L4–L5 and L5–S1 are the most common sites affected.
- Herniation occurs when the nucleus pulposus prolapses through the annulus fibrosis.
- More common in men

The nucleus pulposus is a thick gel. Herniation of the nucleus pulposus is like toothpaste being squeezed out of the tube.

Signs and Symptoms

- Limited spinal flexion
- Pain and paraesthesia with a dermatomal distribution
- Specific signs depend on nerve root involved:
    - L4: Decreased knee jerk, weakness of anterior tibialis
    - L5: Weakness of extensor hallucis longus, decreased sensation over lateral aspect of calf and first web space
    - S1: Decreased ankle jerk, decreased plantar flexion, decreased sensation over lateral aspect of foot

Remember:
L3–L4 herniation affects L4 nerve root
L4–L5 affects L5
L5–S1 affects S1

Treatment

- Nonsteroidal anti-inflammatory drugs (NSAIDs) for symptomatic relief
- Advise smoking cessation.
- Surgical treatment is indicated only for severe cases.

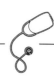

Cigarette smoking is associated with an increased risk of herniation.

ANKYLOSING SPONDYLITIS

Definition

- HLA-B27 antigen associated arthropathy characterized by ossification of the ligaments of the shoulders, spine, hips, and sacroiliac joints
- Most common in men aged 20 to 40.

Signs and Symptoms

- Decreased chest expansion
- Low back pain and stiffness (worse in the morning)
- Kyphosis
- About one fourth of patients develop uveitis as a complication.

Diagnosis

- Elevated erythrocyte sedimentation rate (ESR)
- Rheumatoid factor negative
- X-ray findings: Fusion of vertebral bodies, producing a **bamboo spine** (see Figure 7-1) and **syndesmophytes** (osseous excrescence at insertion of annulus fibrosis)

Treatment

- NSAIDs for symptomatic relief
- Extension exercises to prevent kyphosis
- Recommend sleeping on a firm mattress or hard surface
- Balanced diet; advise smoking cessation
- Surgical treatment includes removing areas of abnormally ossified bone and placing rods to straighten the spine.

Typical scenario:
A young man with stiffness in the lower back that improves with exercise. *Think: Ankylosing spondylitis.*

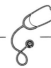

The brittle spine of ankylosing spondylitis is prone to fracture even with minimal trauma. Patients should be restricted from high-risk activities such as skydiving, bungee jumping, and contact sports.

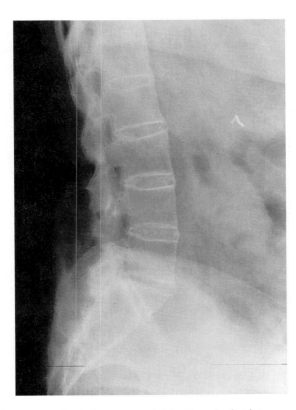

FIGURE 7-1. Bamboo spine of ankylosing spondylitis. Note the bridging syndesmophytes.
(Reproduced, with permission, from Wilson and Lin, *General Orthopedics.* New York, NY: McGraw-Hill, 1997: 454.)

- This is the most common manifestation of osteoporosis.
- It is also seen in patients on long-term steroids and in patients with lytic bony metastases.
- The thoracic spine is the most common site affected (see Figure 7-2).

Signs and Symptoms

- Height loss
- Sudden back pain after mild trauma
- Local radiation of pain—the extremities are rarely affected (unlike a herniated disc).

Diagnosis

Plain radiographs of LS will not show compression fracture until there is loss of 25 to 30% bone height.

Treatment

- Symptomatic relief with NSAIDs
- Treatment of osteoporosis prevents compression fractures:
    - Recommend weight-bearing exercises
    - Estrogen replacement therapy
    - Calcium supplementation
    - Calcitonin (IM) inhibits bone resorption.
    - Bisphosphonates increase bone mass by inhibiting osteoclast activity.

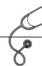

Bisphosphonates such as alendronate (Fosamax) irritate gastric mucosa, so advise patients to eat beforehand and stay upright for 30 minutes after taking it.

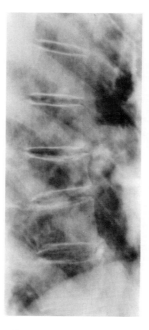

FIGURE 7-2. Compression fracture of osteoporosis. Note the anterior collapse of the vertebra.
(Reproduced, with permission, from Wilson and Lin, *General Orthopedics.* New York, NY: McGraw-Hill, 1997: 489.)

- Spinal abscesses are most commonly found in the immunosuppressed, IV drug users, and the elderly.
- An abscess can form anywhere along the spinal cord and as it expands, it compresses against the spinal cord and occludes the vasculature.

Etiology

- The infection is generally spread from the skin or other tissue.
- *Staphylococcus aureus*, gram-negative bacilli, and *Tuberculosis bacillus* are the leading organisms involved.

Signs and Symptoms

- Presents with a triad of pain, fever, and progressive weakness.
- The pain develops over the course of a week or two and the fever is often accompanied by an elevated white count.

Diagnosis and Treatment

- Magnetic resonance imaging (MRI) can localize the lesion. Lumbar puncture (LP) is not required unless meningitis is suspected.
- Emergent decompressive laminectomy can prevent permanent sequelae. This should be followed up with long-term antibiotics.

SPINAL METASTASIS

- Metastatic lesions invade the spinal bone marrow, leading to compression of the spinal cord.
- Typically involves the thoracic spine
- The most common primary tumors involved include breast, lung, prostate, kidney, lymphoma, and multiple myeloma.

Signs and Symptoms

- Back pain
- Lower extremity weakness
- Hyperreflexia
- Upward Babinski sign
- Urinary incontinence
- Decreased rectal sphincter tone

Diagnosis

MRI is the preferred imaging technique.

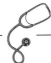

Spinal cord compression is an emergency. Missed diagnosis can lead to permanent paralysis.

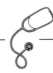

Any cancer patient who develops back pain should be investigated for spinal metastases.

Treatment

Glucocorticoids are used to reduce inflammation and edema. Radiation therapy should be started as soon as possible. Surgery is indicated only if radiation fails to improve the symptoms.

CAUDA EQUINA SYNDROME

Definition

Compression of the lumbar and sacral nerve roots that comprise the cauda equina

Signs and Symptoms

- Motor or sensory loss in lower extremities
- Sciatica
- Urinary incontinence
- Bowel incontinence
- Saddle anesthesia

Etiologies

- Tumor
- Midline disc herniations (rare)
- Congenital narrowing of the lumbar canal

Treatment

- Bed rest on a hard surface and analgesia
- Neurosurgical evaluation for potential laminectomy for acute symptoms

RHEUMATOID ARTHRITIS (RA)

Definition

A systemic inflammatory disease primarily affecting the synovial membranes. Pannus (granulation tissue) develop in the joint spaces and erode into the articular cartilage and bone.

Signs and Symptoms

- Early symptoms are nonspecific: Malaise, anorexia, fatigue, vague musculoskeletal complaints
- Hypertrophy of synovial tissue
- Prolonged morning stiffness
- Joint pain—most common joints affected: Proximal interphalangeal (PIP), metacarpophalangeal (MCP), wrist, knees, ankles
- Subcutaneous painless rheumatic nodules

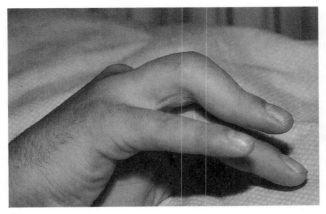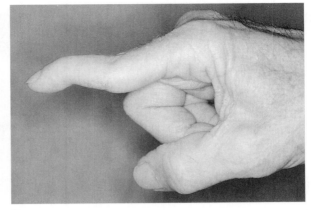

A   B

FIGURE 7-3. Boutonniere (A) and Swan neck (B) deformities of rheumatoid arthritis.
(Reproduced, with permission, from Knoop, Stack, and Storrow, *Atlas of Emergency Medicine*. New York, NY: McGraw-Hill, 1997: 291.)

- Instability of cervical spine due to bone erosion
- Extra-articular involvement also occurs. Common manifestations include: Vasculitis, pleuritis, pulmonary nodules, and secondary amyloidosis

Diagnosis

At least four out of the following seven criteria must be present to diagnose rheumatoid arthritis; criteria 1 through 4 must have been present for ≥ 6 weeks:

1. Morning stiffness for ≥ 1 hour
2. Arthritis of three or more joint areas
3. Arthritis of hand joints
4. Symmetric arthritis
5. Rheumatoid nodules
6. Positive serum rheumatoid factor
7. Radiographic changes

Laboratory

- Rheumatoid factor (RF)—an IgM directed against the Fc fragment of IgG
- Anemia of chronic disease
- Elevated ESR

Treatment

- NSAIDs for symptomatic relief
- Physical therapy to maintain strength and range of motion
- Low-dose steroids
- Disease-modifying, slow-acting antirheumatic drugs (shown to slow or even reverse joint damage) include:
    - Methotrexate

The presence of RF generally signifies more significant disease.

If the WBC count is low, think of *Felty's syndrome:*
- Rheumatoid arthritis
- Splenomegaly
- Leukopenia

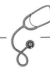

Most arthritis patients (regardless of the type of arthritis) have taken NSAIDs for long periods of time. This places them at high risk for ulcers.

- Gold compounds (adverse effects: stomatitis, nephrotic syndrome, dermatitis)
- Hydroxychloroquine (adverse effect: retinopathy)
- Penicillamine
- Sulfasalazine

OSTEOARTHRITIS (OA)

Definition

Degeneration of articular cartilage followed by new and abnormal bone formation; more common in women

Etiology

- *Primary disease:* No known cause
- *Secondary disease:* Known underlying etiology such as trauma, metabolic (hemachromatosis, Wilson's disease), endocrine (acromegaly), or congenital (congenital hip dislocation)

Signs and Symptoms

- Joint pain relieved with rest
- Morning stiffness that resolves within 30 minutes
- Painless nodules on the hand (see Figure 7-4):
  - **Heberden's nodes** at the DIPs
  - **Bouchard's nodes** at the PIPs
- Loss of range of motion (e.g., decreased internal rotation of hip)
- Joint effusions

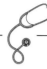

OA is also called "wear-and-tear disease" and "degenerative joint disease" (DJD).

OA can cause morning stiffness but is it usually short-lived (in contrast to RA).
OA affects the **O**uter joints on the hand — the DIPs. RA affects the inner joints — MCPs and PIPs.

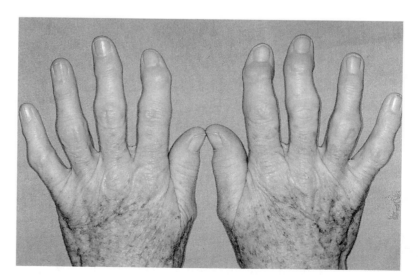

FIGURE 7-4. Heberden and Bouchard nodes of osteoarthritis.
(Reproduced, with permission, from Wilson and Lin, *General Orthopedics.* New York, NY: McGraw-Hill, 1997: 413.)

Diagnosis

Lab findings are normal. X-ray will show joint space narrowing, osteophyte formation, and subchondral cysts.

Treatment

- NSAIDs for symptomatic relief
- Intra-articular injection of lidocaine provides temporary relief
- Joint replacement as necessary
- Strengthen periarticular muscles

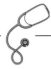

OA is not a systemic inflammatory disease; therefore, lab studies should be normal.

SYSTEMIC LUPUS ERYTHEMATOSUS (SLE)

Definition

- An autoimmune disorder of unknown etiology characterized by autoantibodies
- Associated with HLA-DR2 and HLA-DR3

Epidemiology

- Ninety percent of cases occur in women of childbearing age.
- Blacks are affected more commonly than whites.

Typical scenario:
A 27-year-old black female presents with general malaise, arthralgias, oral ulcers, and a photosensitive rash. *Think: Systemic lupus erythematosus.*

Signs and Symptoms

- Fatigue, malaise, anorexia, weight loss, fever
- Arthralgias, myalgias
- Rash
- Oral and nasopharyngeal ulcers
- Alopecia
- Cognitive dysfunction
- Pericardial rub
- Heart murmur
- Pallor
- Shortness of breath
- Headache
- Visual symptoms

UV light causes flare ups, so many patients are sensitive to sunlight.

Diagnosis

American College of Rheumatology SLE Criteria (1982): Presence of four or more criteria make the diagnosis with 98% specificity and 97% sensitivity.

1. Malar rash: The classic flat, erythematous, nonscarring *"butterfly"* rash on the cheeks and bridge of nose
2. Discoid rash: A scarring, raised erythematous circular facial rash seen in 20% of SLE patients
3. Photosensitivity

4. Oral ulcers
5. Arthritis
6. Serositis (e.g., pleuritis, pericarditis)
7. Renal disorder (e.g., proteinuria)
8. Neurologic disorder (e.g., seizures, psychosis)
9. Hematologic disorder (e.g., pancytopenia)
10. Immunologic disorder (e.g., false-positive VDRL [Venereal Disease Research Laboratories], presence of anti-Sm or anti-dsDNA antibodies)
11. Presence of antinuclear antibodies (ANA)

Laboratory

Typical scenario:
A 24-year-old woman presents with a history of multiple miscarriages. She has no known medical history. Which antibodies would you test for? *Think: Lupus anticoagulant and anticardiolipin.*

Typical autoantibodies in SLE patients include:

- **ANA**—seen in most autoimmune conditions, present in > 95% of patients with SLE
- **Anti-Smith (Sm)**—very specific for SLE, but seen only in one-third of SLE patients
- **Anti-dsDNA**—quite specific for SLE; high titers associated with renal involvement
- **Antihistone**—associated with drug-induced lupus
- **Anticardiolipin** and **lupus anticoagulant**–associated with fetal loss, thrombocytopenia, and valvular heart disease

Active SLE flare up associated with elevated transaminases, anemia, elevated ESR, proteinuria, hematuria, and urinary granular casts

Treatment

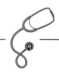

SLE can cause a drop in the RBCs, WBCs, or platelets.

- NSAIDs
- Steroids improve most symptoms
- Immunosuppressive therapy usually reserved for advanced renal involvement

Disease Course and Prognosis

Mean survival rate (from diagnosis):
85% at 5 years
80% at 10 years
75% at 20 years

Most patients with SLE experience remission and flare-ups. Fertility rates are not affected, but the miscarriage rate is high. Patients with renal involvement have the worst prognosis. The terminal event is usually sepsis.

Indicators of renal involvement (poor prognosis):
- Serum creatinine > 1.5
- Hypertension
- Nephrotic syndrome
- Hypoalbuminemia

DRUG-INDUCED LUPUS (DIL)

Definition

A distinct entity from SLE—idiopathic reaction to certain drugs. It is distinguished by:

- Complete resolution of disease once offending drug is discontinued
- Presence of serum antihistone antibodies

Etiology

- Procainamide:
  - Most common offender—used to be used in the old advanced cardiac life support (ACLS) protocols for V-Fib.
- Hydralazine:
  - Second most common offender—used to treat preeclampsia.
- Isoniazid: Used to treat tuberculosis (TB)
- Quinidine: Used to treat malaria and leg cramps
- Methyldopa: Old antihypertensive drug
- Chlorpromazine: Antiemetic also associated with dystonic reactions
- Penicillamine: Used to treat Wilson's disease
- Alpha-interferon: Experimental, used to treat multiple sclerosis (MS) and other autoimmune and viral conditions

Drugs associated with DIL:
H&P, IQ CAMP
Take H&P. If you're smart (in the high IQ CAMP), you'll discontinue these drugs in patients with a malar rash.

Treatment

Discontinue the offending drug; supportive therapy.

SARCOIDOSIS

Definition

- A systemic illness with no known cause, primarily affecting the lungs
- Characterized by noncaseating granulomas
- More common among blacks and in women

Signs and Symptoms

Almost any part of the body can be affected. Some typical extrapulmonary findings are:

Skin—erythema nodosum (erythematous nodes on extensor surfaces of lower extremities, also seen in other conditions)
Kidney—hypercalciuria
Eyes—uveitis (inflammation of uveal tract, iris, ciliary body, choroid)
Cardiac—conduction defects
Nervous—Bell's palsy (self-limited 7th nerve palsy of unknown etiology)

Typical scenario:
A 40-year-old black woman presents with dyspnea, malaise, visual disturbances, and a rash. Chest x-ray shows bilateral hilar adenopathy.
Think: Sarcoidosis.

Staging

I. Bilateral hilar adenopathy
II. Hilar adenopathy plus lung parenchymal involvement
III. Lung parenchymal involvement alone
IV. Pulmonary fibrosis

Remember, when you go from stage II to stage III, you actually lose the hilar adenopathy.

Diagnosis

Requires transbronchial biopsy to prove existence of noncaseating granulomas, but not sufficient on its own to make diagnosis; requires clinical, laboratory, and radiographic adjuncts

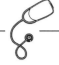

Laboratory

- Lymphocytosis on bronchoalveolar lavage
- Eosinophilia
- False positive RF and ANA
- Elevated angiotensin converting enzyme (ACE)
- Skin anergy to common antigens
- Elevated 24-hour urine calcium
- Chest x-ray shows **bilateral hilar adenopathy** and perihilar calcifications (see Figure 7-5)
- Elevated ESR

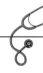

Treatment

Corticosteroids

Prognosis

Most patients have resolution of their disease within 2 years. Death from pulmonary failure occurs in a minority of patients.

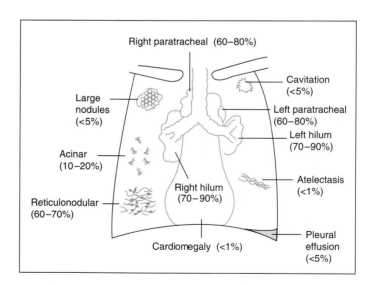

FIGURE 7-5. Abnormal CXR findings in sarcoidosis.

(Reproduced, with permission, from Fauci et al., *Harrison's Principles of Internal Medicine,* 14th ed. New York, NY: McGraw-Hill, 1998: 1925.)

Definition

An autoimmune disorder characterized by widespread fibrosis secondary to overproduction of collagen and other extracellular matrix proteins.

Signs and Symptoms

- Raynaud's phenomenon (vasospasm of arteries in hands in response to cold or emotional stress, resulting in discoloration of hands)
- Thickened, tight skin
- Dysphagia due to esophageal fibrosis
- Renal artery fibrosis
- Pulmonary hypertension
- Telangiectasias

In the limited form of the disease symptoms are generally limited to the **CREST syndrome:**

Calcinosis (calcium deposition forming nodules)
Raynaud's phenomenon
Esophageal dysmotility
Sclerodactyly (stiffness of skin of fingers)
Telangiectasias

Laboratory

- Anti SCl-70 (topoisomerase antibody)
- Antibody to centromere
- Antibody to nucleolar Ag
- Normochromic, normocytic anemia
- Elevated ESR
- Decreased vital capacity on pulmonary function tests (restrictive lung disease)

Treatment

- Penicillamine—may inhibit collagen cross-linking
- Captopril—helps control the renal hypertension
- Calcium channel blockers—diminish the Raynaud's phenomenon
- Steroids—rarely effective in altering the disease course

Definition

Painful compression of the median nerve as it passes through the carpal tunnel; more common in women (see Figure 7-6).

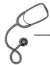

The skin changes in scleroderma at first may actually cause the patient to appear more youthful. The skin becomes tight and wrinkles disappear.

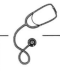

Renal artery fibrosis leads to malignant HTN, the leading cause of death.

HIGH-YIELD FACTS

Rheumatology

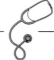
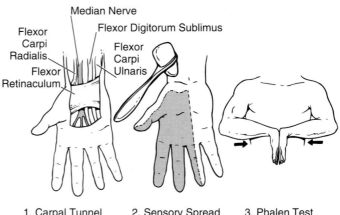

1. Carpal Tunnel   2. Sensory Spread   3. Phalen Test
of Median Nerve

FIGURE 7-6. Carpal tunnel syndrome. 1. The flexor retinaculum in the wrist compresses the median nerve to produce hypoesthesia in the radial 3½ digits. 2. Percussion on the radial side of the palmaris longus tendon oroduces tingling in the 3½ digital region (Tinel sign). 3. Phalen test. Hyperflexion of the wrist for 60 seconds may produce pain in the median nerve distribution; this is relieved by extension of the wrist.

(Reproduced, with permission, from DeGowin's *Diagnostic Examination,* 7th ed. New York, NY: McGraw-Hill, 2000: 720.)

Etiology

Anything that increases pressure within the carpal tunnel can cause it. Most common causes are trauma to carpal bones and flexor tenosynovitis. Can be secondary to systemic illnesses such as RA, sarcoidosis, acromegaly, hypothyroidism, diabetes.

Signs and Symptoms

- Muscle weakness and atrophy—mostly in the thenar eminence
- **Phalen's sign:** Presence of paraesthesias along median nerve distribution after holding wrist flexed at 90° for 30 sec
- **Tinel's sign:** Pain radiating down the fingers following percussion over the carpal tunnel

Treatment

- Rest with wrist splint worn as much as possible and elevation of the hand to reduce inflammation
- Steroids injected into carpal tunnel are suitable for temporary situations.
- Surgical division of the flexor retinaculum

> Patients who work extensively with their hands and pregnant women (due to edema) are at increased risk for carpal tunnel syndrome.

GOUT

Definition

A disorder in purine metabolism, resulting in the deposition of urate crystals in joint spaces. The result is inflammation and exquisite pain.

Epidemiology

Seen most commonly in middle-aged men

Etiology

- Hyperuricemia
- Inborn errors of metabolism (such as Lesch–Nyhan)
- High-protein diet (sweetbreads, sardines, anchovies, liver, kidney)
- Alcohol
- Diuretics (decrease urate excretion)

Hyperuricemia
is caused by:
- Increased urate production
- Decreased urate excretion

Signs and Symptoms

- Acute onset of extreme pain in small joints, accompanied by redness and swelling
- **Tophi** are aggregates of gouty crystals and giant cells. They can erode away at tissue.
- **Podagra** is inflammation of the first metatarsophalangeal joint, and presents in 50 to 75% of all patients as an exquisitely painful nodule on the medial aspect of the foot (see Figure 7-7).

Fifty percent of first gout attacks involve first metatarsophalangeal joint.

Diagnosis

Aspirated joint fluid reveals needle-shaped monosodium urate crystals with **negative birefringence.** Ninety-five percent of patients will have elevated serum uric acid, however many patients can have elevated uric acid levels and never develop gout.

Gout:
Small joints
Negative birefringence
Pseudogout:
Large joints
Positive birefringence

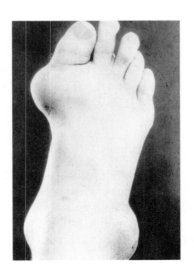

FIGURE 7-7. Podagra.
(Reproduced, with permission, from Fauci et al., *Harrison's Principles of Internal Medicine,* 14th ed. New York, NY: McGraw-Hill, 1998: 2162.)

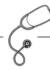

Aspirin is *contraindicated* in acute gout because it decreases urate excretion.

Laboratory

- Hyperuricemia
- Elevated WBC
- Elevated ESR
- Isosthenuria
- Proteinuria
- Normal glomerular filtration rate (GFR)

Treatment

Prophylaxis
- Allopurinol—xanthine oxidase inhibitor
- Probenecid—increases renal urate excretion
- Dietary discretion—reduce intake of high protein and high fat foods, discontinue alcohol.

Acute Attacks
- Indomethacin—NSAID
- Colchicine—inhibits chemotaxis
- Intra-articular corticosteroids—decrease inflammation

PSEUDOGOUT

Definition

Deposition of calcium pyrophosphate dihydrate (CPPD) crystals in joint spaces

Etiology

- Acute inflammatory reaction to the deposition of CPPD in joint spaces
- Changes related to age that make the synovial fluid environment more hospitable to CPPD growth

Signs and Symptoms and Diagnosis

Similar to gout, the affected joints are painful and red. Unlike gout:
- Large joints are affected (knees, wrists, shoulder).
- The crystals are rhomboid (gouty crystals are needle shaped).
- Radiographs demonstrate calcification in the articular cartilage.
- There is **positive birefringence** of crystals.

Treatment

- NSAIDs can alleviate symptoms.
- Aspirating synovial fluid shortens the duration of the attacks.
- No therapy is available to remove CPPD crystals.

Definitions

Connective tissue diseases that result in proximal muscle weakness. Dermatomyositis differs only in that there is a rash, typically affecting the face, neck, and shoulders. There is also a significant risk of an occult malignancy associated with dermatomyositis.

Both polymyositis and dermatomyositis are more common in women.

Etiology

Etiology unknown. Many viruses including toxoplasma, influenza, and coxsackie have been implicated.

Family history of autoimmune disease or vasculitis increases risk.

Signs and Symptoms

- Symmetrical proximal muscle weakness
- Dysphagia
- Difficulty getting out of a chair, climbing or descending stairs, kneeling, raising arms

Diagnosis

Look for the following four criteria:

1. Proximal muscle weakness
2. Elevated creatine phosphokinase (CPK) (from necrotic muscle fibers)
3. Low amplitude action potentials and fibrillations on electromyography (EMG)
4. Increased muscle fiber size on muscle biopsy

Polymyositis and dermatomyositis can be distinguished from myasthenia gravis by the lack of ocular involvement (ptosis).

Laboratory

- Positive antinuclear antibody (ANA)
- Elevated CPK, LDH, SGOT, aldolase
- ESR is elevated in only 50% of cases.
- Abnormal EMG
- Muscle biopsy shows inflammatory infiltrates.
- One fifth of patients have myositis specific antibodies (Anti-Jo-1).
- Chest x-ray may show interstitial pulmonary disease.

Typical scenario:
A 57-year-old woman complains of difficulty getting out of a chair and difficulty combing her hair. *Think: Polymyositis.*

Prognosis

Presentation is usually insidious, progresses slowly, but disease can be fatal. Seventy-five percent survival at 5 years with long-term corticosteroid therapy.

Treatment

- Range of motion exercises
- Daily steroids
- If refractory to steroids, azathioprine or methotrexate are given.

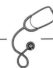

Note both azathioprine and methotrexate suppress the bone marrow. Azathioprine is also hepatotoxic.

HIGH-YIELD FACTS

Rheumatology

Definition

Painful swelling of the costochondral articulations at the anterior chest wall

Etiology

Associated with:
- Recent upper respiratory tract infection
- Trauma
- Overuse

Signs and Symptoms

- Typically affects the second thru fifth costochondral joints.
- Pain is sharp, worse with deep breathing and movement, may radiate to the shoulders and arms.
- Pain is reproducible with palpation

Diagnosis

Diagnosis is clinical. Can do a chest x-ray to look for metastatic lesions to the sternal bone marrow, which can produce similar symptoms.

Treatment

NSAIDs; avoid overuse of muscles.

AVASCULAR NECROSIS (AVN) OF THE HIP

AVN of the hip in children is called Legg–Calvé–Perthes disease.

Definition

The limited blood supply to the head of the femur makes this site particularly vulnerable to AVN.

Etiology

Seen with a variety of conditions such as trauma, long-term steroid therapy, excessive radiation, alcoholism, sickle cell disease, and Gaucher's disease

Signs and Symptoms

Pain, often referred to the **knee,** exacerbated by internal rotation of the hip

HIGH-YIELD FACTS

Rheumatology

Diagnosis

MRI or bone scan are needed for early detection of the disease. Plain radiographs will be positive only in the late stage.

Treatment

Total hip replacement

NONGONOCOCCAL SEPTIC ARTHRITIS

Definition

Nongonococcal septic arthritis is seen when there is previous joint damage or bacteremia. It is monarticular and affects the large joints (knee, hip, shoulder, and wrist).

Etiology

Young Adults
S. aureus, β-hemolytic strep, and gram-negative bacilli

Sickle Cell Anemia Patients
Salmonella and S .aureus (equal)

IV Drug Users and Immunocompromised
Gram-negative organisms such as E. coli and Pseudomonas aeruginosa

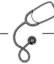

Nongonococcal septic arthritis: Patients will often describe previous **trauma** to the joint.

Risk factors

- Rheumatoid arthritis
- Prosthetic joints
- Immunodeficiency
- Age

Signs and Symptoms

- Pain, swelling, and warmth over the joint
- Limited range of motion
- Fever

Diagnosis

- Blood cultures are positive in 50% of cases.
- ESR will be elevated.
- Gram stain can pick up 75% of S. aureus infections.

Arthrocentesis is both diagnostic and therapeutic. Joint fluid will reveal an elevated white count (need > 1,000,000 cells/mm³), predominantly polymorphonucleocytes and a low glucose level. The arthrocentesis releases fluid thereby lowering pressure within the joint capsule and elevating pain. Arthrocentesis should be avoided if the overlying skin is infected or if there is bacteremia because the procedure introduces a portal of entry for bacteria into the joint.

Treatment

- Systemic antibiotics
- Serial arthrocentesis may be necessary if synovial fluid rapidly accumulates
- Surgical drainage is needed for septic hip, and for septic joints that do not improve with intravenous antibiotics within 72 hours.

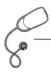

Arthrocentesis should never be attempted in hemophiliacs until the clotting disorder is corrected with the appropriate blood product.

GONOCOCCAL SEPTIC ARTHRITIS

Definition

A disseminated gonococcal infection; more common in women than men.

Etiology

Neisseria gonorrhea

Signs and Symptoms

After 1 to 4 days of a **migratory polyarthritis,** 60% of patients develop a tenosynovitis and 40% a purulent monarthritis. Patients will sometimes have fever but, surprisingly, urethritis is rarely seen. Most patients develop a characteristic skin lesion—**small necrotic pustules**—over their extremities, usually the fingers and toes.

Women are often affected during pregnancy, possibly due to the immunosuppression of pregnancy.

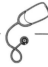

Upper extremities favored in gonococcal arthritis.

Diagnosis

- Synovial fluid shows elevated WBCs.
- Gram stain and blood culture are positive in less than 50% of cases.

Treatment

- Very sensitive to antibiotic therapy (e.g., ceftriaxone)
- Surgical drainage is not usually necessary

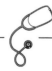

If there is no response to antibiotics, consider Reiter's syndrome.

SERONEGATIVE ARTHRITIDES

Include ankylosing spondylitis, psoriatic arthritis, and ulcerative colitis

Definition

An HLA-B27 associated syndrome involving the musculoskeletal, GU, and ocular systems. Occurs in two forms:

1. Sexually transmitted (1 to 2 weeks after exposure); more common in men
2. Post dysentery (most commonly due to *Salmonella*, *Shigella*, *Yersinia*, and *Campylobacter*); more common in women and children

Signs and Symptoms

- Conjunctivitis
- Urethritis/cervicitis
- Arthritis: Asymmetric, lower extremities
- Oral ulcerations
- Balanitis

Laboratory

- Elevated ESR
- Urethral culture may reveal *C. trachomatis*.

Treatment

- NSAIDs for arthritis
- Doxycycline for urethritis/cervicitis

Reiter's syndrome: "Can't see, can't pee, can't climb a tree"

Definition

Autoimmune disease associated with HLA-B5

Signs and Symptoms

- Aphthous (oral) ulcers
- Genital ulcers
- Deep vein thrombophlebitis
- Arthritis (nondeforming)
- Uveitis
- Colitis
- Psychiatric disturbances

Behçet's syndrome: "Though I enjoyed the experience, I was afterward *beset* with oral and genital ulcers."

HIGH-YIELD FACTS

Rheumatology

Diagnosis

Must have recurrent oral ulcers plus two of the following:

- Recurrent genital ulcers
- Eye lesions
- Skin lesions
- Positive pathergy test

Behçet's ulcers pain the male but spare the female (painless in women).

Laboratory

- Elevated ESR
- Hypergammaglobulinemia
- Cryoglobulinemia

Pathergy test: Inflammatory reaction of skin to any scratches.

Treatment

- Colchicine or interferon-α for arthritis
- Aspirin or antiplatelet agents for thrombophlebitis
- Steroids for uveitis and CNS manifestations

POLYARTERITIS NODOSA (PAN)

Definition

Systemic necrotizing vasculitis of small and medium-sized muscular arteries

Signs and Symptoms

- Nonspecific symptoms predominate: Fever, weight loss, malaise
- Specific symptoms depend on organ involved. Most common ones are:
  - Glomerulonephritis, arthritis, mononeuritis multiplex
  - Other systems that may be involved are GI, skin, cardiac, GU, and CNS. Note conspicuous absence of pulmonary involvement.

Laboratory

- Red cell casts in urine
- One third of patients have hepatitis B antigenemia.

Treatment

- Prednisone
- Cyclophosphamide

Definition

Medium vessel arteritis, also known as allergic angiitis and granulomatosis; it is very similar to PAN except that the pulmonary findings predominate.

Signs and Symptoms

- Bronchospasm (asthma)
- Eosinophilia
- Fever
- Erythematous maculopapular rashes, palpable purpura, and cutaneous nodules

Treatment

Steroids; if steroids fail, consider azathioprine and cyclophosphamide.

WEGENER'S GRANULOMATOSIS

Chronically relapsing small artery vasculitis of upper and lower respiratory tracts and glomerulonephritis

Signs and Symptoms

- Kidney: Glomerulonephritis
- Lungs: Hemoptysis, pulmonary infiltrates
- Nasopharynx: Sinusitis, otitis
- Arthralgias/arthritis
- Fever
- Weight loss

Diagnosis

- Granulomatous vasculitis on lung biopsy
- Postive c-ANCA titer
- Exclusion of Goodpasture's syndrome, tumors, and infectious disease.

Treatment

Steroids, cyclophosphamide

Goodpasture's is the other disease that involves both lungs and kidney. Its triad is:
- Glomerulonephritis,
- Pulmonary hemorrhage
- Anti-GBM Ab

HIGH-YIELD FACTS

Rheumatology

TAKAYASU'S ARTERITIS

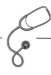

Takayasu's is also called "pulseless disease" and "aortic arch syndrome."

Definition

An arteritis of unknown (possibly autoimmune) etiology that is seen commonly in young people of Asian descent, usually affects medium and large-sized arteries. More common in women.

Signs and Symptoms

- Loss of pulses in arms and carotids bilaterally
- Raynaud's phenomenon
- Signs of transient brain ischemia such as blindness and hemiplegia
- Abdominal pain, atypical chest pain

Diagnosis

Arteriography

Treatment

- Steroids
- Methotrexate

TEMPORAL ARTERITIS

Temporal arteritis is also called giant cell arteritis.

Inflammation of medium and large-sized arteries, commonly the temporal artery. See neurology section.

HLA ASSOCIATIONS

SLE	DR2 and DR3
Multiple sclerosis	DR2
Rheumatoid arthritis	DR4
Ankylosing spondylitis and Reiter's syndrome	B27
IDDM	DR3 and DR4
Behçet's Syndrome	B5
Polymyositis and dermatomyositis	DR3

Nephrology and Acid–Base

Thomas M. Boyd

ACID–BASE DISORDERS

GENERAL LABORATORY STUDIES

Serum Electrolytes

- Plasma bicarbonate (HCO_3): Increased in metabolic alkalosis and compensated respiratory acidosis. Decreased in metabolic acidosis and compensated respiratory alkalosis.
- Serum potassium: Increased in acidemia and decreased in alkalemia.
- Serum chloride: Compare with the serum sodium. In dehydration or overhydration they should be increased or decreased proportional to one another. If there is a nonproportionate change, calculate the anion gap later on.

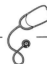

Serum chloride level of 100 mmol/L roughly corresponds to Na of 140 mmol/L.

Arterial Blood Gas (ABG)

Normal values:

pH	7.4	(7.35–7.45)
$PaCO_2$	40	(35–45)
PaO_2	90	(80–100)
HCO_3	24	(21–27)
O_2 sat	98	(95–100)
Base excess	0	(−2 to +2)

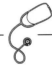

Learn this ABG sequence as these values are frequently reported in this order without labels (e.g., 7.4/40/90/24/98/0).

- **Look for hypoxia** using PaO_2; correlate with the clinical scenario
- **Determine the type of disturbance** using pH, P_aCO_2, and HCO_3 (see Table 8-1)
- **Calculate the degree of compensation:**
  - A change in $PaCO_2$ of 10 mm Hg, up or down, causes pH to increase or decrease by 0.08 units (pH decreases as $PaCO_2$ rises).
  - A pH change of 0.15 is the result of a bicarbonate change of 10 mEq/L.

TABLE 8-1. Acid–base Disturbances

Disorder	Abnormality	Compensation	pH	PaCO₂	HCO₃
Metabolic acidosis	Gain H⁺/lose bicarb	Increase ventilation	↓	↓	↓
Respiratory acidosis	Hypoventilate	Generate bicarbonate	↓	↑	↑
Metabolic alkalosis	Lose H⁺/gain bicarb	Decrease ventilation	↑	↑	↑
Respiratory alkalosis	Hyperventilation	Bicarbonate consumption	↓	↓	

↓ = decreased; ↑ = increased.

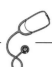

Use Winter's formula to determine if compensation is appropriate in the setting of metabolic acidosis:
$1.5 \times (HCO_3{-}) + 8 \pm 2 = pCO_2$

Isopropyl alcohol (rubbing alcohol) does NOT cause acidosis but it is associated with ketonemia. Ketone bodies are not acids.

Causes of anion gap metabolic acidosis:
MUDPILES
Methanol, Metformin
Uremia
DKA
Paraldehyde
INH, or iron tablets
Lactic acidosis
Ethanol
Salicylates

Anion Gap

- The concentration of serum anions not measured in routine electrolyte profiles (e.g., lactic and keto acids)
- Anion Gap = Na − (Cl + HCO₃) Normal = 9 − 14 mEq/L

METABOLIC ACIDOSIS

Definition

- Decrease in pH with decrease in HCO₃
- Etiology depends on presence or absence of an anion gap

Anion Gap Metabolic Acidosis

ETIOLOGY

- Lactic acidosis
- Ketoacidosis (DKA, ethanol intoxication, starvation)
- Uremia (chronic renal failure)
- Toxic ingestions (ASA, paraldehyde, methanol, ethylene glycol)

DIAGNOSIS

Diagnosis is conveniently divided by the presence or absence of ketonuria.

Ketonuria Present
- Diabetic ketoacidosis (hyperglycemia present)
- Alcoholic ketoacidosis (history of EtOH abuse)
- Paraldehyde poisoning (urine positive for acetaldehyde, positive toxicology screen)
- Starvation or high-fat diet
- Isopropyl alcohol intoxication

Ketonuria Absent
- Renal failure (elevated blood urea nitrogen [BUN]/creatinine)
- Lactic acidosis (elevated serum lactic acid levels)
- Methanol poisoning (elevated osmolal gap, blindness, positive toxicology screen). Methanol is a component of varnish and deicing solutions.

- Ethylene glycol (component of antifreeze) causes elevated osmolal gap, calcium oxalate crystals in urine, positive toxicology screen. Oxalate crystals in the urine is key to diagnosis on the exam.
- Salicylate poisoning (normal osmolal gap, history of ingestion, positive toxicology screen)

Normal Anion Gap Metabolic Acidosis

ETIOLOGY

- Renal tubular acidosis
- Diarrhea, pancreatic fistula
- Carbonic anhydrase inhibitors (acetazolamide)
- Dilutional acidosis (from rapid infusion of bicarbonate-free isotonic saline)
- Exogenous acid ingestion (ammonium chloride, calcium choride)
- Ileostomy
- Medications (spironolactone, beta blockers)

THERAPY FOR METABOLIC ACIDOSIS

- Correct underlying cause
- "Overshoot alkalosis" occurs when sodium bicarbonate is used too quickly. Correct bicarbonate only to 15 mEq/L, and correct no more than half of the deficit in 12 hours.
- Hypernatremia and fluid overload may occur, which can be dangerous in the setting of congestive heart failure (CHF) or renal failure.

RESPIRATORY ACIDOSIS

Definition

Hypoventilation from any cause increases the $PaCO_2$ and decreases the serum pH. There is a compensatory increase in bicarbonate.

Etiology

- Pulmonary (chronic obstructive pulmonary disease [COPD], severe alveolar infiltrates, pulmonary edema, interstitial restrictive lung disease)
- Airway obstruction (foreign body, severe bronchospasm, laryngospasm)
- Thoracic disorders (pneumothorax, flail chest)
- Alveolar hypoventilation (myasthenia gravis, severe hypokalemia causing weak muscles of respiration, muscular dystrophy)
- Peripheral nervous system disorders (Guillain–Barré syndrome, botulism, tetanus, organophosphate poisoning)
- Depression of central respiratory drive (narcotic overdose, general anesthesia, increased intracranial pressure [ICP]).

Signs and Symptoms

- Confusion, encephalopathy, coma

Typical scenario:
A 47-year-old man was binge drinking EtOH 3 days ago. No alcohol consumption for 3 days. He presents with acidosis and ketonemia. Blood EtOH is zero. *Think: Alcoholic ketoacidosis.* Treatment: Glucose-containing fluids (D₅NS). This stimulates the pancreas to secrete insulin and treats the acidosis.

Do not rely on sodium bicarbonate to correct metabolic acidosis. Correct the underlying cause.

Typical scenario:
A 34-year-old diabetic man with renal insufficiency has normal anion gap. K is high; bicarbonate level is low. *Think: Type IV RTA (hyporeninemic hypoaldosteronism).*

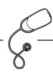

Hyperventilation may be due to tachypnea or hyperpnea.

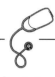

Respiratory alkalosis is a frequent component of mixed acid–base disorders.

Treatment

- Treat underlying cause.
- Mechanical hyperventilation will decrease the amount of CO$_2$ retention in severely hypoxic patients.

RESPIRATORY ALKALOSIS

Definition

Elevated arterial pH, and hyperventilation resulting in decreased PCO$_2$ and compensatory decrease in serum bicarbonate

Etiology

- Most commonly caused by anxiety, which provokes hyperventilation
- Other causes: shock, sepsis, pulmonary disease, CVA, pregnancy, liver disease, hyperthyroidism, salicylates

Signs and Symptoms

- Rapid, deep breathing
- Chest tightness, chest pain, and anxiety
- Circumoral paresthesias, tetany in severe cases

Treatment

- Reassurance
- If patient can be calmed enough, have him or her breathe into a paper bag.
- Decrease the minute volume in the mechanically ventilated patient

METABOLIC ALKALOSIS

Definition

- Elevated pH, increased plasma bicarbonate, and a compensatory increase in PaCO$_2$

Etiology

Divided into chloride-responsive and chloride-resistant forms:
- Chloride-responsive: Urine chloride < 15 mEq/L:
  - Vomiting or prolonged NG tube drainage
  - Pyloric stenosis
  - Laxative abuse
  - Diuretics
  - Post-hypercapnic states

- Chloride-resistant: Urine chloride > 15 mEq/L:
  - Severe Mg or K deficiency
  - Diuretics (thiazides or loops)
  - Increased mineralocorticoids (Cushing's syndrome, primary aldosteronism, renal artery stenosis)
  - Licorice, chewing tobacco
  - Inherited disorders (Bartter's syndrome)

Signs and Symptoms

- Irritability and neuromuscular hyperexcitability
- Concomitant signs of hypokalemia (muscular weakness, cramping, ileus)
- Suspect metabolic alkalosis when the physical exam suggests hypovolemia and chronic GI volume loss

Treatment

- Mild metabolic alkalosis requires no specific treatment.
- Correct the underlying defect that is causing retention of bicarbonate by the kidney (contraction alkalosis).
- Hydration
- In patients who are prone to volume overload (CHF), KCl can be given cautiously instead of normal saline.
- In severe hypokalemia and hypermineralocorticoid states the alkalosis is chloride-resistant and cannot be corrected until potassium is replaced. Specific therapy must address hypermineralocorticoid state.

BODY FLUIDS

Definitions

- Total body water (TBW) is approximately 60% of lean body mass.
- Intracellular fluid (ICF) is two thirds of TBW:
  - The major cations in ICF are K^+ and Mg^{2+}.
  - The major ICF anions are proteins and organic phosphates (ATP, ADP, AMP).
- Extracellular fluid (ECF) is one third of TBW:
  - Consists of interstitial fluid (third space) and plasma
  - The major ECF cation is Na^+.
  - The major ECF anions are Cl^- and HCO_3^-.
- Plasma comprises one fourth of the ECF (one twelfth of TBW). The major plasma proteins are albumin and globulins.
- Interstitial fluid is three fourths of the ECF (one fourth of TBW). The electrolyte composition of interstitial fluid is the same as plasma. However, interstitial fluid contains little protein (ultrafiltrate).

Fluid Shifts Between Compartments

- Water shifts between ECF and ICF so the osmolarities of the two compartments remain equal.

Major toxins that increase the serum osmolarity: EtOH, methanol, ethylene glycol.

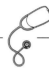

Diarrhea and normal saline hydration (isosmotic volume contraction/expansion) do not change the serum osmolarity.

- Solutes that do not cross the cell membranes freely contribute to ECF osmolarity (glucose, sodium, mannitol, IV contrast materials).

Serum Osmolarity

- Normal range: 280 to 300 mOsm/kg
- Serum osmolarity can be estimated with the following formula:

$$\text{Serum osm} = 2(\text{Na} + \text{K}) + \frac{\text{Glucose}}{18} + \frac{\text{BUN}}{2.8}$$

- Elevated in dehydration, hypernatremia, diabetes insipidus, uremia, hyperglycemia, mannitol therapy, toxin ingestion, hypercalcemia, diuretic therapy
- Decreased in syndrome of inappropriate antidiuretic hormone (SIADH), hyponatremia, overhydration with 5% dextrose solution, Addison's disease, hypothyroidism

HYPONATREMIA

Definition

Plasma sodium < 134 mEq/L

Etiology and Classification

Hyponatremia is subdivided into three categories based on the serum osmolarity:

- Hypotonic hyponatremia is further subdivided into three categories:
  - Isovolemic/hypotonic hyponatremia: Renal failure, SIADH, glucocorticoid deficiency (hypopituitarism), hypothyroidism, and medications
  - Hypovolemic/hypotonic hyponatremia:
    - Renal losses (diuretics, partial urinary tract obstruction, salt-wasting nephropathies)
    - Extrarenal losses (vomiting, diarrhea, extensive burns, third-spacing (pancreatitis, peritonitis)
  - Hypervolemic/hypotonic hyponatremia: CHF, nephrotic syndrome, cirrhosis
- Isotonic hyponatremia (normal serum osmolarity):
  - Pseudohyponatremia (discussed later)
  - Isotonic infusions (glucose, mannitol)
- Hypertonic hyponatremia (increased serum osmolarity):
  - Hyperglycemia: Each 100 mL/dL increase in serum glucose above normal decreases plasma sodium concentration by 1.6 mEq/L.
  - Hypertonic infusions: mannitol, glucose.

Signs and Symptoms

- Moderate hyponatremia or gradual onset: Confusion, muscle cramps, lethargy, anorexia, nausea
- Severe hyponatremia or rapid onset: Seizures or coma

Diagnosis

- Normal osmolarity: Consider pseudohyponatremia and overinfusion of non–sodium-containing isotonic solutions such as glucose and mannitol.
- Low osmolarity: Clinically assess the extracellular fluid volume. Look for tachycardia, hypotension, poor skin turgor (indicative of hypovolemia). Also look for peripheral edema (indicative of hypervolemia). Normal vital signs and no edema usually indicate isovolemia.
- High osmolarity: Measure serum glucose concentration to consider hyperglycemia. Also consider overinfusion of hypertonic, non–sodium-containing solutions (mannitol, glucose, glycine).

Serum Chemistries

See Table 8-2.

Pseudohyponatremia

- Hyponatremia associated with increased or normal serum osmolarity
- Since plasma is 93% water and 7% plasma protein and lipid, and sodium ions are only dissolved in the plasma water, increasing the non-aqueous phase artificially lowers the Na^+ concentration.
- This occurs in multiple myeloma (due to increased plasma protein) or hyperlipidemia.

Pseudohyponatremia is suspected if the measured and calculated serum osmolarities are different.

Treatment

- Treatment approach is twofold: Correction of the serum sodium, and treatment of the underlying disorder
- Serum sodium should be corrected only halfway to the lower range of normal within the first 24 hours.
- Never correct sodium faster than 1 mEq/hr. Central pontine myelinolysis (CPM), seizures, and cerebral edema may occur.

TABLE 8-2. Causes of Hyponatremia

		Urine Osm	Urine Sodium
Hypovolemic	Extrarenal: GI losses, skin losses, lung losses, third-spacing (fistula, burns, vomiting, diarrhea, GI suction, edema, pancreatitis)	↑	↓
	Renal: Diuretics, intrinsic renal damage (including acute tubular necrosis), partial urinary tract obstruction	↑	↑
	Adrenal insufficiency (Addison's)	↑	↑
Isovolemic	Water intoxication	↓	↓
	SIADH	↑	↑
Hypervolemic	CHF, liver cirrhosis, and the nephrotic syndrome	↑	↓

↓ = decreased; ↑ = increased.

- Hypovolemic hyponatremia: 0.9% NaCl (normal saline) infusion to correct volume deficit. Monitor the serum sodium to prevent complications of rapid correction. Hypertonic saline is rarely indicated.
- Hypervolemic hyponatremia: Sodium and water restriction. In CHF, the combination of captopril and furosemide is effective.

Central Pontine Myelinolysis (CPM)

- Sometimes termed osmotic demyelination syndrome, occurs as a treatment complication of severe or chronic hyponatremia (< 110 mEq/L).
- A symmetric zone of demyelination occurs in the basis pontis (and extrapontine areas), leading to stupor, lethargy, quiet and confused delirium, and quadriparesis.
- CPM can be avoided by increasing the serum sodium no faster than 0.5 mEq/hr. Some patients treated symptomatically will recover in 3 to 4 weeks; however, in some, the damage is irreversible.

Definition

Serum Na > 145 mEq/L

Etiology and Classification (see Table 8-3)

Hypovolemic
- Loss of water and sodium (water loss >> than sodium loss)
- Renal losses (diuretics, glycosuria); GI, respiratory, or skin losses; adrenal deficiencies

Isovolemic
- Decreased TBW, normal total body sodium, and decreased ECF
- Diabetes insipidus (neurogenic and nephrogenic), skin losses (hyperthermia), iatrogenic causes, reset osmostat

Hypervolemic
- Increased TBW, markedly increased total body sodium, and increased ECF
- Iatrogenic (hypertonic fluid administration)
- Mineralocorticoid excess (Conn's tumor, Cushing's syndrome)
- Excess salt ingestion

Signs and Symptoms

- Fatigue
- Confusion (can progress to coma and seizures)
- Lethargy
- Edema

TABLE 8-3. Causes of Hypernatremia

		Urine Osm	Urine Sodium
Hypovolemic	Renal loss: Osmotic diuresis (glycosuria, urea), acute/chronic renal failure, partial obstruction	N/↓	↑
	Extrarenal loss: Hyperpnea, excessive sweating	↑	↑
	Extrarenal loss: Diarrhea, burns, moderate sweating	↑	↓
	Iatrogenic (bicarbonate, dialysis, salt tablets)	↑	↑
Isovolemic	Diabetes insipidus (from any cause)	↓	↓
Hypervolemic	Mineralocorticoid excess (eg, Conn's syndrome)	N/↓	N/↓

↓ = decreased; ↑ = increased; N = normal.

Treating Hypernatremia

Hypovolemic
- Fluid replacement with normal saline. Correct plasma osmolarity no faster than 2 mOsm/kg/hr.

Isovolemic
- Fluid replacement with half normal (0.45%) saline. Correct only half of the estimated water deficit in the first 24 hours.
- The correction rate should not exceed 1 mEq/L/hr in acute hypernatremia and 0.5 mEq/L/hr in chronic hypernatremia.
- Vasopressin for central diabetes insipidus

Hypervolemic
- Fluid replacement with half normal (0.45%) saline (to correct hypertonicity
- Loop diuretic therapy (e.g., furosemide) to increase sodium excretion

Water deficit (WD) in hypernatremic patients: WD (in liters) = 0.6 × body weight (kg) × (Measured Na/Normal Na) − 1).

HYPOKALEMIA

Definition

Plasma potassium < 3.3 mEq/L

Etiology and Classification

- Cellular shift (redistribution) and undetermined mechanisms:
  - Alkalosis (each 0.1 increase in pH decreases serum K^+ by 0.4 − 0.6 mEq/L.)
  - Insulin
  - Vitamin B_{12}
  - β-adrenergics
  - Correction of digoxin toxicity with digitalis antibody fragments (Digibind).

- Increased renal potassium excretion:
  - Medications (diuretics, amphotericin B, cisplatin, aminoglycosides, corticosteroids)
  - Renal tubular acidosis type I (distal) or type II (proximal)
  - DKA
  - Ureteroenterostomy
  - Hypomagnesemia
  - Postobstruction diuresis, diuresis stage of acute tubular necrosis
  - Osmotic diuresis (mannitol)
  - Bartter's syndrome: JG-cell hyperplasia causing increased rennin/aldosterone, metabolic alkalosis, hypokalemia, muscle weakness, and tetany (seen in young adults).
  - Interstitial nephritis
  - Increased mineralocorticoid activity (1° or 2° hyperaldosteronism), Cushing's syndrome
  - Chronic metabolic alkalosis from loss of gastric fluid (pyloric stenosis causing hypokalemic, hypochloremic metabolic alkalosis)
- GI losses:
  - Vomiting, nasogastric suctioning
  - Diarrhea, laxative abuse
  - Villous adenoma
  - Fistulas
  - Inadequate dietary intake (anorexia nervosa)
- Cutaneous losses from excessive sweating

Periodic paralysis can be associated with either hypokalemia or hyperkalemia. Both forms are autosomal dominant. However, hypokalemic periodic paralysis first presents in the teenage years, whereas hyperkalemic periodic paralysis presents in infancy.

Signs and Symptoms

- Impaired gastric motility, nausea, and vomiting
- Mild muscle weakness to overt paralysis depending on severity
- Rhabdomyolysis
- Atrial and ventricular dysrhythmias

Patients on dialysis are particularly prone to electrolyte imbalances.

Treatment

Replace potassium (PO or IV, depending on severity). Intravenous infusion of K+ should not exceed 20 mEq/hr.

HYPERKALEMIA

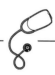

Patients taking digitalis must have their potassium checked regularly because hypokalemia increases the risk and severity of digitalis toxicity.

Definition

Serum K > 5.5 mEq/L

Etiology

- Pseudohyperkalemia is the most common cause.
- Intra- to extracellular potassium shifting occurs in acidosis, heavy exercise, insulin deficiency, and digitalis toxicity.

A 20 mEq infusion will raise the serum K by 0.25 mEq/L.

- Increased potassium load occurs with IV potassium supplementation, potassium containing medications, and increased cellular breakdown.
- Decreased potassium excretion occurs with oliguric renal failure, potassium sparing diuretics, beta blockers, angiotensin-converting enzyme (ACE) inhibitors, aldosterone deficiency, and obstructive uropathies.

Signs and Symptoms

- GI: Nausea, vomiting, diarrhea.
- Neuro: Muscle cramps, weakness, paresthesias, paralysis, areflexia, tetany, focal neurologic deficits, confusion
- Respiratory insufficiency
- Cardiac arrest

Diagnosis

EKG Changes
- 6.5 to 7.5 mEq/L: Tall peaked T-waves (see Figure 8-1), short QT interval, prolonged PR
- 7.5 to 8.0 mEq/L: QRS widening, flattened P-wave
- 10 to 12 mEq/L: QRS may degrade into a "sine-wave" pattern.
- V-Fib, complete heart block, or asystole may occur.

Treatment

- Cardiac membrane stabilization (calcium):
  - Contraindicated in patients on digoxin
- Shifting K$^+$ from ECF to ICF (insulin, albuterol, bicarbonate):
  - This is a temporary fix that wears off after the drugs do.
- Removal of K from the body (cation exchange resin such as Kayexalate, dialysis)

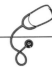

Pseudohyperkalemia is a serum K of > 5.5 due to hemolysis during phlebotomy or from hemolysis that occurs if sample is not analyzed within 30 minutes. Redraw sample if hemolysis and hyperkalemia are present.

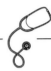

Chronic, slowly developing hyperkalemia is better tolerated than acute changes.

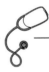

Perform a STAT ECG on patients with moderate to severe hyperkalemia.

Treatments for hyperkalemia:
Calcium
Kayexalate
Insulin and glucose
Dialysis
Albuterol

Controlling **K** Immediately Diverts Arrhythmias

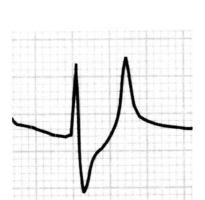

FIGURE 8-1. Peaked T-wave due to hyperkalemia.

217

Definition

- Serum Ca < 8.5 mg/dL
- Calcium is found in ionized (bound to serum proteins) and unionized (free) forms. The free fraction is biologically active.

Etiology

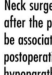

Neck surgery, even long after the procedure, can be associated with postoperative hypoparathyroidism usually due to ischemia of the parathyroid glands.

- PTH insufficiency
- Pseudohypoparathyroidism (Albrights' hereditary osteodystropy)
- Vitamin D deficiency (intestinal malabsorption, cholestyramine, primidone, renal, or liver disease)
- Toxins: Fluoride, cimetidine, ethanol, citrate, phenytoin
- Sepsis
- Pancreatitis
- Rhabdomyolysis, tumor lysis syndrome (increased serum phosphate)
- Severe magnesium deficiency

Parathyroid Hormone (PTH)

Secretion is stimulated by low free calcium and inhibited by increasing free calcium. Three major actions:

- In kidney, PTH facilitates excretion of phosphate and retention of calcium.
- Also in the kidney, PTH stimulates conversion of 25-OH vitamin D to 1,25-dihydroxy vitamin D (active vitamin D).
- PTH activates bone remodeling

Signs and Symptoms

- Circumoral paresthesia is usually the first symptom.
- **Chvostek's sign:** Facial muscle spasm with tapping of the facial nerve
- **Trousseau's sign:** Carpal spasm after occluding blood flow in forearm with blood pressure cuff.

Diagnosis

ECG findings: Prolonged QT and ST intervals (peaked T-waves are also possible, as in hyperkalemia).

Correcting for hypoalbuminemia: The measured Ca should be adjusted upward by 0.8 mg/dL for each 1.0 g/dL of albumin below normal.

Treatment

- For PTH deficiency: Replacement therapy with vitamin D or calcitriol combined with high oral calcium intake. Thiazide diuretics are used to lower urinary calcium and prevent calcium urolithiasis.
- Repletion of magnesium for hypomagnesemia
- Oral calcium supplementation, dietary phosphate restriction, and calcitriol for chronic renal failure
- Vitamin D and calcium supplementation for pseudohypoparathyroidism
- IV calcium for severe, life-threatening hypocalcemia

Definition

Serum Ca > 10.2 mg/dL

Etiology

Drugs
- Calcium supplementation (IV)
- Excess vitamin A
- Excess vitamin D increases intestinal calcium absorption
- Antacid abuse
- Thiazides (inhibit renal calcium excretion)
- Lithium

Malignancies
- Colon, lung, breast, prostate
- Multiple myeloma
- Zollinger–Ellison syndrome (as part of MEN I)
- Metastases
- Milk alkali syndrome

Endocrinopathies
- Hyperparathyroidism
- Hyperthyroidism
- Acromegaly
- Addison's disease
- Paget's disease (of bone)

Other
- Immobility (leads to increased bone turnover with increased bone resorption)
- Granulomatous diseases such as sarcoidosis, tuberculosis (1,25-2OH-vitamin D production by macrophages within granulomatous tissue)

Signs and Symptoms

- Malaise, fatigue, headaches, diffuse aches, and pains
- Patients are often dehydrated and a vicious cycle ensues. Dehydration decreases renal calcium excretion and patients take in less fluids because of vomiting and nausea.
- Lethargy and psychosis occur when hypercalcemia is severe.
- Metastatic calcifications may occur in skin, cornea, conjunctiva, and kidneys.

Diagnosis

Shortened QT interval on ECG

Causes of hypercalcemia:
"CHIMPANZEES"
Calcium supplementation
Hyperparathyroidism
  Hyperthyroidism
Immobility/Iatrogenic
Metastasis/Milk alkali
syndrome
Paget's disease
Addison's disease/
Acromegaly
Neoplasm
Zollinger–Ellison syndrome
Excessive vitamin A
Excessive vitamin D
Sarcoidosis

Primary hyperparathyroidism is the most common cause of hypercalcemia in the outpatient. Malignancy is the most common cause in the inpatient.

Hypercalcemia is a risk factor for kidney stones.

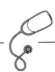

Acute pancreatitis can be precipitated by hypercalcemia.

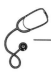

Treatment

- Calcitonin
- Bisphosphonate derivatives
- Parathyroidectomy for decreased creatinine clearance, renal stones, and diminished bone mass

PRIMARY HYPERPARATHYROIDISM

Definition

- Elevated parathyroid hormone and elevated serum calcium.
- May occur in conjunction with MEN I or MEN IIa (all glands are hyperplastic).
- Usually, only one parathyroid gland is enlarged, and hypercalcemia suppresses the function of the remaining glands.

Epidemiology

More common in middle-aged to elderly women.

Hyperparathyroidism: "Stones, bones, groans, and psychiatric overtones"

Signs and Symptoms

- Usual presentation is asymptomatic hypercalcemia noted on routine laboratory examination.
- Patients may also have nonspecific complaints like fatigue, weight loss, depression, abdominal pain, or arthralgias.
- Hypercalciuria from the kidneys' inability to reabsorb the large calcium load may lead to nephrocalcinosis or renal calculi.
- Elevated PTH levels lead to bone remodeling and decreased bone mass.

Diagnosis

- Hypercalcemia
- PTH level in the high-normal range
- Hypophosphatemia
- Hypercalciuria

Hypercalcemic crisis is an uncommon manifestation of 1° hyperparathyroidism presenting with severe hypercalcemia, volume depletion, and altered mental status.

MALIGNANCY AND HYPERCALCEMIA

Definitions

Humoral hypercalcemia of malignancy: From tumor production of PTH-related peptide. Stimulates bone resorption and renal calcium reabsorption. PTH-related peptide is not detected by the usual PTH immunoassay. Specific immunoassay exists for PTH-related peptide.

Local osteolytic hypercalcemia: Malignant cells in multiple myeloma or solid tumors with bone metastases may cause osteoclast stimulation. Osteoclast-activating factors (OAFs) are interleukins, transforming growth factors, and other cytokines.

Management of Severe Hypercalcemia

- Admit to intensive care unit (ICU) setting.
- Rehydration with normal saline to initiate calciuresis.
- Initiate potassium replacement.
- Ambulation should be encouraged if possible.
- IV infusion of **Pamidronate** (bisphosphonate) should be initiated simultaneously.
- May also use calcitonin.

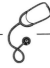

Inpatients with underlying cardiac failure consider furosemide to maintain diuresis and pulmonary artery pressure monitoring to avoid volume overload.

SECONDARY HYPERPARATHYROIDISM/RENAL OSTEODYSTROPHY

Pathophysiology

- Nephron loss reduces phosphate excretion, causing hyperphosphatemia
- This lowers serum calcium (increasing PTH secretion) and impairs calcitriol formation.
- Decreased calcitriol formation (also due to nephron loss) reduces intestinal calcium absorbtion.
- This provides further stimulation for PTH secretion.

Etiology and Classification

Three types of bone lesions are associated with secondary hyperparathyroidism:

1. Osteitis fibrosa cystica: Normal bone is replaced by fibrous tissue, primitive woven bone, and cysts.
2. Osteomalacia: Associated with vitamin D deficiency, characterized by defective osteoid mineralization.
3. Adynamic bone disease: Cause is unknown.

Signs and Symptoms

- Bone pain
- Proximal muscle weakness
- Pruritus
- Soft-tissue ulcerations
- Diffuse soft-tissue calcifications

Treatment

Goal is to normalize the calcium–phosphate balance:
- Reduce intestinal absorption of phosphate with aluminum-containing antacids.
- Vitamin D with calcitriol to increase serum calcium and reverse some of the bone changes
- Subtotal parathyroidectomy may benefit patients who do not respond to medical therapy.
- Renal transplant in selected patients

Definition

Serum phosphate < 2.5 mg/dL

Etiology

- Decreased PO intake: Prolonged IV infusions without phosphate supplementation, alcoholism with poor nutrition
- Renal losses: Renal tubular acidoses (RTAs)
- Intracellular shift: EtOH withdrawal, DKA (recovery phase), glucose/insulin infusion, total parenteral nutrition (TPN), theophylline toxicity
- Malabsorption syndromes
- Phosphate-binding antacids (aluminum containing)
- Acute tubular necrosis (diuretic phase)
- Hyperparathyroidism (1° or 2°)
- Hypokalemia, hypomagnesemia
- Acute volume expansion
- Acetazolamide

Signs and Symptoms

Musculoskeletal
- Rhabdomyolysis
- Proximal muscle weakness
- Altered gait
- Bone pains

Neurologic
- Paresthesias
- Seizures
- Coma
- Ataxia

Hematologic
- Hemolytic anemia
- Leukocyte or platelet dysfunction

Diagnosis

- Exclude presence of glucose/insulin infusions
- Exclude respiratory alkalosis
- Urine phosphate excretion:
  - Low (< 100 mg/day): GI losses or internal redistribution
  - High (> 100 mg/day): Exclude Fanconi's syndrome
- Serum calcium (if Fanconi's has been excluded):
  - High: 1° hyperparathyroidism, hypercalcemia of malignancy
  - Low: 2° hyperparathyroidism, recovery from renal failure, vitamin D resistant rickets, familial hypophosphatemia

Treatment

- Mild to moderate (> 1 mg/dL): Oral phosphate repletion
- Severe, symptomatic (< 1 mg/dL): IV phosphate salt administration until serum phosphate is > 1.5 mg/dL.

HYPERPHOSPHATEMIA

Definition

Plasma phosphate > 5 mg/dL

Etiology

- Iatrogenic (excessive phosphate administration):
  - Excessive oral intake or IV administration
  - Oral laxatives containing phosphate (phosphate tablets, phosphate enemas)
- Decreased renal phosphate excretion:
  - Acute or chronic renal failure
  - Hypoparathyroidism (post-thyroidectomy), pseudohypoparathyroidism
  - Acromegaly, thyrotoxicosis
  - Bisphosphonate therapy
  - Tumor calcinosis
  - Sickle cell anemia
- Extracellular shift:
  - Tumor lysis syndrome (rapid necrosis of tumors sensitive to chemotherapy)
  - Acidosis
  - Rhabdomyolysis, malignant hyperthermia

Signs and Symptoms

- Symptoms of hypocalcemia due to hyperphosphatemia
- Ectopic soft-tissue calcifications (kidneys, cornea, lung, blood vessels, skin) occur in the setting of chronic renal failure if the product of the calcium and phosphate $(Ca^{2+} \times PO_4^-)$ is > 70.

Treatment

Address the underlying condition where possible:
- Oral calcium carbonate binds phosphate in the gut and decreases absorption (slow).
- Insulin and glucose infusion promotes intracellular phosphate shift (rapid, but temporary, carries risk of hypokalemia).
- In severe refractory cases, dialysis may be necessary.

A common cause of high phosphate serum values is *in vitro* hemolysis. Most labs will report that the specimen was hemolyzed, however.

Definition

Serum magnesium < 1.8 mg/dL

Etiology

Gastrointestinal and Nutritional
- Malabsorption (defective GI uptake)
- Inadequate GI intake (most common in alcoholics)
- IV fluid replacement or parenteral nutrition without magnesium supplementation
- Chronic diarrhea, prolonged NG tube suctioning, small bowel or biliary fistulas

Excessive Renal Losses
- Diuretic therapy
- Resolving acute tubular necrosis (diuresis phase)
- Endocrine disturbances inducing excessive renal losses: DKA, hyperaldosteronism, hyperthyroidism, hyperparathyroidism
- Hypokalemia and hypercalciuria induce hypomagnesemia.

Cellular Redistribution
- Hypoalbuminemia/cirrhosis
- Insulin/glucose administration
- Acute pancreatitis
- Miscellaneous causes: Sweating, burns, prolonged exercise, "hungry-bone syndrome"

Hungry-bone syndrome is the rapid transfer of calcium into bones following removal of a hyperactive parathyroid nodule.

Signs and Symptoms

Neuromuscular
- The most common early findings:
  - Weakness, hyperreflexia
  - Fasciculations, tremors, and seizures may occur.
  - Altered mental status may occur.

ECG
- Prolonged QT, flattened T waves, prolonged PR interval
- Atrial fibrillation may occur.
- Torsade de pointes may occur.

Electrolyte Disturbances
- Hypokalemia refractory to potassium replacement
- Hypocalcemia refractory to calcium replacement (Mg necessary for parathyroid function)

Treatment

- Correct deficiency regardless of etiology—cardiac manifestations may be life threatening:
    - Mild and asymptomatic: Oral magnesium oxide
    - Severe (< 1.0 mg/dL) or symptomatic: IV $MgSO_4$
- Address underlying cause.

HYPERMAGNESEMIA

Definition

Serum magnesium > 2.3 mg/dL

Etiology

- Iatrogenic: During treatment of hypomagnesemia or eclampsia/ preeclampsia
- Renal failure (decreased glomerular filtration rate)
- Decreased renal excretion of Mg due to salt depletion
- Magnesium-containing antacid abuse in patients with underlying renal insufficiency
- Deficiency in mineralocorticoid secretion
- Massive cell breakdown (tumor lysis, rhabdomyolysis)
- Redistribution: DKA, pheochromocytoma
- Miscellaneous: Lithium toxicity, volume depletion, familial hypocalciuric hypercalcemia

Signs and Symptoms

- Hypoactive deep tendon reflexes
- Paresthesias
- Hypotension
- Coma, apnea
- Acute, severe hypermagnesemia can suppress parathyroid secretion and cause hypocalcemia
- ECG: Shortened PR interval, heart block, peaked T-waves, widened QRS

Treatment

- Discontinue any IV magnesium infusion
- ECG changes: IV calcium immediately
- Dialysis for refractory hypermagnesemia

- Always check the other electrolytes—isolated electrolyte abnormalities are uncommon.
- Abnormal calcium level is meaningless without an albumin level in an asymptomatic patient.
- Redraw labs if *in vitro* hemolysis is a possibility.
- If severe, place patient on continuous ECG monitoring.
- Neurological exam soon after treatment begun—focus on level of consciousness, presence of confusion, and deep tendon reflexes. Serial neuro exams during treatment can guide therapy while labs are pending.

ACUTE RENAL FAILURE (ARF)

Definition

Clear-cut definition does not exist. Usually rapid onset of oliguria with increasing BUN and creatinine. Often occurs in the hospitalized patient.

Classification

Prerenal, postrenal, or intrinsic renal failure

General Approach

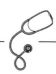

Oliguria: Urine output less than 400 mL/day. Minimum volume needed to excrete daily production of metabolites and waste products.

- Renal failure suspected from oliguria or increasing BUN/creatinine
- Prerenal:
  - BUN rising out of proportion to creatinine (> 20:1)
  - Volume depletion from hemorrhage, dehydration, surgery
  - CHF causing decreased cardiac output and secondary renal hypoperfusion
  - Third-spacing from cirrhosis, nephrotic syndrome, sepsis, burns
  - Most common cause of inpatient renal insufficiency due to decreased renal perfusion
  - Exacerbated by NSAIDs and ACE inhibitors
- Postrenal:
  - Bilateral ureteral obstruction: Urothelial tumor, benign prostatic hypertrophy (BPH), cervical CA
  - Urethral obstruction: Bladder CA
  - Renal sonogram: May show bilateral hydronephrosis, retrograde ureterogram is more sensitive
  - Reversible if obstruction removed in time
  - Postobstructive diuresis: Frequent temporary sequela of obstruction removal—if present, hydrate and follow electrolytes

Intrinsic Renal Failure

- Medication-induced acute tubular necrosis (ATN): Aminoglycosides, cisplatin, pentamidine, lithium, amphotericin

- IV contrast–induced failure
- Acute allergic interstitial nephritis (AIN)
- Vascular disorders and atheromatous emboli
- Acute, subacute, and rapidly progressive glomerular syndromes
- Myeloma kidney/amyloid nephropathy
- Exacerbation of chronic, established renal disease

Urinary Sodium

- Prerenal failure has low urine sodium (< 15 mEq/L) and high urine osmolarity (> 500 mOsm/L). The urine specific gravity is usually around 1.020.
- Intrinsic renal failure has high urine sodium (> 15 mEq/L) and low urine osmolarity (< 400 mOsm/L).
- The fractional sodium excretion (FE Na⁺) is the best discriminator between prerenal and intrinsic renal failure:

$$FE\ Na^+ = \frac{(Urine\ Na/Plasma\ Na)}{(Urine\ creatinine/Plasma\ creatinine)} \times 100\%$$

Prerenal failure: < 1.0%   Intrinsic renal failure: > 1.0%

Dopamine, diuretics, mannitol, and saline confound use of fractional sodium excretion in finding etiology of renal failure.

Urinary Sediment

Intrinsic renal disease shows large amounts of protein and an "active" sediment (blood, protein, and red and white cell casts) that often will point toward the underlying cause of the renal disease:
- Acute glomerulonephritis: Red blood cell casts with hematuria and proteinuria and low urine specific gravity
- Acute tubular necrosis: Many renal epithelial cells and pigmented granular casts

Serologic Testing

Serologic testing can further delineate the cause of the failure:
- Antiglomerular basement membrane Ab in Goodpasture's syndrome
- Antineutrophil Ab (ANCA) in microscopic polyarteritis nodosa or Wegener's syndrome
- Antinuclear Ab (ANA) in SLE

CAUSES OF INTRINSIC ARF

Tubulointerstitial diseases:
- ATN and interstitial nephritis
- Tubulointerstitial causes of renal failure are the most common in the hospital and have the best outcomes if recognized early.

Acute Tubular Necrosis

DEFINITION

Acute necrosis of renal tubules due to ischemic or toxic insult

ETIOLOGY

- Ischemic: Shock, trauma, sepsis, hypoxia
- Toxic: IV contrast media, aminoglycosides, rhabdomyolysis, and tumor lysis

COURSE

- Patients present with dramatic renal failure
- Most survive and recover normal renal function.
- Severity correlates with survival.
- Failure lasts 1 to 2 weeks, during which intensive care is required.
- ~50% have normal urine output (less severe).

DIAGNOSIS

- Muddy brown urine with tubular epithelial casts.
- High urine sodium
- FENa is > 1%.

COMPLICATIONS

- Volume overload and water intoxication with hyponatremia
- Hyperkalemia, hyperphosphatemia, and acidemia (metabolic).
- Infection from indwelling catheters (35 to 70% will have some form of infection), pulmonary and urinary tracts are common foci
- Uremic syndrome: Pericarditis, anemia, coagulopathies, GI disturbances, and CNS abnormalities

Peripheral neuropathies and renal osteodystrophy are features of the uremic syndrome not seen in ATN.

RECOVERY

- BUN/creatinine levels plateau then fall
- Urine output increases
- Hypercalcemia in the diuretic phase of recovery

PREVENTION

- Monitor creatinine in patients receiving nephrotoxic substances.
- Maintain adequate intravascular volumes in patients going to or recovering from surgical procedures.
- Maintain good cardiac output.

TREATMENT

Fever in the patient with acute renal failure:
- CXR, sputum, blood, and urine cultures
- Broad-spectrum empiric antibiotics
- Tailor therapy to culture results

- IV diuretic therapy is frequently used in the early stages of ATN to promote urine flow—there is little evidence that this prevents progression of ATN.
- Match fluid and salt intake to the daily outputs.
- Restrict dietary and intravenous potassium.
- Restrict dietary protein.

- 1,000 to 2,000 Kcal per day observing dietary restrictions
- Treat severe metabolic acidosis, but correct slowly to prevent hypocalcemic complications such as tetany.
- Treat infections aggressively.

Interstitial Nephritis

DEFINITION

Inflammation of the renal parenchyma

ETIOLOGY

- Systemic diseases: Sarcoidosis, Sjögren's syndrome, lymphoma
- Systemic infections: Syphilis, toxoplasma, CMV, EBV
- Medications: Beta-lactam antibiotics, diuretics, and NSAIDs

CLINICAL AND LAB FINDINGS

- Clinical and lab findings similar to ATN
- Drug-induced interstitial nephritis is associated with eosinophils in the urine as well as other signs of systemic hypersensitivity reaction.

TREATMENT

- Address underlying cause.
- Manage renal failure as for ATN.

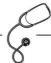

NSAIDs usually do not cause interstitial nephritis, but by inhibiting prostaglandin synthesis they decrease the GFR, which in a patient with underlying renal problems can precipitate renal failure.

Allergic interstitial nephritis is characterized by WBCs, eosinophils, and white cell casts in the urine. Treat with steroids.

CHRONIC RENAL FAILURE

Definition

Slowly progressing loss of renal function, usually over years

Etiology

- Diabetes mellitus: Diffuse glomerulosclerosis, nodular glomerulosclerosis (Kimmelstiel–Wilson lesions)
- Idiopathic failure
- Hypertension: Nephrosclerosis
- Chronic glomerulonephritis: Red blood cell casts
- Chronic tubulointerstitial diseases: Sodium wasting, no proteinuria, prolonged obstructive uropathies
- Polycystic kidney disease

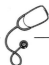

Renal biopsy should be performed before end-stage renal disease occurs because at that point the biopsy is unlikely to uncover a specific cause.

Pathophysiology

- Nephrons are lost and remaining healthy nephrons compensate by increasing their GFR. This process damages the healthy nephrons causing disease progression.
- Loss of renal endocrine function: Decreased synthesis of activated vitamin D, ammonia, and erythropoietin

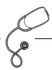

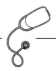

Creatinine is neither secreted nor reabsorbed by the nephron, it is only filtered. Therefore, the creatinine clearance is directly proportional to the GFR.

GFR and creatinine clearance:
For each doubling of the serum creatinine, the GFR has decreased by 50%.

Large kidneys are seen on sonogram in diabetes, amyloidosis, polycystic kidney disease.

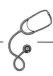

Any patient in renal failure needs special attention to the doses of medications cleared by the kidney.

Renal Function in CRF

- Usually asymptomatic until GFR less than 50% of baseline
- Water and sodium balance:
  - Initially: Decreased urine concentrating ability, easy dehydration, sodium wasting
  - Later: volume overload after the kidneys are unable to excrete dietary sodium
- Potassium: Once GFR becomes markedly diminished the ability to excrete dietary potassium is lost. The distal tubule compensates for the loss of excretory function until there is oliguria.
- Acid-base balance: When GFR < 50% of baseline the tubular excretion of H+ is impaired because renal production of ammonia is impaired, causing anion gap metabolic acidosis.
- Calcium and phosphate:
  - Hypocalcemia, hyperphosphatemia
  - Decreased activation of vitamin D due to loss of 1-hydroxylase activity
  - Secondary hyperparathyroidism
  - Severe bone resorption
  - Ectopic calcifications
- Serum creatinine increases (creatinine clearance decreases with decreased GFR).
- BUN increases, but to a lesser extent than the creatinine.

Signs and Symptoms

- Uremic syndrome, nephrotic syndrome (see individual sections)
- Ultrasound often reveals shrunken kidneys with cortical thinning.
- Rule out urinary tract infection (UTI) with urine culture.

Treatment

- At initial diagnosis, a 24-hour creatinine clearance should be obtained; from then on, the creatinine can be used to follow the GFR.
- Treat reversible causes.
- Diet: Modest protein restriction with near normal caloric intake decreases nitrogen intake and avoids catabolism.
- Fluids and electrolytes:
  - Sodium: Restrict, but sodium and water depletion should be avoided
  - Phosphate: Prevent hyperphosphatemia (minimize uremic osteodystrophy)—minimize dietary phosphate intake (dairy products), decreasing GI absorption (calcium carbonate, nonabsorbable aluminium antacids)
- Dialysis (see below)

DIALYSIS

Chronic hemodialysis (HD) is the mainstay of therapy for chronic renal failure, but chronic ambulatory peritoneal dialysis (CAPD) is also an alternative.

Absolute Indications for Dialysis
- Uremic pericarditis with or without cardiac tamponade
- Progressive motor neuropathy
- Intractable volume overload
- Life-threatening and intractable hyperkalemia or acidosis

Clinical Findings Responding to Dialysis (Relative Indications)
- Fluid and electrolyte imbalances
- Volume-dependent hypertension
- CNS abnormalities
- Anemia and bleeding diatheses
- Anorexia, nausea, and vomiting
- Glucose intolerance
- Weight loss
- Pruritus and ecchymoses

Patients on chronic medications (cardiac meds, warfarin, chemotherapy, etc.) dramatically drop their serum drug levels during dialysis. The timing and dosing of doses must be decided with the dialysis schedule in mind.

Hemodialysis

- The two most commonly used vascular access sites are arteriovenous fistulae (usually in the forearm) and artificial shunts inserted between an artery and a vein. Dialysis needles are placed directly into the shunt.
- Dialysis patients are frequently instrumented and combined with the dialysis patient's impaired immunity, infection is common. Subacute bacterial endocarditis may occur if the infections are not recognized early and treated correctly.
- Viral hepatitis is also a risk of hemodialysis because of the frequent necessity of transfusion.
- Psychologically, dialysis can be extremely burdensome.

Chronic Ambulatory Peritoneal Dialysis

- Permanent catheter is inserted into the peritoneum allowing dialysis to be undertaken by the patient outside the hospital.
- Approximately 2 L of dialysis fluid is infused rapidly and allowed to remain in the peritoneal cavity for 4 to 6 hours. The fluid is then drained and new fluid is immediately infused.
- Peritoneum acts as a dialysis membrane.
- Infusion of hypertonic glucose solution allows for concurrent volume reduction.
- Bacterial peritonitis is more common than with HD.
- Hypoalbuminemia, hypertriglyceridemia, and anemia are common.

Bacterial peritonitis: Fever and abdominal pain are the most common complaints. Treat with intraperitoneal vancomycin for 3 weeks or until culture and sensitivity data are available.

UREMIC SYNDROME

Definition

Uremia is a syndrome associated with chronic renal failure that affects multiple organ systems.

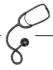

Signs and Symptoms

- Appearance: Pale complexion, wasting, purpura, excoriation
- Complaints: Pruritus, polydipsia, nausea, anorexia, vomiting
- Urinalysis: Isosthenuria, proteinuria, abnormal sediment with tubular casts

Etiology

- Unknown

Systemic Effects

- CNS: Foot drop, carpal tunnel syndrome, clonus, asterixis, seizures
- Cardiac and pulmonary:
  - Hypertension leading to left ventricular hypertrophy (LVH) and diastolic dysfunction
  - Accelerated atherosclerosis, development of ischemic heart disease
  - Pleuropericardial inflammation (pericarditis with effusion and tamponade)
  - Calcification of mitral and aortic valves
  - Pulmonary edema and pleural effusions
- Hematologic:
  - Normochromic, normocytic anemia due to decreased erythropoietin synthesis, among other reasons
  - Defective platelet function—prolonged bleeding time
  - White cell function and absolute counts are reduced, resulting in increased likelihood of infection.
- GI: Mild GI bleeding, nausea/vomiting, anorexia
- Metabolic: Elevated triglycerides, insulin resistance with impaired glucose tolerance is common.

NEPHROTIC SYNDROME

Definition

Glomerular lesion causing proteinuria > 3 g/day

Pathophysiology

- Loss of glomerular impermeability to plasma proteins
- Proteinuria
- Severe decrease in serum proteins, oncotic pressure
- Edema and serosal effusions
- Hypercholesterolemia also common

Common Causes of the Nephrotic Syndrome

- Minimal change disease (nil disease, lipoid nephrosis):
  - Usually idiopathic
  - Electron microscopy shows loss of epithelial foot processes
  - Usually responds to steroid therapy

- Recurs frequently
- Does not progress to chronic renal failure (unlike the other causes of nephrotic syndrome)
- Focal glomerulosclerosis:
    - Glomerular scarring involving limited number of glomeruli
    - Immunoglobulin and complement deposition detected by immunofluorescence
    - Most commonly seen in intravenous drug abusers and HIV patients
    - Leads to hypertension and chronic renal failure
    - Steroids usually not helpful
- Membranous glomerulonephritis:
    - Caused by immune complex deposition
    - Cause of nephritic syndrome in 50% of adult nephrotic syndrome
    - Idiopathic, or associated with SLE or hepatitis B
    - Treat with steroids and cytotoxic agents (chlorambucil)
    - Rule of thirds
- Systemic causes:
    - Sickle cell anemia (papillary damage due to sickling in hyperosmotic medullary interstitium)
    - Diabetic glomerulopathies (diffuse glomerulosclerosis, nodular glomerulosclerosis)
    - Multiple myeloma (Bence Jones proteinuria from immunoglobulin light chains or their breakdown products)

Rule of thirds for membranous glomerulonephritis: One third progress to CRF; one third have spontaneous remission; one third remain nephritic but do not progress.

GLOMERULONEPHRITIS

Definitions and Terminology

- Azotemia: Elevated BUN and creatinine
- Nephritic syndrome: Clinical definition involves abrupt-onset hematuria with RBC casts, mild proteinuria; often includes hypertension, edema, and azotemia
- Acute glomerulonephritis (AGN): Nephritic syndrome (synonym)

Poststreptococcal Glomerulonephritis (PSGN)

ETIOLOGY

Infection with nephritogenic strains of group A, beta-hemolytic streptococcus (usually associated preceding with pharyngitis or impetigo)

EPIDEMIOLOGY

- Incidence decreasing in United States and Europe
- In developing nations, large-scale streptococcal epidemics yield some form of PSGN in 5 to 10% of patients with pharyngitis and 25% with impetigo.

PATHOLOGY AND PATHOGENESIS

- Immune complex deposition with complement (IgG, C3, C4) in a granular pattern
- Complement-mediated inflammatory reaction leads to the glomerular damage.

SYMPTOMS AND SIGNS

- Most commonly asymptomatic hematuria
- More severe: Coca-Cola or smoky urine, hypertension, edema

COURSE

- Ten to 30% of adults and 1% of children with clinically apparent PSGN will develop rapidly progressive glomerulonephritis (RPGN).
- Most children regain normal renal function, but proteinuria and hematuria may continue for an extended period (months to years).

LABORATORY FINDINGS

RBC casts are pathognomonic of any glomerulonephritis.

- 24-hour urine protein usually between 0.5 and 2 g/day
- Urinary sediment: Predominantly RBC casts, WBC casts usually present also
- Anti-streptolysin-O (ASO): Ab positive within 1 to 2 weeks in post-pharyngitis PSGN
- Antihyaluronidase Ab more indicative of postpyodermal PSGN
- Hypocomplementemia of C3 and C4 during active disease, returning to normal within 6 weeks
- If the PSGN is membranoproliferative type, complement level will not return to normal.
- Azotemia after GFR begins to fall, GFR usually returns to normal within 1 to 3 months

PROGNOSIS IN PSGN

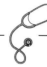

Antimicrobial therapy of the initial streptococcal infection does NOT prevent the onset of PSGN (as opposed to rheumatic fever).

- Prognosis is usually good in younger patients in whom initial renal damage is less severe.
- In severe cases with hypertension, hypertensive encephalopathy can occur.
- Of patients who develop RPGN, 20% will have persistent renal failure.
- The small percentage of patients that present with total anuria, severe hyperkalemia, and hypervolemia will die quickly unless dialysis is initiated.

TREATMENT

- Immunosuppressive drugs are ineffective and steroids may worsen the condition.
- Restrict dietary protein in presence of azotemia.
- Restrict sodium in presence of volume overload, edema, or severe hypertension.
- Treat hypertension aggressively.
- Severe renal failure may necessitate dialysis.

Other Diseases Associated with Acute Nephritic Syndrome

Glomerulonephritis can also occur after other bacterial infections, viral infections, and parasitic infections.

Primary Glomerular Diseases
- Membranoproliferative GN
- Mesangial proliferative GN
- IgA nephropathy

Secondary (Multisystem-Associated) Glomerular Diseases

- Collagen vascular disorders:
  - Polyarteritis nodosa
  - Systemic lupus erythematosus (SLE)
  - Wegener's granulomatosis
  - Henoch–Schönlein purpura (HSP)
- Hematologic disorders:
  - Thrombotic thrombocytopenic purpura (TTP), hemolytic–uremic syndrome
  - Serum sickness
- Glomerular basement membrane diseases:
  - Alport's syndrome
  - Goodpasture's syndrome
  - Thin basement membrane disease

Rapidly Progressive Glomerulonephritis

DEFINITION

- Also called crescentic GN
- Focal and segmental necrosis
- Epithelial cell proliferation (crescents) in most glomeruli
- Characterized by fulminant renal failure with proteinuria, hematuria, and RBC casts

ETIOLOGY, INCIDENCE, AND CLASSIFICATION

- Uncommon
- Pauci-immune RPGN:
  - 50% of RPGN
  - No immune complex or complement deposition
  - ANCA is serologic marker for pauci-immune RPGN associated with systemic vasculitis.
- Immune complex RPGN:
  - 40% of RPGN
  - Idiopathic
  - Can be associated with certain medications, syphilis, some malignancies
  - Usually concurrent systemic disease like SLE or HSP
- Anti-GBM Ab disease:
  - 10% of RPGN
  - Idiopathic
  - Major antigen is a component of type IV collagen.
  - Anti-GBM Ab present in blood—can be seen on GBM with immunofluorescent microscopy
  - Cytotoxic T-cells may contribute to the pathogenesis.

In 60 to 90% of patients, the anti-GBM Ab cross-react with pulmonary alveolar basement membranes.

SYMPTOMS AND SIGNS

- Insidious onset of weakness, fatigue, and low-grade fever
- Nausea, vomiting, and dizziness common
- Fifty percent have history of edema and influenza-like illness within 4 weeks of the onset of renal failure.

Laboratory Findings and Diagnosis

- Mild to severe azotemia
- Hematuria
- RBC casts
- Anemia and leukocytosis common
- Early renal biopsy imperative, as once end-stage renal failure develops, biopsy is rarely diagnostic.

Prognosis and Treatment

- Remission rare in idiopathic disease
- Eighty percent of untreated patients progress to end-stage renal disease within 6 months.
- Irreversible anuria is common.
- Without dialysis, death will ensue in a matter of weeks.
- RPGN due to SLE, polyarteritis nodosa, Wegener's granulomatosis, and PSGN have more favorable prognoses.
- Corticosteroid therapy may reduce serum creatinine levels and delay dialysis for > 3 years in pauci-immune or immune complex GN.
- ANCA-positive patients show some improvement with cyclophosphamide.
- If drug therapy is ineffective, plasmapheresis can delay disease progression.
- Once drug therapies and plasmapheresis have been exhausted and chronic renal failure has occurred, therapy becomes nonspecific and includes dialysis and consideration of renal transplant.
- Renal transplant is somewhat controversial in these diseases because the disease may reoccur in the transplanted organ.

Endocrinology

Thomas M. Boyd

DIABETES MELLITUS (DM)

INSULIN-DEPENDENT DM (IDDM)

Definition

Hyperglycemia resulting from autoimmune destruction of the insulin-producing β cells of the pancreas

Epidemiology

- Most commonly develops in younger patients. Usually diagnosed before age 30.
- Accounts for 10 to 15% of all DM cases

Etiology

- Eighty percent of IDDM patients have HLA phenotypes associated with anticytoplasmic antibodies directed toward pancreatic beta cells (islet cell antibodies) and to glutamic acid decarboxylase (GAD antibodies).
- Glucagon-secreting alpha cells are not involved
- Antibodies detected during the initial stages of the disease usually become undetectable after a few years.
- Environmental factors may also play a role in pathogenesis:
  - Viral infection (congenital rubella, mumps, coxsackie B viruses)
  - Exposure to cow's milk instead of human milk during infancy

Signs and Symptoms

- Usually presents with symptomatic hyperglycemia or diabetic ketoacidosis (discussed later)
- Polyuria
- Polydipsia

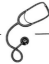

IDDM is also called:
- Juvenile onset DM
- Type I DM

HLA-DR3 and DR4 are the most common HLA genotypes in IDDM.

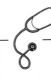

Typical scenario:
A woman presents with a recurrent vaginal candidiasis that is refractory to treatment. *Think: Diabetes mellitus.* Get a blood glucose.

- Weight loss
- Dehydration
- Blurred vision
- Fatigue
- Foot ulcers
- Can get restrictive cardiomyopathy without coronary artery disease

Diagnosis

- Confirmed with a fasting serum glucose of > 126 mg/dL
- Glycosuria (causes an osmotic diuresis that leads to the dehydration)
- HbA_1C is a measure of glucose control over the past 3 months. Most complications can be prevented if the HbA1c level is kept below 8%.

Treatment

- Mainstay of therapy is insulin (see Table 9-1 for types)
- Most IDDM patients require less than 50 units of insulin per day.

Initiating Therapy

- Patients are usually hospitalized at the time of initial diagnosis and are started on a sliding-scale insulin coverage with regular insulin.
- The average total daily dose of regular insulin is used as the initial dose of outpatient insulin therapy (be conservative so as not to induce hypoglycemic episodes).
- Use NPH or 70/30 preparations (not regular insulin alone).
- Divide the total daily dose to give two thirds before breakfast and one third before dinner.
- Initially, the patient should monitor finger stick glucose levels five times a day and keep a record of the levels:
    - Tighter blood glucose control can be obtained with diet and increase in insulin dose.
    - Some patients may be candidates for rapid-acting insulin analogs (Lispro) given right before meals or for continuous subcutaneous insulin infusion (CSII)
    - Choose the regimen that is easiest for the patient to follow while maintaining good blood glucose control.

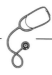

It is important for diabetics to have their feet frequently inspected to look for small cuts that may develop into ulcers. Due to neuropathy, diabetics can often have significant foot pathology and not feel anything.

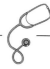

Diabetics have increased susceptibility to infections due to decreased efficacy of granulocytes despite normal number:

- Pseudomonas
- Mucormycoses
- Actinomycoses
- Aspergillosis (eosinophilic pneumonia with asthma; treat with steroids)
- Renal abscesses (with urinary tract infections)

IDDM patients must use insulin. They cannot use oral hypoglycemics because they have no functioning pancreatic β cells.

TABLE 9-1. Insulin Preparations

Preparation	Onset of Action	Peak Action	Duration
Regular insulin	30–60 min	2–4 hr	6–8 hr
Rapid-acting (Lispro)	15 min	30–90 min	2–4 hr
Intermediate-acting (NPH and Lente)	1–3 hr	6–12 hr	18–26 hr
Long-acting (Ultralente and PZI)	4–8 hr	14–24 hr	28–36 hr

Complications of All Diabetes (IDDM and NIDDM)

- Hypoglycemia
- Diabetic ketoacidosis (DKA)
- Nonketotic hyperosmolar coma
- Cataracts
- Retinopathy
- Stroke
- Renal insufficiency
- Charcot joint
- Extremity gangrene leading to amputation
- Neuropathy
- Silent myocardial infarctions (MIs)
- Infections

Dawn Phenomenon

An exaggeration of the normal tendency of the plasma glucose to rise in the early morning hours before breakfast, probably secondary to an increase in growth hormone secretion

Somogyi Effect

- Characterized by nighttime hypoglycemia followed by a dramatic increase in fasting glucose levels and increased plasma ketones
- If Somogyi phenomenon is suspected, patients should check their blood glucose around 3 A.M. Hypoglycemia at this time confirms diagnosis.
- The morning hyperglycemia is a rebound effect.
- Replacement of intermediate-acting insulin with long-acting insulin at bed time can prevent this effect (want to try to avoid peaking of insulin effect in the middle of the night).

NON–INSULIN-DEPENDENT DM (NIDDM)

Definition

Hyperglycemia due to insulin resistance

Epidemiology

- Accounts for 90% of diabetes cases in the United States
- Usually diagnosed in patients > 30 years old, but can occur in adolescents and children.
- Concordance rate for NIDDM in monozygotic twins is > 90% (< 50% in IDDM)
- Commonly associated with obesity, and often presents after period of weight gain

Measure finger-stick glucose levels 5x/day:
- Morning fasting
- Breakfast postprandial
- Lunch postprandial
- Dinner postprandial
- Before bed

Postprandial is 2 hours after the meal.

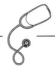

Typical scenario:
A patient presents with persistent morning hyperglycemia, despite steadily increasing his nighttime NPH insulin dose. He also complains of frequent nightmares. His wife brings him now because she witnessed him having a seizure in the middle of the night.
Think: Somogyi effect.

NIDDM is also called:
- Adult-onset DM
- Type II DM

Etiology

- Hyperglycemia is caused by:
  - Impaired secretion of insulin
  - Decreased insulin effectiveness at glucose uptake
  - Impaired inhibition of hepatic gluconeogenesis
- The syndrome of insulin resistance involves hyperglycemia leading to obesity, hypertension, hyperlipidemia, and coronary artery disease.
- Glucose toxicity: Hyperglycemia may cause further glucose intolerance because hyperglycemia decreases insulin sensitivity and increases hepatic glucose production.

Signs and Symptoms

- Patients may be asymptomatic
- Presenting compliant is often a complication of their diabetes, such as a soft tissue infection. Can also present with signs of hyperglycemia.
- Increased susceptibility to fungal infections (cell-mediated immunity is impaired by acute hyperglycemia).
- Patients with NIDDM will suffer from DKA only in rare instances.
- The nonketotic hyperglycemic–hyperosmolar coma (NKHC) is also a rare presenting situation.

DKA is a complication mostly associated with IDDM, while nonketotic hyperglycemic hyperosmolar coma (NKHC) is associated with NIDDM. However, either can occur with either type of DM.

Diagnosis

- Symptomatic patients with random glucose > 200 mg/dL
- Asymptomatic patients require a fasting glucose of > 126 mg/dL on two separate occasions.
- If patients have fasting glucose levels of > 110 mg/dL and < 126 mg/dL, an oral glucose tolerance test is indicated.
- Positive oral glucose tolerance test is a plasma glucose > 200 mg/dL at two hours (or at any time up to two hours) after ingesting 75 g of glucose in solution.

Treatment

- Initial management should consist of education, diet, and exercise to achieve weight control.
- Patient education increases compliance with diet, exercise, and medication therapy. Discussions should involve when to seek medical attention, side effects of medications, proper foot care, and symptoms of hyper- and hypoglycemia.
- If glycemic control cannot be obtained with diet and exercise, start oral hypoglycemic.
  - Combination of low-dose insulin secretogogues (Glyburide) plus low-dose insulin sensitizers (metformin) may improve HbA_{1c} with few side effects.
  - Patients not controlled with oral hypoglycemics alone may require insulin.

- Chlorpropamide: First-generation sulfonylurea.
- Glipizide, Glyburide: Second-generation sulfonylureas.
- Metformin (Glucophage): Most commonly prescribed oral hypoglycemic.

Glucose lowering drugs: See Table 9-2.

TABLE 9-2. Glucose-Lowering Drugs

Sulfonylureas	■ Examples: Chlorpropamide, tolbutamide, glyburide, glipizide ■ Mechanism: Increase postprandial insulin secretion from beta cells. ■ Major side effects: Hypoglycemia is the major side effect. First-generation drugs are bound to plasma protein and may displace other meds. Second-generation are not plasma protein bound and are preferred. Second-generation are also excreted by both the kidney and metabolized by the liver so they are safer in patients with renal insufficiency.
Biguanides	■ Example: Metformin ■ Mechanism: Sensitize skeletal muscle to insulin which promotes glucose uptake. Inhibits hepatic gluconeogenesis. These meds do not cause hypoglycemia. ■ Major side effects: GI side effects. Renally excreted so should not be used in patients with compromised renal function (creatinine > 1.5). Cannot be given within 24–48 hours of injection of radiographic contrast material. Lactic acidosis.
Thiazolidinediones	■ Examples: Troglitazone, rosiglitazone ■ Mechanism: Reduces insulin resistance. Useful addition to insulin therapy in NIDDM patients who need > 30 units of insulin/day. ■ Major side effects: Hepatotoxicity
Alpha-glucosidase inhibitors	■ Example: Acarbose ■ Mechanism: Competitively inhibits monosaccharide and oligosaccharide hydrolysis in the small intestine, thereby decreasing carbohydrate absorption. ■ Major side effects: Transient diarrhea and nausea; abdominal pain

DIABETIC KETOACIDOSIS

Definition

Metabolic acidosis due to ketoacid accumulation due to severely depressed insulin levels

Epidemiology

- Common presenting syndrome in IDDM
- Mostly occurs in IDDM, but can also occur in NIDDM (especially in blacks)

Etiology

- Severe insulin deficiency causes the body to switch from metabolizing carbohydrates to metabolizing and oxidizing lipids.
- Usually precipitated by lapse in insulin treatment, acute infection, or major trauma.

Pathophysiology

- Insulin deficiency causes hyperglycemia, which induces an osmotic diuresis.
- Profound dehydration, sodium loss, and potassium loss occurs.
- Ketosis occurs because of the loss of inhibition of free-fatty acid oxidation in the liver.

DKA is a life-threatening condition and must be recognized early and treated correctly.

Beta-hydroxybuteric acid and acetoacetic acid are the ketones that are produced.

- Metabolic acidosis ketosis results in respiratory compensation.
- Acetone is produced from spontaneous decarboxylation of acetoacetic acid. The acetone is disposed of by respiration and its odor is present on the patient's breath (fruity odor).
- Plasma ratio of beta-hydroxybuteric acid to acetoacetic acid is usually around 3:1 in DKA but can reach levels of 8:1.

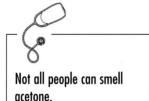

Not all people can smell acetone.

Signs and Symptoms

- Polyuria, nausea, vomiting
- Lethargy and fatigue are later components.
- May progress to coma
- Signs of dehydration are present and patients may be hypotensive and tachycardic.
- Kussmaul respirations (slow deep breaths) may be present.
- Acetone (fruity) odor may be present on the patient's breath.

Diagnosis

- Hyperglycemia
- Hyperketonemia
- Anion gap metabolic acidosis (ketones are unmeasured ions)
- Usually, the diagnosis can be presumed at the bedside if patient's urine is strongly positive for ketones and the finger-stick glucose is high.
- Glucose is usually between 400 and 800 mg/dL.
- Initially, potassium is high due to acidosis, but drops with treatment.
- BUN may be increased because of prerenal azotemia.

Treatment

- Goals of treatment are to remove ketones and correct the acidosis.
- Aggressive fluid resuscitation to correct volume deficit
- Correct hyperglycemia with insulin.
- Prevent hypokalemia during treatment with judicious potassium administration.
- Correct underlying causes (e.g., infection).
- Bicarbonate may be used to correct severe acidosis.
- When serum glucose is reduced to 250 to 300 mg/dL, add 5% glucose to the IV fluids to reduce the risk of hypoglycemia.
- Insulin is required in DKA even after blood glucose returns to normal range. Continue to give insulin and glucose-containing IV fluids.
- Admission to intensive care unit (ICU)

Prognosis

Mortality rate is approximately 10%:
- Hypotension or coma present at admission are negative prognostic indicators.
- Major causes of death are circulatory failure, hypokalemia, and infection.

Definition

A complication of NIDDM characterized by hyperglycemia and altered mental status. Carries a 50% mortality.

Pathophysiology

- Patients usually have a period of symptomatic hyperglycemia before the syndrome develops.
- When fluid intake becomes insufficient, extreme dehydration ensues because of the hyperglycemia-induced osmotic diuresis.

Etiology

- Sepsis
- Dehydration
- Diuretics
- Glucocorticoids

Signs and Symptoms

- Altered mental status
- Signs of profound dehydration
- Seizures and transient hemiplegia may occur.

Diagnosis

- Serum glucose levels are usually > 1,000 mg/dL (much higher than in DKA).
- Serum osmolarity is usually around 385 mOsm/kg.
- Blood urea nitrogen (BUN)/creatinine levels are markedly increased from prerenal azotemia.

Treatment

Goal of treatment is to expand the intravascular volume to stabilize vital signs and improve circulation and urine output:
- Infuse 2 to 3 L of normal saline over 1 to 2 hours.
- Once vital signs have stabilized change fluid to D_5 ½ NS and monitor vital signs, urine output, serum electrolytes, and BUN/creatinine carefully.
- Begin potassium replacement with the initial infusion of D_5 ½ NS.
- Withhold insulin therapy for 30 to 60 minutes, because it drives glucose into the cells, exacerbating volume depletion.
- Monitor patient for signs and symptoms of cerebral edema, which may occur if the osmolarity is corrected too quickly.

NKHC most commonly occurs in patients unable to affect their own environment, e.g., nursing home residents.

HIGH-YIELD FACTS

Endocrinology

If insulin is deemed necessary in the initial resuscitation, 5% glucose should be added to the infusion to prevent hypoglycemia when the serum glucose reaches 250 mg/dL.

Whipple's triad of hypoglycemia:
1. Plasma glucose < 60 mg/dL
2. Symptoms of hypoglycemia
3. Improvement of the symptoms with administration of glucose

Hypoglycemia is the most common cause of altered mental status in most health care environments.

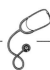

Hypoglycemia due to oral hypoglycemic agents lasts about 24 hours. Patients with sulfonylurea overdose should be admitted to the hospital for 24 hours, for monitoring and continuous glucose administration.

Definition

Abnormally low serum glucose level that causes altered mental status and sympathetic stimulation.

Etiology

- Drug-induced (most common cause): Insulin, alcohol, sulfonylureas
- Islet cell carcinoma/adenoma
- Autoimmune hypoglycemia in nondiabetics
- Insulin receptor antibodies
- Severe liver or renal disease
- Endotoxic shock
- Hypopituitarism with deficiency of both growth hormone and cortisol

Pathophysiology

- Glucose transport across the blood–brain barrier is regulated by adrenergic nervous system activity (resulting in increased growth hormone and cortisol secretion and decreased insulin secretion.)
- Glucagon is secreted by the pancreatic alpha cells and increases plasma glucose levels and stimulates gluconeogenesis in the liver.
- The adrenergic outflow causes the typical sympathetic stimulatory symptoms of hypoglycemia and the lack of glucose to the brain results in altered mental status.

Signs and Symptoms

- History of insulin or sulfonylurea treatment
- Adrenergic symptoms: Diaphoresis, anxiety, tremor, faintness, palpitations, and hunger
- CNS manifestations: Confusion, inappropriate behavior (sometimes mistaken for alcohol intoxication), visual problems, stupor, and coma.

Diagnosis

- Abnormally low serum glucose is < 50 mg/dL.

Treatment

- Once hypoglycemia is confirmed or if serum glucose level is not immediately available, obtain IV access and administer one ampule of 50% dextrose.

- Whenever dextrose is administered for hypoglycemia, and alcoholism or nutritional deficiency is suspected, administer thiamine prior to glucose to prevent Wernicke's encephalopathy.
- If there is not rapid improvement in mental status, repeat D_{50} administration.
- Once mental status has improved, infuse 10% dextrose solution and titrate to maintain a serum glucose level of > 100 mg/dL.
- Finger-stick glucose levels should be obtained every 30 minutes for 2 hours to detect possible rebound hypoglycemia.
- If hypoglycemia is refractory to glucose administration and is associated with signs of adrenal insufficiency, administer hydrocortisone 100 to 200 mg IV.

PITUITARY TUMORS

- Anterior pituitary (adenohypophysis): derivative of Rathke's pouch
- Posterior pituitary (neurohypophysis): composed of hypothalamic neuronal axon terminals, storage and release site for hormones produced by these neurons
- For specific hormones, see Table 9-3.

TABLE 9-3. Pituitary Hormones and Their Functions

Anterior Lobe	Main Stimulatory Actions	Hypothalamic Stimulus
Adrenocorticotropic hormone (ACTH, corticotropin)	- Growth and secretion of adrenal cortex to make cortisol and sex hormones	CRH
Growth hormone (GH, somatotropin)	- Secretion of somatomedin C (insulinlike growth factor) - Body growth	GRH
Thyroid stimulating hormone (TSH, thyrotropin)	- Growth of thyroid gland - Production of T_3 and T_4	TRH
Follicle stimulating hormone (FSH)	- Spermatogenesis in the male - Ovarian follicle growth in the female	GnRH
Luteinizing hormone (LH)	- Testosterone secretion in the male - Ovulation in the female	GnRH
Prolactin	- Milk production - Maternal behavior	PRH (stimulates) Dopamine (inhibits)
Melanocyte stimulating hormone (MSH)	- Skin pigmentation	
Posterior Lobe		**Releasing Stimulus**
Antidiuretic hormone (ADH, vasopressin, AVP)	- Retains sodium and water, producing concentrated urine	Osmoreceptors
Oxytocin	- Milk letdown - Contractions of labor	Touch receptors in uterus, genitalia, and breast

Pathology

- Constitute ~10% of intracranial tumors
- Most are benign, slow growing
- Anterior pituitary: Craniopharyngiomas, adenomas
- Posterior pituitary: No primary tumors
- Metastases and meningiomas are occasionally seen
- Pathology arises from:
    - Excess hormone production
    - Compression of suprasellar structures
    - Destruction of normal pituitary parenchyma
    - Compression of pituitary stalk

Adenomas

- Somatotroph tumors produce growth hormone (GH).
- Corticotroph tumors produce adrenocorticotropic hormone (ACTH).
- Lactotroph tumors produce prolactin.
- Thyrotroph tumors produce thyroid-stimulating hormone (TSH); they are rare.
- Luteinizing hormone (LH) and follicle-stimulating hormone (FSH) producing adenomas occur, but do not cause well-defined clinical syndromes.
- Pituitary microadenomas (< 10 mm) are found in ~15% of asymptomatic women by MRI; in the absence of progression (assessed by f/u MRI), they are clinically insignificant.

Craniopharyngiomas

- Arise from embryologic remnants of Rathke's pouch
- Most common tumors of suprasellar region in children
- Solid or cystic
- Usually calcified

Neurologic Symptoms

- Headache
- Compression of optic chiasm:
    - Superior bitemporal quadrantanopia: Early visual defect, since compression begins on inferior surface of chiasm
    - Bitemporal hemianopia ("tunnel vision"): Classic finding, occurs when tumor has reached significant size
- Signs of increased intracranial pressure (ICP) are rare as tumors are usually diagnosed before they reach the requisite dimensions

Diagnosis

- X-ray: May show enlargement of sella; craniopharyngiomas may show calcifications in suprasellar regions
- Computed tomography (CT): More sensitive than x-ray

- MRI: More sensitive than CT, can detect microadenomas; use with gadolinium contrast
- Hormone studies: Detect excesses or deficiencies, give information about type of tumor; useful when tumor cannot be detected radiographically

Treatment

- Surgery: Indicated whenever there are neurologic symptoms
- Radiotherapy: Can reduce size of tumor without surgery, sometimes used as surgical adjunct
- Hormone replacement for hypopituitarism
- Bromocriptine may be useful for lactotroph tumors (prolactinomas)

HYPOPITUITARISM

Etiology

- Tumors causing dysfunction either by invasion, replacement, or compression affecting:
  - Normal pituitary parenchyma
  - Pituitary stalk
  - Hypothalamic parenchyma
- Surgical destruction of pituitary or hypothalamus: Either therapeutic or as a casualty of an unrelated neurosurgical procedure
- Sheehan's syndrome: Pituitary gland enlarges during pregnancy due to hyperplasia of lactotrophs without commensurate increase in blood supply; if hypotension occurs during childbirth, pituitary infarction can result
- Systemic (rare): Hemochromatosis, sarcoid
- Infectious (rare): Tuberculosis (TB), neurosyphilis

Signs and Symptoms

- ACTH deficiency: See section on adrenal insufficiency
- GH deficiency: Growth retardation in children
- Prolactin:
  - Deficiency: Failure to lactate after childbirth
  - Excess: Amenorrhea and galactorrhea in women, decreased libido and gynecomastia in men
- TSH deficiency: See section on hypothyroidism
- LH and FSH deficiency: Amenorrhea and genital atrophy in women, decreased libido in men
- In slow-growing tumors, GH, FSH, and LH levels are affected early; ACTH and prolactin levels decline only with advanced disease.
- Antidiuretic hormone (ADH) deficiency known as diabetes insipidus (discussed in separate section below).

Typical scenario:
A 29-year-old woman presents with inability to lactate after childbirth. Delivery was complicated by blood loss and hypotension. *Think: Sheehan's syndrome.*

Typical scenario:
A 36-year-old woman complains of amenorrhea for 1 year, increasingly bad headaches, clumsiness, and sporadic nipple discharge; beta-HCG levels are normal. *Think: Prolactinoma.*

Drugs that inhibit dopamine activity also cause hyperprolactinemia: TCAs, prochlorperazine, haloperidol, methyldopa, metoclopramide, cimetidine.

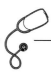

Unlike other pituitary hormones prolactin secretion is controlled by **inhibitory** hypothalamic input. Destruction of the pituitary stalk or hypothalamus results in release from dopaminergic inhibition causing lactotroph hyperplasia. This results in hyperprolactinemia in the setting of hypopituitarism.

Diagnosis

- Pituitary hormone levels must be considered with other factors:
    - ACTH levels must be taken with serum cortisol levels, if cortisol is normal or high ACTH is probably low due to feedback inhibition. Insulin-induced hypoglycemia stimulates ACTH secretion and is an effective test of the entire hypothalamic–pituitary–adrenal axis. Test is administered similarly to GH provocation described below.
    - Prolactin levels are normally elevated in the third trimester and in breast-feeding mothers.
    - GH levels cycle daily, peaking in the evening, and decline to minimal levels by age 30. Evaluation requires stimulation testing: Insulin or levodopa stimulate a burst in serum GH, serum levels are drawn at 30, 60, and 90 minutes post-stimulus and compared to normal values.
    - TSH must be taken with serum T_3 and T_4; if they are normal or high, TSH is probably low due to feedback inhibition.
    - In women, LH and FSH levels vary with the menstrual cycle so the timing of the levels is important; postmenopausal women have high LH and FSH levels normally.
    - ADH levels normally vary according to plasma osmolality; testing is discussed in section on diabetes insipidus.
- Evaluation of target organ function is usually required: Tests include imaging studies, hormone levels, and response to exogenous pituitary hormones

Treatment

- Address underlying cause: Tumor, infection, systemic disease
- Hormone replacement:
    - Cortisol for ACTH deficiency
    - Prolactin:
        - No treatment for deficiency
        - Bromocriptine (dopamine agonist), surgery, or radiation for excess
- GH for GH deficiency in children
- Thyroxine for TSH deficiency
- FSH and LH deficiency can be treated with estrogen/progesterone replacements in women (fertility is usually not restored) and testosterone replacements in men.
- dDAVP for ADH deficiency

Psychogenic polydipsia:
Psychiatric disorder of compulsive water drinking most common in young to middle-aged women. Presents with polyuria and dilute urine, distinguished from DI by low plasma osmolality.

DIABETES INSIPIDUS (DI)

Definitions

- Central DI: Inadequate pituitary secretion of ADH
- Nephrogenic DI: Lack of renal response to ADH

Etiology

Central DI
- Idiopathic: Accounts for 50% of cases

- Posterior pituitary or hypothalamic damage (tumor, trauma, neuro-surgery)
- Systemic: Sarcoidosis, neurosyphilis, encephalitis

Nephrogenic DI
- Familial
- Chronic renal disease
- Sickle cell anemia (renal papillary necrosis)
- Hypokalemia
- Hypercalcemia
- Drugs: Lithium, demeclocycline, methoxyflurane

Signs and Symptoms

- Polyuria (3 to 15 L/day)
- Thirst
- Dilute urine (specific gravity < 1.005)

Diagnosis

- High plasma osmolality (280 to 310) due to incomplete compensation for the inability to resorb free water
- Water deprivation followed by exogenous ADH:
  - Central DI: Low urine osm → high urine osm
  - Nephrogenic DI: Low urine osm → low urine osm
  - Normal: High urine osm → high urine osm
- Infusion of hypertonic saline normally results in a sharp decrease in urine output; patients with DI do respond.

Treatment

- Desmopressin (dDAVP): Analog of ADH, useful in central DI
- Thiazide diuretics: Paradoxically decrease urine output in patients with DI by increasing sodium and water resorption in the proximal tubule. They are the only therapy useful in nephrogenic DI.
- Chlorpropamide: Oral hypoglycemic with side effect of potentiating secretion and action of endogenous ADH. Partial function must exist for this therapy to be of use.

SYNDROME OF INAPPROPRIATE ANTIDIURETIC HORMONE SECRETION (SIADH)

Definition

Excess production of ADH

Etiology

- Idiopathic overproduction via the hypothalamic-posterior pituitary axis: often associated with disorders of the CNS (encephalitis, stroke, head trauma) and pulmonary disease (TB, pneumonia)

Other causes of excess ADH secretion:
- Adrenal failure
- Renal failure
- Edema
- Fluid loss

- Ectopic production by malignant tumors, particularly small cell lung cancer and pancreatic carcinoma
- Pharmacologic stimulation of the hypothalamic–pituitary axis: Carbamazepine, chlorpropamide, clofibrate, vincristine

Signs and Symptoms

Attributable to hyponatremia—see chapter on Fluid and Electrolytes

Diagnosis

- Hyponatremia
- Low serum osmolality
- High urinary sodium
- Osmolality of urine > serum

Treatment

- Fluid restriction
- Hypertonic saline in severe hyponatremia
- Demeclocycline: Has side effect of decreasing collecting duct response to ADH

ACROMEGALY

Definition

Disorder marked by progressive enlargement of peripheral body parts resulting from excess pituitary GH production.

Etiology

Pituitary somatotroph adenoma

Signs and Symptoms

- Progressive enlargement of peripheral body parts, particularly head, hands, and feet
- Decreased glucose tolerance due to the anti-insulin actions of GH
- Hyperphosphatemia due to GH's influence on tubular resorption of phosphate
- Gigantism in children due to excess linear growth

Diagnosis

- Serum GH levels: Should be measured in the morning while still in bed as GH levels are raised by stress and exercise; may still be normal.
- Lack of GH suppression by glucose load.
- Serum IGF-I levels: Insulin-like growth factor-I is made by the liver under stimulation by GH, elevated in acromegalics

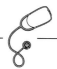

Acromegaly: The changes in a patient's appearance occur over many years, and may not be apparent to the patient or his family. Old photos may suggest the diagnosis.

Treatment

- Adenectomy
- Radiotherapy
- Octreotide: GH analog that has no GH effects, but suppresses GH levels in acromegalics

Definition

Increased synthesis and secretion of free thyroid hormones resulting in hypermetabolism

Epidemiology

- Ten times more common in women than in men
- Annual incidence is 1 in 1,000 women.

Etiology

- Graves' disease (most common cause, 80% of cases in the United States)
- Toxic multinodular goiter
- Toxic adenoma (Plummer's disease)
- Iatrogenic (lithium therapy), inadvertent toxic ingestion, or factitious (thyrotoxicosis factitia)
- Transient hyperthyroidism (subacute thyroiditis)

Pathophysiology

High levels of free thyroid hormones increase levels of cellular metabolism and cause multiple effects, resulting in a general state of hypermetabolism.

Signs and Symptoms

- Heat intolerance
- Palpitations (hyperthyroidism is a common cause of atrial fibrillation)
- Weight loss
- Sweating
- Tremor
- Nervousness and anxiety
- Weakness and fatigue
- Hyperdefacation

Diagnosis

Measure TSH, free T_4, and free T_3 (if the T_4 level is normal) (see Table 9-4)

TABLE 9-4. Laboratory Evaluation of Thyroid Function

Thyroid state	T_4	FT_{4I}	T_3	FT_{3I}	TSH	TRH
Hypothyroidism						
1°	↓	↓	↓	↓	↑	↑
2°	↓	↓	↓	↓	↓/N	↓
3°	↓	↓	↓	↓	↓/N	N
Peripheral unresponsiveness	↑/N	↑/N	↑/N	↑	↓/N	↑/N
Hyperthyroidism						
Pituitary tumor (secretes TSH)	↑	↑	↑	↑	↑	↓
Graves' disease	↑	↑	↑	↑	↓	↓
T_3 thyrotoxicosis	N	N	↑	↑	↓	↓
T_4 thyrotoxicosis	↑	↑	N	N	↓	↓
Toxic nodular goiter	↑	↑	↑	↑	↓	↓

Treatment

Depends on underlying disorder

THYROID STORM

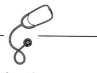

Thyroid storm is a medical emergency.

Definition

Exaggerated manifestation of hyperthyroidism

Epidemiology

Mortality is high (20 to 50%) even with the correct treatment.

Etiology

- Infection
- Trauma and major surgical procedures
- DKA
- MI, cerebrovascular accident (CVA), pulmonary embolism (PE)
- Withdrawal of antihyperthyroid medications, iodine administration, thyroid hormone ingestion
- Idiopathic

Signs and Symptoms

Overactivated sympathetic nervous system causes most of the signs and symptoms of this syndrome:
- Fever > 101°
- Tachycardia (out of proportion to fever)

- High-output congestive heart failure (CHF) and volume depletion
- Exhaustion
- GI manifestations: Diarrhea, abdominal pain
- Continuum of CNS alterations (from agitation to confusion when moderate, to stupor or coma with or without seizures when most severe)
- Jaundice is a late and ominous manifestation.

Diagnosis

- This is a clinical diagnosis, and since most patients present in need of emergent stabilization, treatment is initiated empirically.
- Patients may have improperly treated hyperthyroidism.
- May also occur in the setting of unintentional or intentional toxic ingestion of synthetic thyroid hormone in the hypothyroid patient.

Treatment

- Primary stabilization:
  - Airway protection
  - Oxygenation
  - Assess circulation (pulse/BP) and continuous cardiac monitoring
  - IV hydration
- Beta-blocker therapy (e.g., propranolol) to block adrenergic effects
- Treat fever with acetaminophen (not aspirin, which displaces T_4 from thyroid binding protein).
- Propylthiouracil (PTU) or methimazole to block synthesis of new thyroid hormone
- Iodine to decrease release of preformed thyroid hormone. Do not give iodine until the PTU has taken effect (1.5 hours) because more thyroid hormone will be produced.
- Treat any possible precipitating factors that may be present.

In initial stabilization of thyroid storm, cooling blankets can be applied to treat hyperpyrexia, if present.

Never send any thyroid storm patient for a procedure involving iodine contrast before giving PTU.

GRAVES' DISEASE

Definition

Autoimmune disease causing hyperthyroidism due to antibody, which stimulates TSH receptor

Graves' disease is the most common cause of hyperthyroidism.

Pathophysiology

- Antibody is produced that interacts with the receptor for TSH resulting in continuous excess secretion.
- Cause of the exophthalmos (infiltrative opthalmopathy) in Graves' is unknown, but is thought to be due to immunoglobulins that interact with self-antigens in the extraocular muscles and on orbital fibroblasts. These antibodies are not the same antibodies as those interacting with the TSH receptor.

Graves' (and Hashimoto's thyroiditis) are sometimes associated with other autoimmune diseases (Type I diabetes mellitus, vitiligo, myasthenia, pernicious anemia, collagen diseases).

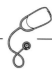

Signs and Symptoms

- Diffusely enlarged thyroid
- Exophthalmos
- Pretibial myxedema
- Tachycardia
- Palpitations
- In elderly patients the presentation is less classic. Apathy can be present without the common hyperactivity signs (apathetic hyperthyroidism). Cardiovascular features may be prominent and hyperthyroidism may not be suspected initially.

Diagnosis

- High radioactive iodine uptake on a radionuclide scan. (If uptake is present but low, then diagnosis is thyroiditis or factitious hyperthyroidism.)
- Elevated free thyroid hormones (T_3, T_4)
- Undetectable TSH levels
- High thyroglobulin level

Treatment

Long-Term Antithyroid Therapy
- Usually accomplished with propylthiouracil (PTU)
- Methimazole is as effective as PTU when administered at one tenth of the PTU dosage.
- PTU has the advantage of inhibiting the peripheral conversion of T_4 to T_3, thus there is usually a more rapid symptomatic improvement.
- Twelve- to 24-month course is usually used and one third to one half of patients remain well indefinitely.
- *Complications:* Leukopenia (check CBC before initiating therapy). Stop medication if absolute PMN drops below 1,500 cells/μL. If patient develops fever or sore throat, he or she should be instructed to return.

Radioactive Iodine Ablation Therapy (Preferred Treatment)
- Can produce the same effects as surgery without the surgical complications
- Tends to produce hypothyroidism over time. Forty to 70% for patients will develop hypothyroidism within 10 years of therapy.
- Some prefer to reserve radioactive iodine ablation therapy for patients over 30 years of age because of a higher incidence of hypothyroidism in younger patients.
- *Complications:* Radiation thyroiditis commonly appears within 7 to 10 days after therapy and is associated with accelerated release of thyroid hormone into the blood. Rarely, this results in thyrotoxic crisis.

Adrenergic Agonists
- Propranolol is the agent of choice.
- Should be used only as adjunctive therapy because it does not treat the underlying problem.

Subtotal Thyroidectomy
- Still used for younger patients or when ablation therapy is unsuccessful

- Prior to surgery, patients should be euthyroid (pre-treated with PTU); then give iodine to cause involution of thyroid gland.
- Immediate complications include hemorrhage, which can result in airway compromise.
- Delayed complications include hypoparathyroidism (can be life threatening) and hypothyroidism.

HYPOTHYROIDISM

Definition

- TSH levels greater than twice the upper limit of normal in primary hypothyroidism
- Can be clinically evident hypothyroidism with classic physical findings or subclinical hypothyroidism detectable only upon laboratory analysis

Epidemiology

- Clinically evident hypothyroidism occurs in 1.5 to 2% of women and in 0.2% of men.
- The incidence increases with age, usually between 40 and 60.
- In people over age 60, 6% of women and 2.5% of men have TSH levels greater than twice the upper limit of normal.

Etiology

Primary Hypothyroidism (Thyroid Gland Dysfunction)
- Hashimoto's thyroiditis
- Previous treatment for hyperthyroidism
- Subacute thyroiditis
- Radiation therapy to the neck (for other malignancy)
- Iodine deficiency or excess
- Medications (lithium is the most common)
- Prolonged treatment with iodine containing substances

Hashimoto's thyroiditis (chronic lymphocytic thyroiditis) is the most common cause of hypothyroidism in patients older than eight years of age.

Secondary Hypothyroidism (Pituitary Dysfunction)
- Postpartum necrosis (Sheehan's syndrome)
- Space-occupying pituitary neoplasm
- Infiltrating disease (TB) causing TSH deficiency

Tertiary Hypothyroidism (Deficiency in TRH [Thyroid-Releasing Hormone] Secretion)
- Granuloma
- Neoplasm
- Hypothalamic radiation

Signs and Symptoms

- Fatigue, lethargy, weakness
- Constipation, weight gain (usually > 15 pounds)
- Muscle weakness, cramps, arthralgias

Muscle weakness and cramps occur in both hyper- and hypothyroidism. In hyperthyroidism, CPK will be normal. In hypothyroidism, it will be elevated.

- Cold intolerance
- Slow speech with hoarse voice (from myxedematous changes in vocal cords)
- Slow thinking with poor memory
- Skin: Dry, coarse, thick, and cool; nonpitting edema of the skin and eyelids
- Hair: Brittle and coarse; loss of outer one-third of eyebrows
- Thyroid gland: May or may not be palpable (depending on the etiology of the hypothyroidism)
- Heart: Distant heart sounds may be present if pericardial effusion is present. Bradycardia may occur.
- Neurologic: **Delayed relaxation phase of deep tendon reflexes** (very specific). Cerebellar ataxia can be present. Peripheral neuropathies with paresthesias; carpal tunnel syndrome.
- Musculoskeletal: Muscular stiffness and weakness

Consider evaluating thyroid function tests in any patient with hypercholesterolemia.

Diagnosis

- See Table 9-4 for results of thyroid tests.
- Serum cholesterol, triglycerides may be elevated.
- LDH, AST, ALT, and the MM fraction of CPK may be elevated.
- Hematocrit and hemoglobin may be decreased.
- Hyponatremia may be present.
- Hashimoto's thyroiditis: May show increased antithyroglobulin and antimicrosomal antibody titers.

The TRH stimulation test is useful in distinguishing secondary from tertiary hypothyroidism.

Treatment

Therapy
- Start therapy with low-dose levothyroxine and increase dose every 6 to 8 weeks, depending on the patient's response (start low, go slow).
- Elderly patients and patients with coronary artery disease should be started on a low dose of levothyroxine because high doses may precipitate angina pectoris.

Monitoring Therapy
- In 1° hypothyroidism, it is adequate to measure the TSH level, which should fall well within the normal range.
- In 2° hypothyroidism, measure the T_4 level, which should fall well within the normal range.

SUBCLINICAL HYPOTHYROIDISM

Definition

Elevated TSH level with normal thyroid hormone levels in the absence of overt clinical symptoms

Clinical Course

This is not usually a precursor to 1° hypothyroidism. There are usually two distinct patterns:

- Patients who will eventually develop 1° hypothyroidism: Women who have both elevated TSH and detectable antithyroid antibodies have a 5% annual incidence of overt hypothyroidism. Patients over age 65 with this combination will usually develop clinical hypothyroidism within 4 years.
- Euthyroidism with reset thyrostat: Permanent state without definitive progression to 1° hypothyroidism. Probably due to subtle damage to the thyroid gland from another cause.

Treatment

Replacement therapy:

- All patients with TSH > 10
- Patients with TSH > 5 and goiter or antithyroid Ab
- All patients with a history of iodine therapy

MYXEDEMA COMA

Definition

Life-threatening complication of hypothyroidism with profound lethargy or coma usually accompanied by hypothermia. Mortality is 20 to 50% even if treated early.

Etiology

- Sepsis
- Prolonged exposure to cold weather
- CNS depressants (sedatives, narcotics)
- Trauma or surgery

Signs and Symptoms

- Profound lethargy or coma is obvious.
- Hypothermia: Rectal T < 35°C (95°F)
- Bradycardia or circulatory collapse
- Delayed relaxation phase of DTRs, areflexia if severe (this can be a very important clue).

Diagnosis

Lab tests for the patient presenting with profound altered mental status:

- CBC with differential
- Blood and urine cultures
- Serum electrolytes
- BUN and creatinine
- Blood glucose

Hypothermia
is often missed by tympanic thermometers. Use a rectal probe if hypothermia is suspected.

Differential diagnosis of myxedema coma:
- Severe depression or primary psychosis
- Drug overdose or toxic exposure
- CVA
- Liver failure
- Hypoglycemia
- CO_2 narcosis
- CNS infection

- Urine toxicology screen
- Serum transaminases and LDH
- Arterial blood gas (ABG) to rule out hypoxemia and CO_2 retention
- Cortisol level
- Carboxyhemoglobin
- Chest radiograph
- Brain CT

Treatment

- Airway management with mechanical ventilation if necessary.
- Prevent further heat loss.
- Monitor patient in intensive care unit.
- Pharmacologic therapy:
  - Intravenous levothyroxine
  - Glucocorticoids (until coexisting adrenal insufficiency is excluded)
  - IV hydration (D_5 ½ NS)
  - Rule out and treat any precipitating causes (antibiotics for suspected infection).

THYROIDITIS

Definition

- Inflammation of the thyroid
- Can be divided into three common types (Hashimoto's, subacute, and silent), and two rarer forms (suppurative and Riedel's)

Etiology

- Hashimoto's thyroiditis: Autoimmune disorder that involves CD_4 lymphocyte-mediated destruction of the thyroid. The lymphocytes are specific for thyroid antigens. Cause for activation of these cells is unknown.
- Subacute thyroiditis: Possibly a postviral condition because it usually follows a viral URI. Not considered an autoimmune reaction.
- Silent thyroiditis: Usually occurs postpartum and is thought to be autoimmune mediated
- Suppurative thyroiditis: Usually, a bacterial infection, but fungi and parasites have also been implicated in some cases. Commonly seen in HIV+ patients with PCP.
- Riedel's thyroiditis: Also called fibrous thyroiditis, fibrous infiltration of the thyroid of unknown etiology.

Signs and Symptoms

- Hashimoto's: There may be signs of hyper- or hypothyroidism depending on the stage. Usually, there is diffuse, firm enlargement of the gland, but it may be of normal size if the disease has progressed.

The thyroid in Hashimoto's is nontender, which distinguishes it from other forms of thyroiditis.

Typical scenario:
A 35-year-old man with a history of hyperthyroidism and a recent flu presents with neck pain and an elevated ESR. *Think: Subacute thyroiditis.*

- Subacute: Tender, enlarged gland. Fever, and signs of hyperthyroidism are initially present. Hypothyroidism may develop.
- Silent: Similar to subacute except there is no tenderness of the gland (painless thyroiditis).
- Suppurative: Fever with severe neck pain. Focal tenderness of involved portion of the gland.
- Riedel's: Slowly enlarging rock-hard mass in the anterior neck. Tight, stiff neck. Must differentiate from thyroid CA. Hypothyroidism may occur if advanced. Fibrosis may involve mediastinum.

Diagnosis

History
- Presentation following viral URI is suggestive of subacute thyroiditis.
- Presentation after penetrating injury to the neck is suggestive of suppurative processes.
- Postpartum presentation is suggestive of silent thyroiditis.

Laboratory Examination
- TSH and free T_4 may be normal or indicative of hypo- or hyperthyroidism.
- WBC with differential should be obtained to look for leukocytosis and left shift (subacute and suppurative).
- Antimicrosomal antibodies are present in > 90% with Hashimoto's and 50 to 80% with silent thyroiditis.
- Serum thyroglobulin levels are elevated in subacute and silent thyroiditis (test is very nonspecific).

Imaging Studies
- Radioactive iodine uptake (RAIU) can be useful to distinguish Graves' disease (increased RAIU) from Hashimoto's thyroiditis (decreased RAIU).

Treatment

- Treat hypothyroidism, if present, with levothyroxine for 6 to 8 weeks. Reevaluate the TSH level.
- Control symptoms of hyperthyroidism, if present, with propranolol.
- Pain management in patients with subacute thyroiditis should be accomplished with NSAIDs. If ineffective, begin steroids.
- IV antibiotics and abscess drainage, if present, should be performed in suppurative thyroiditis.
- Do not give PTU or methimazole in thyroiditis.

Prognosis

- Hashimoto's: Most patients do not completely recover their total thyroid function.
- Subacute: Hypothyroidism persists in 10%.
- Silent: Hypothyroidism persists in 6%.
- Suppurative: Full recovery is common.
- Riedel's thyroiditis: Hypothyroidism occurs when the entire gland undergoes fibrosis.

Differential diagnosis of thyroiditis:
- The hyperthyroid stage of Hashimoto's, subacute, or silent, may mimic Graves' disease.
- Riedel's must be differentiated from thyroid CA.
- Subacute can be mistaken for oropharyngeal or tracheal infections or for suppurative thyroiditis.

EVALUATION OF THE THYROID NODULE

Epidemiology

- Common (0.8% of men and 5.0% of women)
- Incidence increases after age 45

Signs and Symptoms

- History of neck irradiation (increased CA risk)
- Family history of pheochromocytoma, thyroid CA, or hyperparathyroidism (MEN II)
- Dysphagia, hoarseness
- Physical exam: Likelihood of malignancy increases with nodule larger than 2 cm, regional lymphadenopathy, fixation to tissues, age less than 40, male sex.

If thyroidectomy is planned, obtain a thyroglobulin level. A return to normal following thyroidectomy suggests the absence of metastatic thyroid tissue.

Diagnosis

- Fine-needle aspiration is the best initial study. Accuracy can be > 90%.
- Thyroid ultrasound is performed to evaluate the size and number of thyroid nodules. It also evaluates whether the nodules are cystic or solid.
- Thyroid scan with technetium 99m classifies nodules as hyperfunctioning (hot nodules, less likely to be malignant) or hypofunctioning (cold nodules, more likely to be malignant).

HYPERPARATHYROIDISM

Definitions

- Primary: Hypersecretion of PTH by the parathyroid glands; *the rest of the section refers to 1° only.*
- Secondary: Glandular hyperplasia and elevated PTH in an appropriate response to hypocalcemia (due to renal failure, GI disturbances, etc.)
- Tertiary: Continued elevation of PTH after the disturbance causing 2° hyperparathyroidism has been corrected

Epidemiology

- Most common in middle-aged and elderly women
- Common: Present in 0.1% of the population

Etiology

- Parathyroid adenoma: 85%, 1 gland involved
- Parathyroid hyperplasia: 14%, all four glands involved
- Parathyroid carcinoma: 1%, 1 gland involved
- Associated with MEN II and III
- Neck irradiation increases risk.

Pathophysiology

- Parathyroid hormone (PTH) increases serum Ca^{2+} levels:
  - Stimulates renal hydroxylation of vitamin D (necessary for GI absorption of Ca^{2+})
  - Increases renal resorption of Ca^{2+}
  - Decreases renal resorption of PO_4^-
  - Increases resorption of bone (increases osteoclastic activity)
- PTH secretion is stimulated by decreased serum levels of Ca^{2+} and inhibited by high levels, except in adenomas and carcinomas in which feedback inhibition is lost.

Signs and Symptoms

Attributable to hypercalcemia: See chapter 8

Diagnosis

- Elevated serum Ca^{2+}, low serum PO_4^-
- High serum PTH
- Hypercalciuria

Treatment

- Older asymptomatic patients with serum $Ca^{2+} < 12$ should just be followed for progression.
- Surgery:
  - Adenomas should be completely excised.
  - In hyperplasia, all four glands are removed and a small portion is reinserted in an easily accessible place such as the sternocleidomastoid so that it can function, but if hyperplasia recurs, subsequent surgical intervention is simplified.
- Emergency measures:
  - Hydration with furosemide diuresis
  - Bisphosphonates to block bone resorption
  - Calcitonin acts rapidly but loses its efficacy after several days

Other causes of hypercalcemia:
- Bone metastases
- Sarcoidosis
- Hyperthyroidism
- Thiazide diuretics
- Immobilization
- Paget's disease

HYPOPARATHYROIDISM

Mg deficiency is seen in alcoholism, SIADH, and pancreatitis.

Definition

Condition characterized by PTH deficiency

Etiology

- Idiopathic
- DiGeorge syndrome (see Chapter 10)
- Postsurgical
- Infiltrative carcinoma
- Irradiation
- Hypomagnesemia (magnesium is necessary for parathyroid gland to secrete PTH)

Typical scenario:
A 30-year-old woman presents with perioral paresthesias and a long QT interval on ECG. She recently had surgery for a thyroid goiter. *Think: Hypoparathyroidism* (due to neck surgery with probable accidental resection of the parathyroids).

Vitamin D acts on the intestines to increase absorption of calcium and phosphate. It enters the skin via sunlight as a previtamin and is converted to an inactive intermediate (25-OH vit D) in the liver before being converted to its active form 1,25-(OH)2 vit D (calcitriol) in the kidney.

Pseudohypoparathyroidism presents the same as hypoparathyroidism, except that the pathophysiology in pseudohypoparathyroidism is tissue resistance to PTH, so that PTH is high (distinguishing feature). Pseudohypoparathyroidism is associated with Albright's hereditary osteodystrophy.

Primary adrenal insufficiency is known as Addison's disease.

Epidemiology

Equal incidence in men and women

Signs and Symptoms

Signs and symptoms of hypocalcemia (see chapter 8):
- Seizures
- Perioral paresthesia
- Fasciculations, tetany, and muscle weakness
- CNS depression, irritability, confusion
- Chvostek's and Trousseau's signs
- Faint heart sounds
- Bronchospasm
- Anxiety, psychosis

Diagnosis

- QT prolongation on ECG
- Low serum calcium
- High serum phosphorus
- Normal or low PTH
- Normal 25-OH vit D
- Low 1,25-$(OH)_2$ vit D

Treatment

- Treat severe, life-threatening hypocalcemia with intravenous calcium.
- Maintenance therapy with calcitriol and oral calcium supplementation

ADRENAL INSUFFICIENCY

Definition

- Primary insufficiency is due to a problem with the adrenal gland itself, in which it does not produce hormones.
- In secondary insufficiency, the adrenal gland is intact, but the pituitary does not produce ACTH, so that there is no stimulus for the adrenal gland to secrete its hormones.
- Tertiary insufficiency is due to hypothalamic failure

Epidemiology

More common in women (2:1)

Etiology

Primary Insufficiency
- Autoimmune (80%)
- Tuberculosis (15%)

- Neoplastic disease
- Sarcoidosis
- Amyloidosis
- Blastomycosis
- Hemochromatosis
- AIDS
- Adrenal hemorrhage due to trauma, anticoagulants, or coagulopathies
- Congenital adrenal hyperplasia
- Waterhouse–Friderichsen syndrome (fulminant septicemia in newborns)
- Adrenalectomy

Secondary Insufficiency
- Suppression of hypothalamic–pituitary–adrenal axis by exogenous steroids (most common)
- Sheehan's syndrome (postpartum pituitary necrosis)
- Pituitary infarct
- Autoimmune destruction of pituitary

Anatomy

The adrenal cortex consists of three zones:
- Zona glomerulosa—produces aldosterone.
- Zona fasciculata and zona reticularis—produce cortisol and androgens (sex hormones)

The adrenal medulla produces catecholamines.

Pathophysiology

Aldosterone
- Produced when angiotensin II acts on the zona glomerulosa to convert corticosterone to aldosterone
- Principal function is to increase renal sodium reabsorption in the distal tubule and collecting ducts, causing secretion of potassium and hydrogen ions
- Deficiency results in hyperkalemia and hyponatremia.

Cortisol
- Stimulates gluconeogenesis by increasing protein and fat catabolism and decreasing utilization of glucose and tissue sensitivity to insulin
- Promotes anti-inflammatory state via inhibition of arachidonic acid, inhibition of interleukin-2 production, and inhibiting release of histamine from mast cells
- Has widespread effects on carbohydrate and protein metabolism
- Acts to counteract the effects of insulin and maintain blood glucose levels
- Governs body water distribution
- Enhances the pressor effects of catecholamine on heart muscle
- Inhibits inflammatory and allergic reactions
- Deficiency results in impairment of body's ability to handle stress

Addisonian or adrenal crisis is an acute complication of adrenal insufficiency characterized by shock, dehydration, confusion, vomiting, hyperkalemia, and hypoglycemia. It is precipitated by sepsis, hemorrhage, trauma, and other stressors.

Primary insufficiency results in increased levels of ACTH. Melanocyte-stimulating hormone (MSH) and ACTH are cleaved from the same propeptide, so elevated ACTH results in increased skin pigmentation.

Typical scenario: An 18-year-old man with hemophilia A who was recently mugged (receiving multiple blows to the back and abdomen) is now complaining of dizziness, abdominal pain, dark patches on his elbows and knees, and uncontrollable cravings for pizza and french fries. *Think: 1° adrenal insufficiency.*

Signs and Symptoms

- Hyperpigmentation of mucosa, areolae, hand creases, knees, elbows, and knuckles (1° only)
- Salt craving (1° only)
- Orthostatic hypotension (1° only)
- Weakness
- Amenorrhea, loss of axillary hair (due to absence of androgens)
- Anorexia
- Weight loss
- Abdominal pain

Diagnosis

ACTH (Cortrosyn) Test

- Give test dose of ACTH and measure serum cortisol levels at 0 and 30 minutes. A level < 20 μg/dL at 30 minutes suggests adrenal insufficiency.
- Measuring the plasma ACTH after test will tell you whether it is primary (high ACTH) or secondary (low or normal ACTH).
- Hyperkalemia, hyponatremia, extracellular fluid (ECF) volume contraction and metabolic acidosis due to aldosterone deficiency (1° only)
- Hypoglycemia
- Anemia
- Elevated BUN and creatinine
- Elevated ACTH, low serum cortisol

Treatment

- Glucocorticoid replacement for all patients
- Instruct patients to increase their glucocorticoid dose in times of stress and infection.
- Patients with Addison's disease should also receive mineralocorticoid replacement therapy.

ADRENAL EXCESS: CUSHING'S SYNDROME

Definition

- Cushing's syndrome: Symptoms caused by excess cortisol production
- Cushing's disease: Cushing's syndrome caused by excess ACTH secretion by pituitary

Epidemiology

More common in females

Etiology

- Exogenous corticosteroid therapy
- Adrenal neoplasm

- Ectopic ACTH production
- Cushing's disease

Signs and Symptoms

- Hypertension
- Facial plethora
- Hair loss
- Central obesity (apple-shaped habitus, moon facies, thin extremities)
- Hump on back of neck (Buffalo's hump)
- Fragile, easily bruised skin
- Abdominal purplish striae
- Proximal muscle weakness
- Hirsutism
- Emotional lability
- Osteoporosis

Diagnosis

Overnight Dexamethasone Suppression Test
- 1 mg dexamethasone is given at night, plasma cortisol measured in the A.M.
- If < 5 µg/100 mL, excludes Cushing's as a diagnosis

High-Dose Dexamethasone Suppression Test
- Give 8 mg dexamethasone, then measure ACTH.
- If ACTH is undetectable or decreased and there is no suppression, likely adrenal etiology
- If ACTH normal or increased and there is no suppression, likely ectopic ACTH etiology
- If ACTH high with partial suppression, likely pituitary etiology

Other Findings
- Increased 24-hour urinary free cortisol (> 100 µg/24 hr)
- Hypokalemia, hypochloremia, metabolic alkalosis
- Hyperglycemia, hypercholesterolemia
- CT of adrenals to look for mass
- MRI of pituitary to look for mass
- Malignancy workup if ectopic ACTH production is suspected

Treatment

Pituitary Adenomas (see Figure 9-1)
- Transsphenoidal surgery
- Radiation for children and cases refractory to surgery

Adrenal Adenoma
- Unilateral resection, followed by 3 to 12 months of glucocorticoid replacement (normal adrenal needs time to come out of suppression)

Patients with ectopic ACTH production often do not have all the mentioned symptoms; they usually only have weight loss and weakness because the ACTH they secrete is usually an inactive form.

Cushing's disease can be distinguished from Cushing's syndrome by the presence of hyperpigmentation.

Typical scenario:
A 42-year-old woman on long-term steroids for asthma has excess adipose tissue in her neck and upper trunk, a wide "moon face," and very fine hair. *Think: Cushing's syndrome (due to exogenous steroids).*

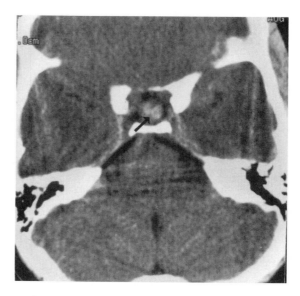

FIGURE 9-1. Pituitary adenoma (arrow).

(Reproduced, with permission, from Lee, Rao, and Zimmerman, *Cranial MRI and CT,* 4th ed. New York, NY: McGraw-Hill, 1999: 653.)

Bilateral Adrenal Hyperplasia
- Bilateral resection with lifelong replacement of glucocorticoids and mineralocorticoids

Ectopic ACTH Production
- Remove source of neoplasm if possible

HYPERALDOSTERONISM

Definition
- Isolated excess production of aldosterone
- Also called Conn's syndrome

Epidemiology
- One to 2% of all patients with hypertension
- Most frequent in ages 30 to 60
- Adrenal tumor more common in women

Etiology
- Unilateral aldosterone producing adenoma (most common cause)
- Bilateral hyperplasia of zona glomerulosa (idiopathic)

Signs and Symptoms
- Usually asymptomatic
- Hypertension

- May see signs of hypokalemia (muscle cramps, palpitations)
- May see signs of glucose intolerance (polyuria, polydipsia)

Diagnosis

Captopril Test
- Administer 25 to 50 mg captopril and measure plasma rennin and aldosterone levels after 2 hours.
- Plasma aldosterone > 15 ng/dL confirms primary hyperaldosteronism.

Other Findings
- Hypokalemia, hypernatremia, and metabolic alkalosis
- High serum aldosterone, low rennin levels
- Glucose intolerance
- 24-hour urine high in potassium and aldosterone
- Evidence of adrenal mass on abdominal CT

Typical scenario:
A 44-year-old woman has hypertension, muscle cramps, and excessive thirst. *Think: Hyperaldosteronism.*

Treatment

- Adrenalectomy for tumor
- Medical management for hyperplasia:
  - Spironolactone (potassium sparing) or ACE inhibitors to control blood pressure
  - Low-sodium diet
  - Maintenance of ideal body weight, regular exercise, smoking cessation

PHEOCHROMOCYTOMA

Definition

Tumor of the adrenal medulla resulting in catecholamine excess

Epidemiology

Equal incidence in men and women. Tumors in women are three times as likely to be malignant.

Etiology

- Multiple endocrine neoplasia types II and III
- MEN II: Pheochromocytoma, parathyroid tumor, and medullary thyroid tumor
- MEN III: Pheochromocytoma, parathyroid tumor, and mucosal neuromas
- Neurofibromatosis
- Von Hippel–Lindau disease: Pheochromocytoma, retinal angiomas, CNS hemangioblastomas, renal cell carcinoma, pancreatic pseudocysts, ependymal cystadenoma

Pheochromocytoma:
Rule of 10s:
10% are extra-adrenal
10% are bilateral
10% are malignant
10% are familial
10% are pediatric
10% calcify
10% recur after resection

Signs and Symptoms

Patients experience "paroxysmal attacks" of high blood pressure. Physical exam usually normal outside of an attack. Symptoms of catecholamine (sympathetic) excess will predominate during an attack.

5H's
- Headache
- Hypertension
- Hot (diaphoretic)
- Heart (palpitations)
- Hyperhidrosis

Other Symptoms
- Tremor
- Anxiety
- Weight loss

Diagnosis

- Elevated urine vanillylmandelic acid (urine catecholamines)
- Hypercalcemia
- Hyperglycemia
- CT to look for adrenal mass

Treatment

- Surgical resection
- Alpha-adrenergic blockade (may also add beta blocker)

OSTEOMALACIA

Definition

- Disease of impaired bone mineralization
- Termed *rickets* in the pediatric population

Etiology

- Decreased Ca^{2+} absorption
- Dietary calcium deficiency: Rare, avoidance of dairy products:
  - GI disorders: Malabsorption syndromes, gastrectomy, dumping syndrome
- Vitamin D deficiency:
  - Hepatobiliary and pancreatic disease: Loss of bile acids or pancreatic lipase reduce absorption of fat soluble vitamins
  - Extremely low-fat diets
  - Renal osteodystrophy: Decreased renal hydroxylation of vitamin D
- Decreased serum PO_4^-:
  - More common cause than calcium deficiency in United States
  - Renal tubular acidosis, Fanconi's syndrome, hypophosphatasia

Signs and Symptoms

- Bone pain
- Weakness
- Difficulty walking: Broad-based waddling gait with short strides
- Thoracic kyphosis

Diagnosis

Radiographs
- Show diffuse, nonspecific osteopenia
- Vertebrae may be biconcave from compression by intervertebral disks
- Pseudofractures (radiolucent lines perpendicular to bone cortex)

Labs
- Ca^{2+} and PO_4^- low to normal
- High alkaline phosphatase
- PTH may be elevated in response to low Ca^{2+}

Treatment

- Address underlying disorder
- Calcium, vitamin D supplements

OSTEOPOROSIS

Definition

Systemic disorder resulting in a reduction of bone mass that leads to increased risk of fracture.

Classification

Two varieties of osteoporosis are commonly recognized:
- Type I:
  - Typically seen in postmenopausal women
  - Manifested by trabecular bone loss
  - Increased incidence of vertebral and distal radius (Colles') fractures.
- Type II:
  - Usually occurs in people over 75 years of age
  - Both trabecular and cortical bone are lost.
  - Increased incidence of hip and vertebral fractures

Epidemiology

Risk factors for osteoporosis include:
- Female and elderly
- Postmenopause
- Family history of osteoporosis
- Cigarette smoking

- Thin body habitus
- Sedentary lifestyle

Pathophysiology

- Reduction in bone mass occurs due to an imbalance between bone acquisition and bone reabsorption.
- There is no change in the ratio of mineral to organic bone.
- Histology: Decreased cortical thickness and decreased number and size of cancellous bone trabeculae (especially horizontal).

Clinical Findings

- Osteoporosis is asymptomatic until fracture occurs (see Figure 7-1).
- Vertebral body fractures:
  - Pain in the lumbar region
  - Acute in onset
  - Radiating to the flank
  - Usually occur after sudden bending or lifting
  - Radiation of the pain down one leg is common
  - Spinal cord compression is rare
- Hip fractures:
  - Most serious complication
  - Most resulting from a fall from a standing position
  - Incidence of fracture increases with age in both men and women

Laboratory Findings

- Serum calcium and phosphorous usually normal
- Alkaline phosphatase is increased after fractures but is usually normal if fractures aren't present.
- Bone-specific alkaline phosphatase assays are useful for monitoring response to therapy.
- Twenty percent of postmenopausal women have hypercalciuria.

Diagnosis

- Since bone loss is a universal process of aging, pathologic osteoporosis should be diagnosed definitively and other causes should be ruled out.
- Biconcavity of vertebral bodies with pathologic fractures is highly suggestive of osteoporosis.
- Bone densitometry establishes the diagnosis.

Prevention and Therapy

- Prevention of low bone mass by adequate dietary calcium and weight-bearing exercise. These measures increase peak bone mass earlier in life and prevent accelerated bone loss later in life.
- Estrogen replacement therapy prevents rapid bone loss and subsequently decreases rate of fractures.
- Calcitonin decreases bone reabsorption.

Differential in osteoporosis:
- Malignancy: Multiple myeloma, lymphoma, leukemia, and metastatic carcinoma
- Hyperparathyroidism
- Osteomalacia
- Paget's disease of bone

- Bisphosphonates (alendronate) increase density of spinal bone and decreases incidence of fractures when used in conjunction with vitamin D and calcium supplementation.

PAGET'S DISEASE OF BONE

Definition

Chronic disease of adult bone in which localized areas of bone become hyperactive, and the normal bone matrix is replaced by softened and enlarged bone.

Etiology

Cause is unknown, but it is suspected that a viral infection plays a role.

Epidemiology

- 3% of people > 40 years
- 3:2 male predominance

Pathophysiology

- Hyperactive bone turnover
- Increased bone formation
- Pelvis, femur, skull, tibiae, and vertebrae all affected
- Enlarged multinucleated osteoclasts

Clinical Findings

- Most patients asymptomatic, diagnosis made at autopsy
- Incidental radiographic findings: Area of hyperlucency surrounded by a hyperdense border
- Elevated alkaline phosphatase
- Symptomatic patients:
    - Increasing hat size due to skull involvement
    - Swelling or lengthening of a long bone causing gait disturbance
    - Dull aching pain, usually in the back, may radiate to the buttocks or lower extremities.
    - Rarely hearing loss due to involvement of the ossicles or auditory canal impinging on CN VIII
- Complications:
    - Pathologic fractures
    - Rarely "high-output" cardiac failure due to high vascularity of lesions
    - Urinary stones due to high calcium excretion
    - Sarcoma occurs in 1% of patients, poor prognosis

Alkaline phosphatase of bony origin is heat labile, whereas the hepatic variant is not.

Typical scenario:
A patient is found to have an elevated alkaline phosphatase during a routine blood test. No other abnormalities were found. Further work up revealed the enzyme to be heat labile. *Think: Paget's disease.*

Treatment

- Most patients require no treatment.
- Indications for therapy are excessive pain, neural compression, profound alteration in posture or gait, high-output heart failure, hypercalcemia, and excessive calciuria, with or without renal calculi.
- Indomethacin is usually satisfactory for pain relief.
- Osteotomy is useful in selected cases of anatomic deformity or impingement.
- Bisphosphonates decrease bone reabsorption and are usually well tolerated.
- Calcitonin may be instituted in cases with cardiac failure or neurologic deficits. Calcitonin also has an analgesic effect.

Urology

Jonathan Posner

PRINCIPLES OF SAFE SEXUAL PRACTICE

Several practices can help prevent the spread of STDs. Important methods include:
- Using latex condoms (oral contraceptives do not protect against STDs)
- Limiting the number of sexual partners
- Eliciting a sexual history from partners
- Routine physical exams
- Seeking out medical care when needed

It is important for all physicians to make patients feel comfortable talking about sex. Taking a sexual history should be routine.

ESTROGEN DEFICIENCY CHANGES

- Increased bone resorption
- Vaginal dryness
- Thinning of the urethral mucosa (increases risk of urinary incontinence)
- Decreased high-density lipoprotein (HDL) cholesterol
- Hot flashes
- Mood changes
- Skin wrinkling

Hormone replacement therapy can combat the undesirable changes of estrogen deficiency. Women with a uterus are given both estrogen and progesterone; women who are s/p hysterectomy need only estrogen.

LEADING CAUSES OF DYSURIA

In Women
- Cystitis
- Pyelonephritis
- Vaginitis:
  - *Trichomonas vaginalis*
  - *Candida albicans*
  - Bacterial (*Gardnerella*) vaginosis
- Urethritis:
  - *Chlamydia trachomatis*
  - *Neisseria gonorrhea*
- Herpes simplex

In Men
- Cystitis
- Prostatitis
- Pyelonephritis
- Inflammation of the bladder trigone
- Carcinoma of the bladder trigone
- Carcinoma of the urethra

CYSTITIS

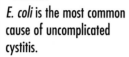

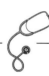
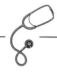
Definition

Infection of the bladder

Causes

Most commonly from colonic bacteria: *Escherichia coli, Proteus, Klebsiella, Enterobacter*

Signs and Symptoms

- Urinary frequency and urgency
- Dysuria
- Suprapubic tenderness

Treatment

Asymptomatic bacteriuria is treated if:
- Patient is pregnant or immunocompromised
- Patient is due to undergo urologic instrumentation
- There are $> 10^5$ colonies in the urinalysis

Uncomplicated cases can be treated with a short course of trimethoprim–sulfamethoxazole (TMP-SMZ) (3 to 5 days).

SYPHILIS

Definition and Pathophysiology

- A sexually transmitted or congenital disease with variable clinical manifestations, depending on stage of the disease.
- Syphilis is transmitted primarily through sexual contact but can be spread through any mucosal or epithelial abrasion.
- The causative organism is *Treponema pallidum,* a spirochete.
- Once the spirochete has entered the body, it spreads throughout most organ systems and the disease then progresses through three active stages.

Signs and Symptoms

All patients develop a painless chancre at inoculation site. If untreated, some patients progress to a disseminated (2°) stage, during which the organism is spread throughout the entire body and is highly infectious.

Primary Syphilis
- Appears 3 to 6 weeks after exposure
- A **painless "buttonlike" chancre** with indurated borders develops at inoculation site within 2 to 6 weeks after exposure.
- Usually develop genital chancre, but may have an extragenital lesion.
- Accompanied by regional lymphadenopathy **("bubo")** within 1 week.
- Chancre can last up to 6 weeks if untreated.

Secondary Syphilis
- Appears 4 to 6 weeks after 1° syphilis resolves, lasts for 6 to 8 weeks
- Maculopapular rash (multiple, discrete, firm, "ham-colored" papules scattered symmetrically over trunk, **palms and soles,** and genitals)
- **Condylomata lata**—soft, flat topped pink papules on anogenital region that are painless wartlike lesions
- Flulike symptoms—fever, malaise, arthralgia, generalized lymphadenopathy, and splenomegaly

Latent Phase
- This stage can last for several years.
- Patients are asymptomatic but remain seropositive.

Tertiary Syphilis
- Develops at any time during the latent phase and continues indefinitely if not treated
- **Gummas**—rubbery granulomatous lesions in subcutaneous tissues of central nervous system (CNS), heart, aorta
- Cardiovascular—vasa vasorum vasculitis, aortic insufficiency
- Neurosyphilis—seizures, personality changes, psychosis, **tabes dorsalis** (posterior column degeneration). The syphilitic pupil is also known as the **Argyll–Robertson pupil.**

Laboratory

- Venereal Disease Research Laboratory (VDRL) and rapid plasma reagin (RPR)—good screening tests but nonspecific
- Fluorescent treponemal antibody-absorption test (FTA-ABS)—done when VDRL or RPR is positive. Good sensitivity and specificity. Remains positive for life, regardless of treatment.
- Darkfield microscopy—smear of exudate from primary chancre or secondary papular lesions reveal a 5 to 20 μm in length spirochete, with kinking and contractile movements but without locomotion.
- *T. pallidum* does not grow in regular blood cultures.

Treatment

Penicillin G

RPR screening is part of dementia workup.

The syphilitic pupil is like a prostitute: It accommodates but doesn't react.

VDRL/RPR false positives are seen in:
- Systemic lupus erythematosus (SLE)
- Infectious mononucleosis
- Hepatitis C

If maternal infection is untreated by 16 weeks' gestation, child may be born with congenital syphilis and is at risk of stillbirth.

HIGH-YIELD FACTS

Urology

URETHRITIS

Divided into gonococcal (GC) and nongonococcal

Causes

C. trachomatis is a predisposing factor for pelvic inflammatory disease (PID) and infertility.

- Gonococcal urethritis is caused by *Neisseria gonorrhea*.
- The leading cause of nongonococcal urethritis is *Chlamydia trachomatis* types D–K. *Chlamydia* is difficult to culture and may be asymptomatic. This can make it very difficult to detect.
- Other causes of nongonococcal urethritis are *Ureaplasma urealyticum* and *Mycoplasma genitalium*.

Signs and Symptoms

- Dysuria
- Purulent urethral discharge

Treatment

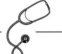

Co-infections are very common; therefore, treatment is generally given for both *N. gonorrhea* and *C. trachomatis*.

GC
- Single dose of ceftriaxone, cefixime, ciprofloxacin, ofloxacin, azithromycin, or spectinomycin

Chlamydia
- Single dose of azithromycin or
- Doxycycline, ofloxacin, or erythromycin × 7 days

BALANITIS

Definition

Inflammation of the glans penis

Causes

- *Candida albicans*
- Allergic reaction (often to latex condoms)
- Reiter's syndrome

Treatment

Any patient who presents with balanitis should be screened for diabetes.

- Candidal infections are treated with nystatin.
- Reiter's syndrome is treated with NSAIDs.
- Antichlamydial treatment may also be useful.

Definition

Infection with herpes virus. Type I usually associated with oral lesions, and type II with genital lesions, but not always.

Signs and Symptoms

- **Painful** vesicular lesions on erythematous base
- Local lymphadenopathy
- Neuralgia often precedes an outbreak

Laboratory

- Tzanck smear test and culture
- Herpes serology

Treatment

Antiviral agents acyclovir, famciclovir, and valacyclovir are not curative but effective in reducing the severity and frequency of outbreak as well as the degree of viral shedding

Infections can remain dormant for years, but the herpes virus is continuously shed and can be transmitted during latent phases.

Adverse effects of acyclovir:
- Renal crystals
- Allergic interstitial nephritis

Divided into bacterial and nonbacterial

Bacterial Prostatitis

DEFINITION

Inflammation of the prostate due to bacteria ascending the urethra and then passing into the prostate through the prostatic ducts.

CAUSES

Most common agents:
- *E. coli*
- *Pseudomonas*

SIGNS AND SYMPTOMS

- Perineal and suprapubic pain
- Dysuria and urinary frequency
- Fever
- Tender prostate on physical exam

Care must be taken during the rectal exam. Vigorously massaging the prostate can lead to bacteremia.

LABORATORY

- Leukocytosis with neutrophil predominance
- Urinalysis (U/A) shows bacteriuria and pyuria.

TREATMENT

- Outpatient therapy consists of TMP-SMZ or ciprofloxacin for 21 days.
- Indications for hospitalization include severe comorbidities, poor patient compliance, or sepsis.

Nonbacterial Prostatitis

An inflammatory process in the prostate from an unknown etiology. Viral agents or an autoimmune reaction are possible causes.

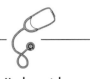

Nonbacterial prostatitis usually causes chronic prostatitis.

SIGNS AND SYMPTOMS

- Urinary frequency and dysuria
- Nontender, enlarged prostate on physical exam

LABORATORY

- U/A and urine culture are negative.
- Leukocytes can be seen in prostatic secretions.

TREATMENT

- A trial of antibiotics is often given.
- Anti-inflammatories for symptomatic relief

VAGINITIS

The normal flora of the vagina creates an acidic environment (pH 3.5 to 4.5) in large part through the colonization of lactobacilli. This protects the vagina from pathogenic organisms. When this environment is disturbed, infections become possible.

Lactobacilli are used to make yogurt. A Yoplait a day keeps vaginitis away.

Causes

- Bacterial vaginosis (BV)—primarily *Gardnerella*
- *Trichomonas vaginalis*
- Yeast—*Candida albicans*

The "whiff" test: Application of KOH to the wet mount will enhance the odor of both *Gardnerella* and *Trichomonas*.

Signs and Symptoms

General
- Vaginal itch and burning sensation
- Abnormal odor

- Increase in discharge:
  - BV: Fishy odor of discharge
  - *Trichomonas:* Fishy odor of discharge, strawberry cervix
  - Yeast: Cheese-like discharge

Diagnosis

Seen on wet mount:
- BV: Clue cells (epithelial cells coated with bacteria)
- *Trichomonas:* Motile trichomonads
- Yeast: Pseudohyphae

Treatment

- Metronidazole for BV and *Trichomonas*
- Nystatin for yeast infection
- Treat sexual partners as well.

Metronidazole is contraindicated in first-trimester pregnancy. Use clotrimazole instead.

Warn patients against having any alcohol while on metronidazole. It can cause a disulfiram-like reaction when co-ingested with alcohol.

HUMAN PAPILLOMA VIRUS (HPV)

Definition

Sexually transmitted disease (STD) caused by the HPV, of which there are many subtypes

Epidemiology

- Most common sexually transmitted disease
- Commonly asymptomatic in men

Signs and Symptoms

- Bowenoid papules on penis
- Condyloma acuminata (papillomatous growths with a soft, macerated surface)
- Warts grow on mucous membrane of penis, perineum, vulva, vagina, and vaginal canal.

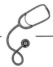

HPV: Mother may infect newborn during delivery, causing **laryngeal papillomatosis.**

Diagnosis

Most HPV warts are flat and invisible to the unaided eye. Coating them with 1% acetic acid turns them white. All white lesions on colposcopy are biopsied for HPV.

Treatment

Lesions are removed via cryosurgery, laser ablation, or chemical ablation (podophyllin).

HPV types 16, 18, 31, 45, 51, 52, and 53 are associated with cervical cancer.

Definition

- An uncommon STD, caused by *Chlamydia trachomatis* serotypes L1, L2, or L3

Signs and Symptoms

- Lesions on genitals and thighs
- Tender inguinal lymphadenopathy
- Cellular inclusion bodies
- Proctitis

Diagnosis

Via serologic complement fixation or microimmunofluorescence test

Treatment

- Doxycycline for 3 weeks
- Erythromycin for pregnant women

Adverse effects of tetracyclines:
- **Photosensitivity**
- **Increase preexisting prerenal azotemia**
- **Brown/yellow deposits in teeth and brittle bones (children)**

INFECTIOUS PROCTITIS

Definition

Inflammation of anal mucosa with concomitant symptoms

Causes

- *Chlamydia* spp.
- *N. gonorrhea*
- Herpes simplex virus

Signs and Symptoms

- *Chlamydia* and *Gonococcus*—confined to distal rectum, no systemic symptoms
- HSV—systemic involvement, high fever

Treatment

Antibiotics or antivirals

HIGH-YIELD FACTS

Urology

Definition

Calculi in the urogenital system

Epidemiology

- One of the most common diseases of the urinary tract
- 2 to 5% of the population will form a urinary stone at some point in their lives.
- Majority of stones form between the ages of 20 and 50.
- Male to female ratio of 3:1
- Familial tendency in stone formation
- Tendency for recurrence—36% of patients with a first stone will have another stone within one year.

Types of Stones

Calcium Oxalate Stones (75%)
- Strongly radio-opaque
- Treat with thiazides.
- Increased incidence in inflammatory bowel disease (increased oxalate), hypercalcemia (hyperparathyroidism), decreased citrate (forms stable soluble complex with calcium), uricosurea (small urate crystals serve as nidi for larger calcium stones)

Struvite (Mg NH$_4$ PO$_4$) Stones (15%)
- Moderately radio-opaque
- Common in *Proteus* UTIs due to high urinary pH (*Proteus* makes urease, which cleaves urinary urea yielding two molecules of ammonia—the conjugate base of ammonium ion)
- Treat by lowering urine pH.

Uric Acid Stones (< 1%)
- Radiolucent
- Increased incidence in myeloproliferative diseases and gout (due to increased purine turnover)
- Treat by raising urine pH.

Cystine Stones (< 1%)
- Moderately radio-opaque
- Seen in congenital cystinuria (NOT homocystinuria)
- Hexagonal crystals, positively birefringent
- Treat by raising urine pH.

Predisposing Factors

- Dietary history—large calcium and alkali intake
- Prolonged immobilization
- Residence in hot climate
- History of urinary tract infections
- History of calculus in the past and in family members

- Drug ingestion (analgesics, alkalis, uricosuric agents, protease inhibitors)
- Prior history of gout
- Underlying gastrointestinal disease (Crohn's, ulcerative colitis, PUD)

Signs and Symptoms

- Severe, abrupt onset of colicky pain which begins in the flank and may radiate toward the groin. In males, the pain may radiate toward the testicle. In females, it may radiate toward the labia majoris.
- Nausea and vomiting are almost universal with acute renal colic.
- Abdominal distention from an ileus
- Gross hematuria

Diagnosis

Urinalysis (see Table 10-2)
- Vast majority of patients (about 85%) will have RBCs in the urine. However, its absence does not rule out renal stones.
- Urinary pH can aid in differentiating the type of stone present. Normal urinary pH is about 5.85. If the pH is > 6, one should suspect the presence of urea-splitting organisms (proteus). A low urine pH (≤ 5) suggests uric acid stones.
- WBCs or bacteria may suggest underlying urinary tract infection and should be aggressively treated.

Radiographic Studies (see Table 10-1)
- Plain abdominal film (KUB) will reveal only radio-opaque stones (60 to 70%)
- Renal ultrasound is useful to detect hydronephrosis and is easy, cheap, and doesn't require subjecting the patient to intravenous contrast. It misses small stones
- Noncontrast renal computed tomography (CT) is most useful to diagnose small stones. It can accurately locate stones in the renal system and detect the presence of hydronephrosis. Overall sensitivity is about 95%.
- Intravenous pyelogram has been the gold standard for the diagnosis of renal and ureteral calculi. It can clearly outline the entire urinary system making it easy to see hydronephrosis and the presence of any type of stones. In addition, an intravenous pyelogram (IVP) can demonstrate renal function and allow for verification that the opposite kidney is functioning properly.

Treatment

- Analgesia
- Hydration

Passage of Stones
- Ninety percent of stones < 5 mm will pass spontaneously.
- Fifteen percent of stones 5 to 8 mm will pass.
- Five percent of stones > 8 mm will pass.

Typical scenario:
A 39-year-old man presents with severe back pain and hematuria. He is writhing around, unable to find a comfortable position, and is nauseous.
Think: Renal colic due to urolithiasis.

For Stones Unlikely to Pass Spontaneously

- Extracorporeal shock lithotripsy has been effective for stones located in the kidney with 85% success rate.
- Percutaneous nephrolithotomy, which establishes a tract from the skin to the collecting system, is used when stones are too large or too hard for lithotripsy.

ACUTE PYELONEPHRITIS

Infection of the renal pelvis and parenchyma

Causes

E. coli, Proteus, Klebsiella, Enterobacter

Signs and Symptoms

- Fever
- Chills
- Urinary frequency and urgency
- Dysuria
- Flank (costovertebral angle) tenderness

Laboratory

- Leukocytosis
- Urine dip shows positive leukoesterase and nitrates.
- U/A will show bacteriuria, pyuria, and possibly hematuria.
- Urine cultures with heavy growth
- Blood cultures sometimes positive

Treatment

Consists of empiric antibiotic therapy.
Indications for hospitalization:
- Inability to tolerate oral hydration or medications
- Poor patient compliance
- Uncertainty about diagnosis
- Single kidney
- Pregnant patient
- Severe co-morbidities

Typical scenario:
A 27-year-old woman presents with dysuria, costovertebral angle (CVA) tenderness and fever. *Think: Pyelonephritis.*

TABLE 10-1. Common Genitourinary Procedures

Test	Description	Uses
Intravenous pyelography	Contrast is injected into a peripheral vein, followed by radiographs, allowing visualization of the renal parenchyma and the ureters.	■ Kidney or urethral trauma ■ Kidney or urethral tumors ■ Urethral diverticulum ■ Assessment of renal damage from pyelonephritis
Voiding cystourethrogram	Contrast medium is placed into the bladder via catheter and visualized with x-ray during active micturition.	■ Congenital abnormalities: ■ Posterior urethral valves ■ Ectopic drainage of ureters ■ Neurogenic bladder ■ Strictures ■ Vesicouretral reflux ■ Stress urinary incontinence ■ Ureteroceles
Cystometry	Bladder is filled with water via catheter. Bladder is emptied into a measuring device. The pressure is recorded during this whole time.	■ Benign prostatic hypertrophy ■ Congenital anomalies ■ Incontinence
Cystoscopy	Introduction of either a flexible or rigid scope into the urethra	■ Biopsy ■ Resection of tumors ■ Crushing of stones ■ Catheterization of ureters
Renal ultrasound	Advantage is that it is noninvasive.	■ Renal calculi ■ Urinary obstruction ■ Renal tumors ■ Renal vein thrombus ■ Evaluating renal failure—the size of the kidneys give an idea of the chronicity of the failure.

TABLE 10-2. Interpretation of the Urinalysis

Finding	Significance
Color/clarity	■ Pus, blood
Specific gravity	■ Inability to concentrate urine is often the first sign of kidney disease. ■ High in dehydration and SIADH
pH	■ Alkaline urine seen in Type I RTA, *Proteus*, and *Ureaplasma* UTIs. ■ Acidic urine is seen in salicylate overdose.
Protein/Albumin	■ Marker of glomerular function—albumin will leak through diseased glomeruli.
Glucose	■ Diabetes mellitus—glucose will spill into the urine.
Ketones	■ Seen in DKA, isopropyl alcohol intoxication, and starvation ketosis
Hemoglobin	■ Intravascular hemolysis
Bilirubin/Urobilinogen	■ Extravascular hemolysis
Nitrite/Leukocyte Esterase	■ UTI, nitrites only from gram-negative spp.
RBCs	■ Stones, glomerulonephritis, tumors
WBCs	■ UTI, vaginitis, prostatitis
Casts	■ Kidney disease
Crystals	■ Renal stones, ethylene glycol intoxication
Squamous epithelial cells	■ Measure of the degree of contamination

Immunology

Thomas M. Boyd

IMMUNITY

Humoral Immunity

- Branch of immune system composed of circulating or cell-bound proteins
- Facilitates and directs cell destruction
- Inactivates toxins
- Two main components:
    - Immunoglobulins: produced by B lymphocytes and plasma cells (see Table 11-1)
    - Complement: produced by the liver

TABLE 11-1. Immunoglobulins and Their Functions

Immunoglobulins

IgG	■ ~70% of total immunoglobulins ■ Predominant antibody in secondary immune response ■ Fixes complement ■ Crosses placenta ■ Four subtypes
IgA	■ ~20% of total immunoglobulins ■ Present in serum, colostrum, saliva, tears, and respiratory and intestinal mucosa ■ Dimer in secretions, monomer in serum
IgM	■ ~10% of total immunoglobulins ■ Predominant antibody in primary immune response ■ Fixes complement best ■ Is a pentamer
IgD	■ ~1% of total immunoglobulins ■ B cell surface receptor
IgE	■ 0.01% of total immunoglobulins ■ Trigger histamine release from mast cells: Immediate hypersensitivity reactions (allergy, anaphylaxis, asthma) ■ Also rises in parasitic infections

Cellular Immunity

- Branch of immune system composed of cells (see Table 11-2)
- Multiple components:
  - T lymphocytes:
    - Cytotoxic T cells: Kill cells expressing foreign antigens, CD8+
    - Helper T cells: Enhance activity of other T cells, B cells, and macrophages, CD4+
    - Suppressor T cells: Inhibit cellular immune response, CD8+
  - Neutrophils
  - Eosinophils, mast cells
  - Reticuloendothelial system (monocytes, macrophages, histiocytes, Langerhan's cells, Kupffer cells, etc.)
  - Natural killer cells

CELL-MEDIATED IMMUNODEFICIENCY (CMI)

Major Diseases Causing CMI

- AIDS
- Hodgkin's disease and other lymphomas
- Hairy cell leukemia
- Advanced solid tumors
- Diabetes mellitus
- Tuberculosis
- Sarcoidosis

Iatrogenic CMI

- High-dose corticosteroids
- Cytotoxic chemotherapy
- Radiation therapy

Other Conditions Associated with CMI

- Uremia
- Malnutrition
- Old age

CMI-Associated Infections

- Bacteria: *Listeria, Nocardia, Mycobacterium tuberculosis,* nontuberculous mycobacteria, *Legionella, Salmonella*
- Viruses: Varicella-zoster, herpes simplex, cytomegalovirus (CMV), human papillomavirus (HPV), human herpes virus (HHV)-6, hepatitis B virus (HBV)
- Fungi: *Cryptococcus, Candida, Histoplasma, Coccidioides, Aspergillus, Pneumocystis carinii*
- Protozoa: *Toxoplasma, Cryptosporidium, Giardia lamblia*
- Helminths: *Strongyloides stercoralis*

TABLE 11-2. Immune Deficiency Disorders

Immune disorders

Bruton's congenital agammaglobulinemia	<ul><li>X-linked</li><li>Absence of B cell, tonsils, and germinal centers</li><li>< 10% of all immunoglobulins present</li><li>Normal cell mediated immunity</li><li>Presents with recurrent bacterial infections once mother's passive immunity is depleted</li><li>Treated with immunoglobulin administration (passive immunity)</li></ul>
Common variable hypogammaglobulinemia	<ul><li>Can be acquired at any age by men and women</li><li>Low levels of IgG, IgA, and IgM</li><li>Normal numbers of B cells, but are defective</li><li>Patients usually well until 15 to 30 years of age</li><li>Increased susceptibility to infections and autoimmune diseases</li></ul>
DiGeorge's congenital thymic aplasia	<ul><li>Absence of T cells and hypocalcemia result from intrauterine insult to developing thymus and parathyroid glands (third and fourth pharyngeal pouches)</li><li>Increased susceptibility to opportunistic and viral infections.</li><li>Patients can die from live virus vaccines</li><li>Normal B cells, normal immunoglobulins</li></ul>
Wiskott–Aldrich syndrome	<ul><li>X-linked</li><li>Characterized by thrombocytopenia, eczema, and recurrent infections</li><li>Depressed cell mediated immunity</li><li>Low IgM, high IgA, normal IgG, and IgE.</li></ul>
Chronic mucocutaneous candidiasis	<ul><li>T cell defect specifically against *Candida albicans*</li></ul>
Severe combined immunodeficiency	<ul><li>No thymus, no T cells, no B cells</li><li>Causes may include missing enzyme adenosine deaminase which prevents DNA synthesis, failure to make MHC class II proteins, or defective IL-2 receptors</li><li>Very short life span</li></ul>
Ataxia–teleangiectasia	<ul><li>Autosomal recessive</li><li>Associated with IgA deficiency</li><li>Hypoplastic thymus</li><li>Presents with cerebellar ataxia and cutaneous teleangiectasia</li><li>High incidence of skin cancer</li></ul>
Chronic granulomatous disease	<ul><li>X-linked</li><li>Decreased respiratory burst due to deficient NADPH oxidase function</li><li>Manifests by age 1 with hepatosplenomegaly, aphthous ulcers, seborrhea</li><li>Infections with *S. aureus*, *Proteus* common</li></ul>
Chédiak–Higashi disease	<ul><li>Autosomal recessive defect in chemotaxis</li><li>Recurrent infections with *Staphylococcus* and *Streptococcus*</li></ul>
Selective IgA deficiency	<ul><li>Most common of the selective immunoglobulin deficiencies.</li><li>Present with mucous membrane infections (URI, UTI, GI)</li><li>Low molecular weight IgM increased in partial compensation</li><li>Serum may contain anti-IgA IgE</li><li>IgA replacement is useless, may cause anaphylaxis</li></ul>
Job's syndrome	<ul><li>Autosomal recessive</li><li>Decreased chemotaxis</li><li>Frequent sinus and pulmonary infections and cold skin *Staphylococcus* abscesses</li><li>High IgE levels</li></ul>
X-linked lymphoproliferative disease	<ul><li>Decreased Ab to Epstein–Barr virus (EBV) nuclear antigen</li><li>EBV infection is fatal</li></ul>

- Fever is a red flag in the neutropenic patient.
- Fever equals life-threatening infection in the patient with absolute neutropenia (< 500 PMN/mm^3).
- Neutropenia of < 10 days' duration is less dangerous than prolonged neutropenia.

RISK FACTORS FOR INFECTION IN THE IMMUNOCOMPROMISED

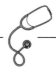

Cancer patients are more often immunocompromised due to cancer treatment (chemotherapy, radiation) than the disease itself.

In Cancer Patients

- Presence, severity, and duration of absolute neutropenia
- Indwelling catheters
- Mucositis from radiotherapy (inflamed mucous membranes provide portal of entry)
- Coexisting defects in humoral immunity increase the risk of infection.

In Transplant Patients

Bone Marrow
- All of risk factors stated above for cancer
- Immunoablation (marrow is completely wiped out with radiation prior to transplant)
- Prior CMV infection
- Graft-versus-host disease

Solid Organ
- Site of transplant
- Presence and status of underlying disease
- Nutritional status
- Age
- Immunosuppressive therapy

In Splenectomy Patients

- Extremes of age
- Reason for splenectomy (e.g., trauma vs. immune mediated)
- Underlying disease (e.g., hematologic, immunologic, neoplastic)
- Defects in humoral immunity and complement

MAJOR CAUSES OF FEVER IN THE IMMUNOCOMPROMISED

In Cancer Patients

- Fever of unknown origin
- Bacteria: Gram-positive or -negative aerobes, anaerobes at site of mixed infection

- Viruses: Respiratory syncytial virus (RSV), parainfluenza, adenoviruses, herpes simplex virus (HSV), CMV
- Fungi: *Candida, Aspergillus, Cryptococcus, Trichosporon*
- *Pneumocystis carinii* and *Toxoplasma* also seen

In Transplant Patients

Bone Marrow
- Similar causes to cancer patients
- Infection is influenced by time since transplant and type of procedure (allogenic vs. autogenic).

Solid Organ
- Influenced by time since transplant, and type of transplant
- Bacteria: Includes gram positive and negative
- Viruses: CMV, EBV, HBV, hepatitis C virus (HCV), adenovirus
- Fungi: Aspergillus, *Pneumocystis carinii*

In Splenectomy Patients

Encapsulated organisms, especially:
- *Streptococcus pneumoniae*
- *Neisseria meningitidis*
- *Hemophilus influenzae*
- *Klebsiella pneumoniae*
- *Salmonella* sp.

Parasites: Malaria, *Babesia*

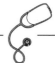

Functionally asplenic patients (sickle cell disease) or postsplenectomy patients (especially from Hodgkin's disease) are at increased risk for infection even if they are not neutropenic.

GENERAL PRINCIPLES OF EVALUATION AND MANAGEMENT

- Determine whether patient is at risk for a systemic or localized infection based on the clinical history:
  - *Pneumocystis carinii* pneumonia (PCP) in HIV+ patients
  - CMV interstitial pneumonitis in allogenic bone marrow transplant patients (30 to 60 days post-transplant)

Diagnostic Studies
- Complete blood count (CBC) with manual differential and coagulation studies
- Culture urine and blood.
- Chest x-ray (CXR) regardless of physical exam findings
- Culture sputum with cough or if CXR warrants.
- Culture stool and cerebrospinal fluid (CSF) in AIDS patients, look for cryptococcal antigen.
- In AIDS and transplant patients, obtain CMV antigen.

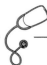

Neutropenic patients are vulnerable to more than one infection at a time. More than one organism may emerge during a single febrile episode. Be aggressive with broad-spectrum antibiotics.

Diagnosis

- Infiltrate may represent infection, extension of tumor, chemotherapy complication, fluid overload, pulmonary infarction, or a combination of factors.
- Leukemia patients within 3 days of initiating chemotherapy are very vulnerable to pneumonia, particularly *Pneumocystis carinii*.
- In any cell-mediated immunodeficiency, a pulmonary infiltrate is usually *Pneumocystis carinii*.
- Biopsy should be considered if other diagnostic methods fail, empiric antibiotic therapy is ineffective, or if persistent hypoxia is present.

Treatment

Choice of Antibiotic
- Combination therapy (e.g.: piperacillin/tazobactam)
- Monotherapy (e.g.: third-generation cephalosporins or carbapenem)
- Adjust therapy based on culture results.

HIV DISEASE: AIDS AND RELATED DISORDERS

AIDS Definition

Any HIV-infected individual with:
- A CD4 count of < 200/μL, regardless of the presence of symptoms or opportunistic diseases
- An AIDS-defining clinical condition, regardless of CD4 count

Major AIDS-Defining Clinical Conditions

- Candidiasis (pulmonary or esophageal)
- Cervical cancer (invasive)
- Cryptococcus (extrapulmonary)
- CMV retinitis with vision loss
- Encephalopathy, HIV-related
- Herpes simplex (chronic ulcers, pulmonary, or esophageal)
- Kaposi's sarcoma
- Lymphoma (Burkitt's or 1° brain)
- *Mycobacterium avium* complex
- *Mycobacterium tuberculosis*
- Atypical mycobacteriosis
- PCP
- Recurrent pneumonias
- Central nervous system (CNS) toxoplasmosis
- Wasting syndrome due to HIV

Life Cycle of HIV

- HIV gp120 binds CD4 molecule on a CD4+ human leukocytes.

- Fusion with host cell via gp41 molecule on HIV
- HIV RNA internalized into host cell
- HIV reverse transcriptase transcribes HIV RNA into dsDNA.
- DNA translocates to nucleus.
- DNA integrated randomly into host genome by virally encoded integrase
- Activation of host cell needed to transcribe the integrated DNA
- mRNA translated into long HIV polypeptides
- Virally encoded protease cleaves polypeptides at specific sites to generate functional proteins
- New infective virus particle (proteins plus genomic viral RNA) assembles at host cell membrane.
- Budding of new virus particle

Antiretroviral medications work against reverse transcriptase and proteases that cleave the newly formed viral proteins after translation.

Transmission of HIV

- Sexual contact
- Blood products
- HIV$^+$ mothers to infants intrapartum, perinatally, or via breast milk

There is no evidence that HIV can be transmitted by casual contact or insects.

SEXUAL CONTACT

- Worldwide HIV is predominantly transmitted by heterosexual sex.
- One-half of U.S. cases are still among homosexual men.
- Incidence of heterosexual transmission in the United States is increasing, mainly among women and minorities.
- HIV is present in infective quantities in seminal fluid and vaginal and cervical secretions.
- Strong association of HIV transmission with receptive anal intercourse.
- Vaginal intercourse: 20-fold greater chance of transmission from man to a woman than woman to a man
- Oral sex: Much less efficient mode of transmission, but cases have been reported.
- Genital ulceration increases chances of transmission (both infectivity and susceptibility to infection).
- Lack of circumcision is associated with higher risk of infection.

BLOOD

Common Modes of Blood Transmission
- Sharing contaminated injection drug paraphernalia
- Transfusion of contaminated blood products

Blood Products Capable of HIV Transmission
- Whole blood and packed RBCs
- Platelets and WBCs
- Plasma

An estimated 10,000 individuals in the United States were infected by contaminated blood products before spring 1985.

Blood Products Incapable of HIV Transmission
- Hyperimmune gamma globulin
- Hep B immune globulin
- Plasma-derived Hep B vaccine
- Rh-immune globulin

Blood Product Screening (United States)
- p24 HIV antigen and HIV antibody by enzyme-linked immunosorbent assay (ELISA), positives confirmed by Western blot

HIV-1 screening of donated blood began in 1985. Risk of infection in the United States from screened blood transfusion is 1 in 450,000 donations.

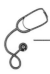

Centers for Disease Control and Prevention (CDC) recommendations for HIV postexposure prophylaxis: Zidovudine, lamivudine, and indinavir for 4 weeks.

Gamma globulin infusion
- Pooled serum immunoglobulin G (IgG) from many donors
- Half-life 27 days
- Very expensive
- Slow infusion—risk of anaphylaxis
- Used to treat idiopathic thrombocytopenic purpura (ITP) (not thrombotic thrombocytopenic purpura [TTP]), AIDS

African Americans and Hispanic Americans constitute a disproportionately high number of HIV cases.

- Self-deferral of donors based on risk behavior
- Screening out of HIV blood based on Hep B or Hep C positivity
- Serologic testing for syphilis

Occupational Transmission
- Transmission risk after skin puncture from blood contaminated sharp object from person with documented HIV infection is 0.3%.
- Transmission for Hep B following similar exposure is 20 to 30%.
- The higher the viral load of the infected patient, the greater the chances of transmission.
- Postexposure prophylaxis and wound cleansing after exposure decrease rate of HIV seroconversion by 79% (to 0.06% for HIV).

MATERNAL–FETAL TRANSMISSION

- HIV can be transmitted from mother to fetus during pregnancy, delivery, or through infected breast milk.
- Transmission rate from untreated mother to newborn is approximately 25% in the United States.
- Zidovudine treatment of HIV-infected pregnant women from the beginning of the third trimester through delivery, with treatment of the infant for 6 weeks after birth, decreases transmission rate to 8%.
- Breast milk transmission (7 to 22%) is most important in developing countries where other means of infant nutrition are not readily available.

TRANSMISSION BY OTHER BODY FLUIDS

- HIV can be identified in almost any body fluid.
- Transmission risk via saliva, sweat, tears, and urine is very small.

AIDS Epidemiology

AIDS WORLDWIDE

- Approximately 36.1 million adults and 1.4 million children were infected worldwide as of December 2000.
- In some sub-Saharan African countries, such as Zimbabwe, approximately 25% of the population is infected.

AIDS IN THE UNITED STATES

Incidence
- AIDS was the fifth leading cause of death in Americans aged 25 to 44 years in 1998.
- The rate of infection is increasing dramatically among heterosexual men and women, especially women and minorities.
- The overall incidence of AIDS has declined in the United States since 1995.

Prevalence
- Overall prevalence of HIV infection in the United States is 0.3 to 0.4%.

AIDS Disease

0 to 12 Weeks
- Virus enters bloodstream and is cleared by lymphoid organs or spleen.
- Virus replicates to critical level in lymphoid organs.
- Burst of viremia occurs, disseminating virus throughout body.
- Partial immunologic control of virus replication occurs.

12 Weeks to 8–10 Years
- HIV evades immune system by:
  - Killing off most the HIV-specific cytotoxic T cells with an overwhelming burst of HIV antigen
  - Saturating the antigen presenting cells in lymphoid tissue with HIV antigen (these cells would otherwise help create more virus specific cytotoxic T cells)
- Clinical latency is the disease-free state when opportunistic infections do not occur, but continued decline of CD4 T cells occurs due to viral cytotoxicity.
- CD4 counts fall approximately 50 cells/μL/yr.

More than 10 Years
- CD4 count falls below critical level (usually about 200 cells/μL)
- Patient becomes highly susceptible to opportunistic diseases.
- CD4 counts may drop to < 10 cells/μL, yet patients can survive for months.
- Patient eventually succumbs to opportunistic infection or neoplasm.

Acute HIV Syndrome

- Approximately 60% experience acute viral syndrome within 3 to 6 weeks of primary infection.
- Symptoms (usually last ~1 week):
  - General: Fever, pharyngitis, lymphadenopathy, headache, lethargy, nausea, vomiting, diarrhea
  - Neuro: Meningitis, encephalitis, peripheral neuropathy
  - Dermatologic: Erythematous maculopapular rash and mucocutaneous ulceration
- Ten percent have fulminant course—clinical and immune deterioration immediately after the initial viral syndrome subsides.
- Ninety percent become asymptomatic (clinically latent phase).

AIDS Symptoms

- Clinical aspects of early symptomatic disease:
  - Generalized lymphadenopathy
  - Enlarged nodes (> 1 cm) in two or more extrainguinal sites for > 3 months
  - Differential diagnosis includes adenopathic Kaposi's sarcoma early in disease.
  - Lymph node biopsy is indicated in patients with fever, weight loss, or if nodes become more enlarged or fixed.

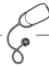

Overall rate of AIDS is declining in the United States. The decline is due in part to the increased rate of HIV reporting and the longer time period from seroconversion to AIDS since effective retroviral therapy has become available.

AIDS progression:
- Status of disease: CD4 count
- Rate of progression: viral load (measure of HIV RNA)

Loss of lymphadenopathy is a marker of disease progression.

HIGH-YIELD FACTS

Immunology

TABLE 11-3. Diseases Associated with CD4 Thresholds in AIDS

350	200	100	50
▪ Pneumococcal pneumonia	▪ Kaposi's sarcoma ▪ TB ▪ Oral thrush ▪ Oral hairy leukoplakia ▪ PCP ▪ Lymphoma	▪ Toxoplasmosis ▪ Disseminated *Candida* ▪ Cryptococcosis	▪ MAC ▪ CMV ▪ PML

PML = progressive multifocal leukoencephalopathy (JC virus)

- Oral lesions: Thrush, oral hairy leukoplakia usually occur at less than 300 CD4 cells/μL
- Reactivation herpes zoster (shingles):
  - Seen in 10 to 20% of patients
  - Usually precedes the appearance of thrush and oral hairy leukoplakia by approximately 1 year
- Thrombocytopenia:
  - Ten percent of patients with counts < 400/μL have platelet counts < 150,000/μL.
  - Most effective treatment of thrombocytopenia in HIV⁺ patients is to decrease viral load through antiretrovirals.

NEUROLOGIC DISEASE

- Opportunistic infections: Toxoplasmosis, cryptococcosis, PML, CMV, syphilis, TB,
- Neoplasms: 1° CNS lymphoma, Kaposi's sarcoma
- Result of HIV infection:
  - Aseptic meningitis, HIV encephalopathy, myelopathies, peripheral neuropathies, myopathies
  - Twenty-five percent of patients will have HIV encephalopathy (AIDS dementia complex) at some time during their course. AIDS dementia results from direct infection of neurons.

OPPORTUNISTIC INFECTIONS

- Leading cause of morbidity and mortality in HIV patients
- Specific infections occur below certain CD4 thresholds (see Table 11-3).
- Eighty percent will die as a direct result of an infection other than HIV.

PNEUMOCYSTIS CARINII PNEUMONIA (PCP)

- PCP is the initial AIDS-defining illness in 20% of patients.
- Half of patients will have at least one bout of PCP.
- PCP is most common in those with a previous episode of PCP.

Clinical Findings

- Often indolent course
- Nonproductive cough
- Retrosternal pain (worse on inspiration)
- Dyspnea on exertion
- Unexplained weight loss
- Breath sounds are usually clear
- Extrapulmonary manifestations: Acute otitis, retinitis, visceral cystic calcifications, intestinal obstruction, lymphadenopathy, bone marrow involvement, ascites, thyroiditis

Spontaneous pneumothorax complicates PCP in 2% of cases.

Diagnosis

- PaO_2 decreases, a-A gradient increases
- CXR usually normal or shows faint, bilateral interstitial infiltrate
- Lactate dehydrogenase (LDH) is often elevated
- Bronchoalveolar lavage
- Induced sputum sample
- Transbronchial biopsy

The probability of death from a single incident of PCP has decreased from 50% to 2% since effective treatment has been implemented.

Treatment

- Trimethoprim–sulfamethoxazole (TMP-SMZ):
  - Fifty to 60% have side effects including rash, fever, leukopenia, thrombocytopenia, and hepatitis
  - 21-day course
  - Patients get worse before they get better and will not improve until the end of the first week of treatment.
  - May give pentamidine for patients intolerant of TMP-SMZ
- Glucocorticoids:
  - Initiate in any AIDS patient with PCP if PaO_2 < 70 mm Hg or a-A gradient > 35 mm Hg
  - Start no later than 36 to 72 hours after starting TMP-SMZ
  - 21-day course (with subsequent taper)
  - Decreases mortality by approximately 50%
- Prophylaxis:
  - TMP-SMZ, dapsone in sulfa-allergic pts.
  - Aerosolized pentamidine for those unable to take systemic prophylaxis
  - HIV+ patients with previous episode of PCP or with CD4 < 200 cells/μL
  - Patients with history of oropharyngeal candidiasis
  - Unexplained fever (> 100.0°F) for > 2 weeks

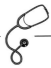

It is advisable to withhold myelotoxic drugs when treating *Pneumocystis* (AZT, ganciclovir).

TOXOPLASMOSIS

- Most common cause of secondary CNS infection in AIDS
- Seen in 15% of all AIDS patients
- Late complication
- Represents a reactivation syndrome

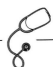

Patients on PCP prophylaxis with TMP-SMZ have a decreased incidence of toxoplasmosis.

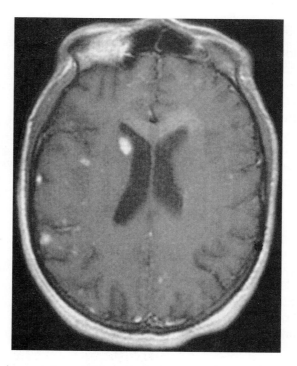

FIGURE 11-1. Toxoplasmosis in an AIDS patient. Note ring-enhancing lesions.
(Reproduced, with permission, from Lee, Rao, and Zimmerman. *Cranial MRI and CT.* New York: McGraw-Hill, 1999: 505.)

Clinical Presentation

- Fever, headache, and focal neurological deficits (90%)
- Also, seizure, hemiparesis, and aphasia occur

Diagnosis

- Magnetic resonance imaging (MRI) or head computed tomography (CT) with contrast shows **multiple ring-enhancing lesions** (see Figure 11-1)
- IgG antibodies to *Toxoplasma*

Treatment

- Pyrimethamine and sulfadiazine: Leukopenia is the major side effect (treat leukopenia with folinic acid).
- Lifelong treatment for toxoplasmosis is necessary, due to relapse rate of 50% within 6 months.
- No prophylactic regimen with an acceptable side effect profile exists.

PROTOZOAL DIARRHEA

Etiology

Cryptosporidia, microsporidia, and *Isospora belli* are the most common agents.

Treatment

- Cryptosporidia and microsporidia: Symptomatic treatment
- *Isospora:* TMP-SMZ

MYCOBACTERIUM AVIUM COMPLEX (MAC)

Epidemiology

- In the United States, disseminated *Mycobacterium avium* is the most common cause of death due to AIDS.
- Median survival after MAC diagnosis is 6 to 8 months.

Symptoms

- Fever
- Weight loss
- Night sweats
- Lymphadenopathy
- Abdominal pain
- Diarrhea

Diagnosis

- 85% of MAC patients have mycobacteremia
- Alkaline phosphatase level often elevated
- Long, slender, acid-fast bacilli (AFB) seen in biopsy specimens or sputum
- CXR: 25% have bilateral lower lobe interstitial infiltrate.
- Blood culture confirms diagnosis (turns positive within 2 weeks)

Typical scenario:
A 29-year-old HIV+ patient presents with CD4 count of 100, unexplained fever, and elevated alkaline phosphatase. *Think: MAC.*

Treatment

- Clarithromycin and ethambutol
- Prophylaxis: Rifabutin when CD4 drops below 100

TUBERCULOSIS

See respiratory chapter for full description.

Epidemiology

- Very common in AIDS patients (approximately 5%)
- HIV increases risk of developing active TB 15 to 30 times.
- HIV disease progresses more rapidly in patients with active TB.

OTHER BACTERIAL INFECTIONS IN AIDS

HIV patients are prone to infection with encapsulated organisms because of impaired B cell function.

FUNGAL INFECTIONS

Candidiasis

- *Candida* infections are the most common fungal infections in HIV+ patients, and virtually all patients experience some form of *Candida* infection during their illness.
- Infections occur early: They are often the first sign of immunosuppression.

THRUSH

- Very early finding in immunocompromise
- White, cheesy exudates on posterior oropharynx
- Pseudohyphae detectable on wet-mount KOH preps

AIDS-DEFINING *CANDIDA* INFECTIONS

- *Candida* infections of lungs, esophagus, trachea, and bronchi
- Esophagitis is most common:
  - Presents with retrosternal pain and odynophagia
  - Diagnosed with upper GI endoscopy

TREATMENT

- Oral and vaginal candida: Topical nystatin or clotrimazole troches
- Severe cases can be treated with systemic therapy (oral ketoconazole or fluconazole)

Cryptococcosis

- *Cryptococcus neoformans* is the leading cause of meningitis in AIDS patients.
- 12% of AIDS patients
- Serious, life-threatening infection

SIGNS AND SYMPTOMS

Subacute Meningoencephalitis
- Fever (virtually all patients)
- Nausea and vomiting (40%)
- Altered mental status
- Headache
- Meningeal signs

DIAGNOSIS

- Cryptococcomas: Seen as multiple ring-enhancing lesions on MRI
- Pulmonary disease shows interstitial pattern on CXR.

- CSF or serum cryptococcal antigen
- Identification of organisms on India ink stain of CSF
- Positive culture of *C. neoformans* from any site

TREATMENT

- Amphotericin B for 6 weeks in combination with flucytosine
- Since 50% of patients relapse after therapy is stopped, fluconazole should be given indefinitely.

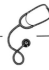

Fluconazole prophylaxis can be given to all patients once CD4 < 100/μL to prevent both cryptococcosis and candidal infections.

VIRAL INFECTIONS

Cytomegalovirus (CMV)

- Ninety-five percent of HIV⁺ patients are CMV positive, and clinical syndromes most often represent reactivation of latent infection (see Figure 11-2).
- CMV retinitis:
  - 25 to 30% of HIV⁺ patients
  - Presents with painless, progressive vision loss; may complain of "floaters"
  - Diagnosis: Funduscopy shows perivascular hemorrhage and exudates
  - Clinical course/complications: Vision loss is irreversible; may be complicated by retinal detachment
  - Treatment:
    - Ganciclovir (ocular implants can be used)

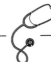

Ganciclovir causes bone marrow suppression and cannot be given with TMP-SMZ or AZT.

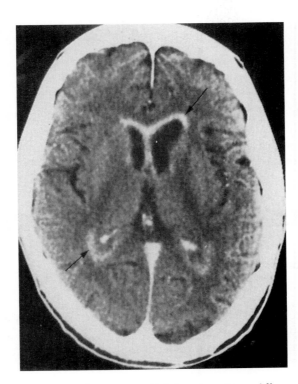

FIGURE 11-2. Cytomegalovirus infection in an AIDS patient. Note diffuse periventricular enhancement.

(Reproduced, with permission, from Lee, Rao, and Zimmerman. Cranial MRI and CT. New York: McGraw-Hill, 1999.)

Foscarnet is associated with electrolyte disorders.

- ■ Foscarnet
  - ■ Works in 80 to 90% of patients
  - ■ Recurrence is common; maintenance therapy with foscarnet
- ■ CMV also causes esophagitis and colitis.
- ■ CMV Ab-negative patients should receive blood products from CMV negative donors if at all possible.

Herpes Simplex (HSV)

- ■ HSV in HIV manifests as recurrent orolabial, genital, and perianal lesions.
- ■ Can cause herpetic esophagitis (beefy red and painful esophagus)
- ■ Can cause recurrent herpetic whitlow (painful nodular lesions usually found on fingers)
- ■ Treat with acyclovir, famciclovir, or valacyclovir.

Typical scenario: An HIV+ patient presents with a painful, poorly healing, perirectal lesion. *Think: HSV.*

Varicella-Zoster (VZV)

- ■ Shingles:
  - ■ Reactivation of latent infection
  - ■ Usually an early complication of HIV
  - ■ Painful, vesicular skin eruptions
  - ■ Extensive involvement of several dermatomes
  - ■ Treatment with acyclovir may shorten course of disease.
- ■ Primary VZV infection (chickenpox) may be *lethal* in the HIV patient: Treat aggressively with acyclovir and hyperimmune globulin.
- ■ Acute retinal necrosis syndrome:
  - ■ Pain, keratitis, and iritis
  - ■ Associated with trigeminal VZV or orolabial HSV
  - ■ Fundus exam shows widespread, pale gray peripheral lesions
  - ■ Often complicated by retinal detachment

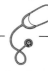

Shingles in any patient under 50 years of age mandates workup for underlying immunodeficiency.

Hepatitis

- ■ Ninety-five percent of HIV+ patients have serologic evidence of HBV or HCV infection.
- ■ Patients with HBV and HIV have less severe inflammatory liver disease because of immunosuppression.

NEOPLASTIC DISEASE AND HIV

Kaposi's Sarcoma

EPIDEMIOLOGY

- ■ Incidence has been decreasing since first recognized as an HIV-associated neoplasm
- ■ 96% of HIV-associated cases occur in homosexual men

CLINICAL FINDINGS

- ■ Multiple vascular nodules appearing in the skin, mucous membranes, and viscera

HIV-associated malignancies:
- ■ HHV-6,8: Kaposi's sarcoma
- ■ HPV: Cervical CA
- ■ HBV: Hepatocellular CA

- Appearance is purplish macular or papular nodule on skin, or discoloration of the oral mucosa
- Lesions often occur in sun-exposed areas.
- Pulmonary involvement can occur; presents as shortness of breath
- May be seen with a normal CD4 count

Diagnosis

Biopsy of suspicious lesion reveals spindle cells, endothelial cells, and extravasation of red blood cells.

TREATMENT

- Indicated when a single or multiple lesions are causing significant pain or discomfort and for lesions in the posterior oropharynx that interfere with swallowing
- Localized irradiation
- Intralesional vinblastine
- Cryotherapy effective in some cases

Lymphomas

EPIDEMIOLOGY

- Six percent of patients develop lymphoma at some point during their disease.
- 120-fold increased incidence in HIV compared with general population
- Three main types occur in HIV:
  - Grade III or IV immunoblastic (60%)
  - Burkitt's lymphoma (20%)
  - Primary CNS lymphoma (20%)

Most are B cell lymphomas (T cells too compromised).

CLINICAL PRESENTATION

- Dependent on the site of tumor
- Persistent unexplained fever
- Focal seizures
- Rapidly growing mass lesion in the oral mucosa
- 80% have extranodal disease

TREATMENT

- Standard intensive regimens have been abandoned due to low response rate.
- Patient's with higher CD4 counts do better with chemotherapy than do those with lower counts.
- Primary CNS lymphoma has the poorest prognosis, though none of the HIV-associated lymphomas have favorable prognoses.

TREATMENT OF HIV INFECTION

General Patient Management

- Disease necessitates patient education about complications, transmission, and prognosis.

- All patients with HIV (especially those with CD4 counts < 200) should designate an individual with durable power of attorney.

Initial and Follow-Up Studies

- Routine chemistry, CBC, and CXR
- CD4 counts
- Two separate HIV RNA levels
- VDRL (Venereal Disease Research Laboratory)
- Anti-Toxoplasma Ab titer
- Purified protein derivative (PPD) skin test
- Mini mental status exam

Antiretroviral Therapy

- Major drug classes for HIV therapy are reverse transcriptase inhibitors (nucleoside analogs and non-nucleoside) and protease inhibitors.
- Nucleoside analog reverse transcriptase inhibitors:
  - Zidovudine (AZT):
    - First drug approved for HIV treatment
    - Acts as DNA chain terminator
    - Most appropriately used as part of combination retroviral therapy for patients with CD4 counts < 500
    - Also used as monotherapy for prevention of maternal–fetal transmission of HIV
    - Side effects:
      - Headache, malaise, nausea, fatigue (often subside with extended therapy)
      - Macrocytic anemia secondary to low erythropoietin (can be managed with recombinant erythropoietin injections)
      - Proximal myopathy
  - Lamivudine (3TC):
    - Licensed only for use in combination with AZT
    - Strains of HIV that are resistant to lamivudine are sensitive to zidovudine
    - Toxicities: Pancreatitis, peripheral neuropathies
- Non-nucleoside reverse transcriptase inhibitors:
  - Nevirapine and delavirdine
  - Bind to reverse transcriptase outside the active site and cause conformational changes that decrease enzyme activity
  - Monotherapy causes rapid resistance
  - Main toxicity is maculopapular rash
- Protease inhibitors:
  - Saquinavir, ritonavir, indinavir, nelfinavir inhibit the activity of HIV protease.
  - Less toxic than the reverse transcriptase inhibitors
  - Monotherapy results in rapid emergence of drug-resistant strains:
    - Indinavir:
      - Main side effects are nephrolithiasis and asymptomatic indirect hyperbilirubinemia

Combination zidovudine and lamivudine (Combivir) is the most potent *(in vitro)* combination of nucleosides.

Lamivudine is one of the best tolerated nucleoside analogs.

- Indinavir is potent and well-tolerated compared to saquinavir and ritonavir.

TREATMENT RECOMMENDATIONS

- Initiate therapy with two nucleoside reverse transcriptase inhibitors (AZT, 3TC) and a protease inhibitor (indinavir) in any one of these conditions:
  - Symptomatic
  - Plasma HIV RNA > 20,000 copies/mL
  - CD4 count < 500
  - Disease is progressing.

Dermatology

Robin R. Blum

TOP CAUSES OF RASH WITH FEVER

- Rubella
- Measles
- Staphylococcal scalded syndrome
- **Toxic shock syndrome**
- Scarlet fever
- **Meningococcemia**
- **Disseminated gonococcal infection**
- **Bacterial endocarditis**
- **Rocky Mountain spotted fever (RMSF)**
- Kawasaki's disease
- **Erythema nodosum**
- **Hypersensitivity vasculitis**

Rashes that can be seen on palms and soles: **Mrs. E**
- **Meningococcemia**
- **RMSF**
- **Syphilis**
- **Erythema multiforme**

TOXIC SHOCK SYNDROME (TSS)

Definition

A toxin-mediated disease characterized by acute onset of fever, hypotension, diarrhea, and generalized skin and mucous erythema, followed by failure of multiple organ systems.

Epidemiology

- Ages 20 to 30
- Increased incidence in women using high-absorbency tampons, and in patients with burns, ulcers, surgical wounds, and nasal packs

Etiology

- *Staphylococcus aureus* producing TSS toxin-1 (TSST-1)
- Group A beta-hemolytic streptococci (rare)

Signs and Symptoms

- Acute onset of fever, hypotension, tingling sensation in hands and feet, myalgia, headache, confusion, disorientation, and diarrhea.
- A generalized erythematous macular eruption occurs most intensely at affected site followed by desquamation of palms and soles 1 to 2 weeks after onset of illness with edema of face, hands, and feet.
- Erythema of oral mucosa, bulbar conjunctiva, vagina, and tympanic membrane

Diagnosis

Centers for Disease Control and Prevention (CDC) Criteria for Diagnosis

- Fever > 102 F
- Hypotension (systolic blood pressure < 90 mm Hg for adults or an orthostatic decrease in blood pressure > 15 mm Hg)
- Involvement of three or more of the following organ systems:
  1. Gastrointestinal: vomiting or diarrhea at onset of illness
  2. Muscular: myalgia or creatine phosphokinase (CPK) > 2 times upper limit of normal
  3. Mucous membrane: vaginal, oropharyngeal, and conjunctival hyperemia
  4. Renal: blood urea nitrogen (BUN) or creatinine > 2 times upper limit of normal, or 5 WBC/HPF
  5. Hepatic: total bilirubin, SGOT, SGPT > 2 times upper limit of normal
  6. Hematologic: platelets < 100,000/μL
  7. Central nervous system (CNS): disorientation or alteration in consciousness
- Gram stain reveals gram positive cocci in clusters.
- Culture grows TSST-1–producing staphylococcus.

Treatment

- Admission to intensive care unit
- Removal of potential foreign bodies
- IV anti-staphylococcus antibiotics
- Management of organ system failure

MENINGOCOCCEMIA

Definition

A potentially fatal disease resulting from meningococcal bacteremia

Epidemiology

- Highest incidence in 6 months to 1-year-old children
- Increased incidence in alcoholics, asplenic, and complement-deficient patients

Etiology

Neisseria meningitidis

Signs and Symptoms

- Prodrome of spiking fever, cough, headache, sore throat, nausea, and vomiting followed by chills, arthralgias, myalgias, and hypotension
- Patients appear **acutely ill** and **listless.**
- Seventy-five percent of patients have discrete **pink macules, papules,** and **petechiae,** which can be distributed over trunk, extremities, and palate (see Figure 12-1), (see Table 12-1 for definitions of primary skin lesions).
- With fulminant disease, patients have **purpura,** ecchymosis, and confluent area of gray-black necrosis.
- Signs of meningeal irritation

Diagnosis

- Blood cultures reveal meningococci 100% of the time.
- Cerebrospinal fluid (CSF) culture is usually positive.
- Skin biopsy cultures are positive 85% of the time.
- Gram stain reveals gram-negative diplococci.

Complications

- Meningitis (50 to 90%)
- Waterhouse–Friderichsen syndrome (fulminant meningococcemia with adrenal hemorrhage)

Treatment

- Admission to intensive care unit
- Vancomycin and ceftriaxone IV at first clinical suspicion of meningococcemia.

> Meningococcemia is fatal if untreated. Treat empirically prior to completion of tests if suspected on clinical grounds.

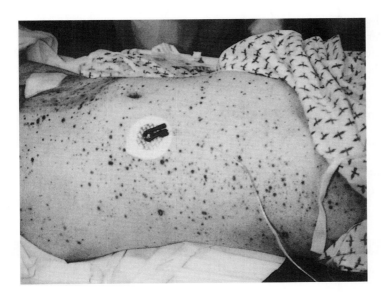

FIGURE 12-1. Meningococcemia.

(Reproduced, with permission, from Knoop, Stack, and Storrow. *Atlas of Emergency Medicine.* New York: McGraw-Hill, 1997: 404.)

Definition

A sexually transmitted infection characterized by fever, petechial lesions, and arthralgia, following hematogenous dissemination from mucosal sites

Epidemiology

Increased incidence among young, sexually active people

Etiology

Neisseria gonorrhea

Signs and Symptoms

- Prodrome of fever, malaise, anorexia, and chills
- Erythematous macules over arms and legs evolve into hemorrhagic painful pustules within 2 to 3 days.
- Tenosynovitis—erythema, edema, and tenderness along acral tendon sheaths
- Asymmetric, red, hot, tender joint of knee, elbow, ankle, hand, shoulder, or hip

Diagnosis

- Confirmed by culture of gonococcus from mucosal site
- Gram stain reveals gram-negative diplococci.

Complications

- Hepatitis
- Perihepatitis (Fitz-Hugh–Curtis syndrome)
- Endocarditis
- Meningitis

Treatment

- Hospitalization for initial therapy
- Ceftriaxone, cefotaxime, or ceftizoxime for 24 to 48 hours. Switch to outpatient cefixime or ciprofloxacin for 1 week.
- Treat presumptively for concurrent *Chlamydia trachomatis*.

Covered in cardiovascular chapter

Typical scenario:
A 20-year-old college student has a low-grade fever, chills, and migratory polyarthralgias accompanied by a tender rash. The rash initially consisted of erythematous macules that have now evolved into hemorrhagic pustules. *Think: Disseminated gonococcal infection.*

HIGH-YIELD FACTS

Dermatology

Definition

- A potentially life-threatening disease due to a tick bite
- The infected tick adheres to vascular endothelium, resulting in vascular necrosis and extravasation of blood.

Epidemiology

- Highest incidence in children aged 5 to 10 years old.
- Ninety-five percent of cases occur from April through September.
- Occurs only in the Western hemisphere, primarily in southeastern states and most often in Oklahoma, North and South Carolina, and Tennessee
- Rarely occurs in the Rocky Mountains
- Only 60% of patients report a history of a tick bite.

Etiology

Rickettsia rickettsii, transmitted via female *Dermacentor* tick

Signs and Symptoms

- Sudden onset of high **fever,** myalgia, severe headache, rigors, nausea, and photophobia within first 2 days of tick bite.
- Fifty percent develop rash within 3 days. Another 30% develop the rash within 6 days.
- Rash consists of 2- to 6-mm pink **blanchable macules** that first appear peripherally on wrists, forearms, ankles, **palms,** and **soles** (see Figure 12-2).

RMSF rash spreads from extremities to trunk.

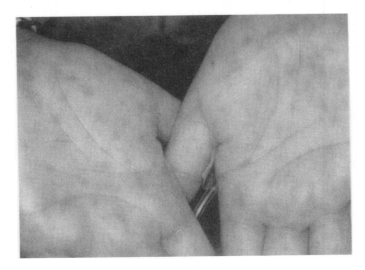

FIGURE 12-2. Rocky Mountain spotted fever.

(Reproduced, with permission, from Fauci, et al. *Harrison's Principles of Internal Medicine,* 14th ed. New York: McGraw-Hill, 1998:10–48.)

- Within 6 to 18 hours the exanthem spreads centrally to trunk, proximal extremities, and face.
- Within 1 to 3 days the macules evolve to deep red papules, and within 2 to 4 days the exanthem is hemorrhagic and no longer blanchable.
- Up to 15% have no rash.
- Many patients have exquisite tenderness of the gastrocnemius muscle.

Diagnosis

- Indirect fluorescent antibody (IFA) assay:
  - Titer > 1:64 is diagnostic.
  - Most sensitive and specific test
- Other, less sensitive tests include:
  - Indirect hemagglutinin, Weil–Felix, complement fixation, and latex agglutination tests
- Biopsy would demonstrate necrotizing vasculitis.

In real time, RMSF is a clinical diagnosis (because current diagnostic tests aren't back fast enough). It is important not to delay treatment.

Complications

Some patients develop long-term sequelae lasting > 1 year, including paraparesis, hearing loss, peripheral neuropathy, bladder/bowel incontinence, and cerebellar, vestibular, and motor dysfunction.

Treatment

- Most patients, except those with very mild disease, require intravenous antibiotics.
- Doxycycline considered drug of choice
- Chloramphenicol for pregnant patients, children younger than 8 years (due to concern of staining the teeth), and severe disease
- Treatment is continued until patient is afebrile for 48 hours.

A delay in treatment of RMSF is associated with increased morbidity and mortality. Increased risk of death with delayed diagnosis and older age of patient.

ERYTHEMA NODOSUM

Definition

- An inflammatory disorder of subcutaneous fat (panniculitis) characterized by painful erythematous nodules on lower legs
- Thought to be an immunological reaction precipitated by multiple etiologies

Epidemiology

Occurs more often in women, age 15 to 30

Etiology

- Forty percent of cases are idiopathic.
- Drugs: Sulfonamides, oral contraceptives

- Infectious: Streptococci, tuberculosis, leprosy, histoplasmosis, coccidiomycosis, blastomycosis, *Chlamydia*, *Yersinia*
- Autoimmune: Sarcoidosis, inflammatory bowel disease, Behçet's disease

Signs and Symptoms

- Fever, malaise, and arthralgias
- Painful, deep-seated, indurated erythematous nodules scattered over lower legs, bilaterally but not symmetrically
- May also occur on forearms, thighs, or any other area with fat

Diagnosis

Confirmed by a careful history and laboratory evaluation including a complete blood count (CBC), throat culture, antistreptolysin-O titre, and chest x-ray

Treatment

- Removal and/or treatment of causative agent
- Bed rest and elevation of legs
- Anti-inflammatory medication for pain
- Systemic corticosteroids (only if etiology is known)

HYPERSENSITIVITY (LEUKOCYTOCLASTIC) VASCULITIS

Definition

- A group of vasculitides in which immune complexes lodge in small blood vessels, resulting in inflammation, fibrinoid necrosis, and painful, palpable purpura
- Patients have a hypersensitivity to antigens in the immune complex: Drugs, infectious agents, or other sources.
- Henoch–Schönlein is a classic example.

Henoch–Schönlein purpura:
- Associated with strep infection + penicillin
- Small-vessel vasculitis
- Purpura of lower extremities and buttocks
- Abdominal pain
- IgA deposits in glomeruli
- More common in children

Signs and Symptoms

- Pruritus and pain, associated with fever and malaise
- **"Palpable purpura"**—multiple, scattered nonblanchable red papules distributed over lower extremities, arms, and buttocks (see Figure 12-3)
- May be crusted due to necrosis of tissue overlying the blood vessel

Diagnosis

American College of Rheumatology criteria for diagnosis includes at least three of the following:

1. Age > 16 at disease onset (development of symptoms)
2. Medication taken at disease onset
3. Palpable purpura
4. Maculopapular rash
5. Biopsy demonstrating eosinophilic material (fibrinoid) deposited in venule walls and necrotic vessel walls

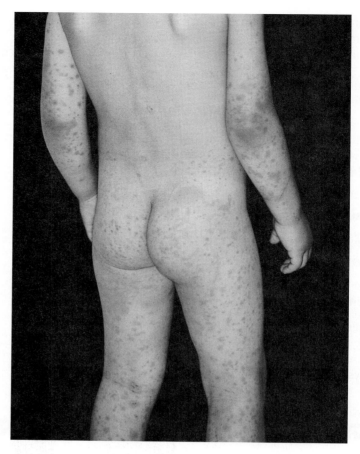

FIGURE 12-3. Henoch–Schönlein purpura.
(Reproduced, with permission, from Knoop, Stack, and Storrow. *Atlas of Emergency Medicine.* New York: McGraw-Hill, 1997: 345.)

Complications

Renal insufficiency, bowel ischemia, central nervous system (CNS) involvement

Treatment

- Eliminate and/or treat causative agent
- Systemic corticosteroids
- Immunosuppressive agents (cyclophosphamide or azathioprine)

SKIN CANCERS

BASAL CELL CARCINOMA

Definition

- The most common type of skin cancer due to a malignancy of the epidermal basal cells
- Basal cells invade locally but almost never metastasize.

Epidemiology

> 40 years of age. Occurs mainly in white males.

Risk Factors

- Fair-skinned people with poor tanning capacity
- Chronic sun exposure
- Radiation therapy

Signs and Symptoms

Physical exam is variable, depending on type of basal cell cancer:
- Nodular type: A single translucent waxy nodule or papule with telangiectasias and a rolled border, distributed on face and neck. May develop central necrosis with adherent crust (rodent ulcer).
- Superficial spreading type: Multiple erythematous scaly plaques with a well-defined border distributed primarily on trunk, with no relation to sun exposure
- Sclerosing type: Yellowish white sclerotic waxy plaques with poorly defined borders, resembling scar tissue or morphea
- Pigmented type: May have any of the above characteristics with pigmentation and is easily confused with malignant melanoma

Typical scenario:
A 47-year-old white male presents with pearly, painless, ulcerated nodules with overlying telangiectasias.
Think: Basal cell carcinoma.

Diagnosis

Clinical, confirmed by biopsy that reveals a palisading pattern of cells at the tumor's periphery

Treatment

Depends on type and location:
- Curettage and desiccation
- Surgical excision
- Radiation therapy (if surgery is contraindicated)
- Regular follow-up to detect recurrences

Definition

- A tumor of malignant keratinocytes accounting for the second most frequent type of skin cancer
- Growth may arise de novo, from an actinic keratosis, or from an underlying skin lesion.
- Lesions arising from an actinic keratosis have the least potential of metastasizing.

Epidemiology

> 55 years of age, commonly occurs in men, people with sun exposure, and outdoor workers

Risk Factors

- Sun and x-ray exposure
- Radiation therapy
- Tar, pitch, mineral oil, or arsenic exposure
- Immunosuppression
- Topical nitrogen mustard
- Human papillomavirus (HPV) infection
- Xeroderma pigmentosum.

Signs and Symptoms

- An erythematous scaling plaque that may be eroded or ulcerated with crust
- Hyperkeratotic center
- Distributed primarily on sun exposed skin of lips, cheeks, helix of ears, scalp, and dorsum of hand

Diagnosis

Clinical, confirmed by biopsy demonstrating malignant keratinocytes invading the dermis with keratin pearls

Treatment

- Surgical excision
- Radiotherapy (if surgery is contraindicated)

Definition

- A malignant proliferation of melanocytes (pigment cells), accounting for 3% of all cancers

- May arise from normal-appearing skin (70%) or from a preexisting melanocytic nevi (mole) or skin lesion (30%)

Pathophysiology

- Characterized by two different growth phases: horizontal and vertical
- During the horizontal growth phase there is lateral extension within the epidermis and dermis, without metastasizing.
- When the tumor enters the vertical phase, it penetrates downward into the dermis, with a high risk of metastasis.
- Prognosis is based on the thickness of the primary tumor, measured histologically according to the depth of invasion from the surface to the deepest part of the tumor (Breslow's classification) or according to the depth of penetration in relation to the different layers of the dermis (Clark's classification).

Melanomas can be brown, black, white, or blue.

Epidemiology

Incidence has been increasing worldwide, possibly related to increased exposure to sunlight.

Risk Factors

- Sunlight exposure
- Fair skin
- Positive family history (5%)

Signs and Symptoms

Commonly recognized clinical variants of melanoma include:

1. *Superficial spreading melanoma*—accounts for 70% of melanomas and is characterized by a prolonged horizontal growth phase. May develop as a new mole or as a change in a preexisting mole. During its horizontal growth phase, it appears as an elevated plaque with irregular borders and variegated colors, but it evolves into a nodule with bleeding and ulceration during its vertical phase.
2. *Nodular melanoma*—accounts for 15% of melanomas and is characterized only by a vertical growth phase. Develops as a blue, gray, or black papule or nodule that may ulcerate or bleed. Associated with a poor prognosis because metastasizes early.
3. *Lentigo maligna melanoma*—accounts for 10% of melanomas and occurs on sun exposed areas of the skin in elderly patients. During its vertical growth phase it develops as a slow growing macule that gradually forms irregular borders, indistinct edges, or variable shades of color. May be present for years as a macule (lentigo maligna) before development of melanoma.
4. *Acral lentiginous melanoma*—accounts for < 5% of melanomas, and is common in black and Asian people. Develops as a flat, variably pigmented macule on the palms, soles, and nail beds that enlarges peripherally during its horizontal growth phase, and becomes nodular during its vertical growth phase.

Suspicious features of malignant melanoma include the ABCDEE's:
- **Asymmetry**
- **Border (irregular)**
- **Color (variegated and mottled)**
- **Diameter (> 0.6 cm)**
- **Elevation**
- **Enlargement**

Diagnosis

Clinical, based on change in size and color or development of bleeding and ulceration

Treatment

- Surgical excision with margins of at least 1 cm, depending on depth of lesion
- Follow-up

Prognosis

Bad Prognostic Factors
- Tumors with a prolonged vertical growth phase
- Proximal tumors
- Palpable nodes

Good Prognostic Factors
- Tumors with < 0.76 mm in depth have almost a 100% cure rate.
- Women have a better prognosis than men.

PAPULOSQUAMOUS REACTIONS

PSORIASIS

Definition

- A chronic, noninfectious hyperproliferative inflammatory disorder characterized by thick adherent scales (see Table 12-2 for definitions of secondary skin lesions)
- Presents with multiple exacerbations and remissions

Pathophysiology

Increased epidermal cell proliferation due to a shortened epithelial cell cycle results in keratinization defects, forming thick adherent scales.

Psoriasis is worse in winter.

Epidemiology

Affects 1 to 3% of the population. Common among ages 15 to 40. Rare under the age of 10. Forty percent have a positive family history.

Risk Factors

Trauma, infection, emotional stress, and drugs (lithium, beta blockers, iodine, and antimalarials)

Signs and Symptoms

- Mild pruritus
- Well demarcated, thick, "salmon-pink" **plaques** with an adherent silver-white scale
- Distributed bilaterally over **extensor surface** of extremities, often on elbows and knees, and trunk and scalp
- Nails are commonly involved: Pitting of nails, oil spots (yellow-brown spots under nail plate), onycholysis (separation of distal nail plate from nail bed), subungual hyperkeratosis (thickening of epidermis under nail plate)
- Can occur at site of injury (Koebner phenomenon)
- Pinpoint capillary bleeding occurs if scale is removed (Auspitz sign).

Typical scenario:
A 35-year-old has salmon colored papules covered with silvery white scale on his scalp, elbows, and knees. *Think: Psoriasis.*

Complications

Psoriatic arthritis, a destructive arthritis of the distal interphalangeal joints of hands and feet **(rheumatoid factor negative)**

Treatment

For mild psoriasis, the following can be applied to plaques:
- Topical coal tar or anthralin (inhibit DNA synthesis)
- Topical corticosteroids
- Calcipotriene (Dovonex is a synthetic vitamin D analog that decreases cellular proliferation)
- Combination therapy

Psoriasis is a chronic disease and complete remission is often not achieved. Goal is to decrease scale and achieve a better cosmetic result.

If the plaques fail to improve, or if psoriasis is extensive and affects > 20% of body surface area, systemic treatment should be implemented:
- UV B phototherapy
- PUVA (psoralen + UV A; psoralen is taken orally 1 to 2 hours prior to UV exposure and is photoactivated in the skin by UV radiation)
- Retinoids (etretinate, tazarotene, acitretin)
- Methotrexate (inhibits DNA synthesis)
- Combination therapy of retinoids or methotrexate with PUVA
- Cyclosporine

PITYRIASIS ROSEA

Definition

A common self-limiting eruption of a **single herald patch** followed by a generalized secondary eruption within 2 weeks.

Epidemiology

Affects children and young adults, primarily ages 10 to 35. Clusters of cases in spring and fall.

Typical scenario:
A young person presents with a pruritic, spotted rash on the trunk that began as one solitary larger patch. *Think: Pityriasis rosea.*

Signs and Symptoms

- Mild pruritus
- 2 to 10 cm solitary, oval erythematous "herald plaque" with a collarette of scale precedes the generalized eruption in 80% of patients
- Within days, multiple smaller pink oval scaly patches appear over trunk and upper extremities.
- Secondary eruption occurs in a Christmas tree distribution, oriented parallel to the ribs.

Treatment

Symptomatic. No treatment shortens disease course:
- Cool baths
- Calamine lotion
- Topical corticosteroids
- Oral antihistamines
- UV B phototherapy or sunlight

LYME BORRELIOSIS (LYME DISEASE)

Definition

- A multisystem disease transmitted by the bite of an *Ixodes* genus deer tick infected with a spirochete
- Characterized by three stages of disease: localized, disseminated, and chronic
- Patients are often unaware of tick bite.

Etiology

Borrelia burgdorferi

Epidemiology

- More frequent in late May through early fall
- Increased prevalence in Northeast and North Central regions, primarily Connecticut, Rhode Island, New York, New Jersey, Delaware, and Pennsylvania

Lyme disease: If untreated, lesions fade within 28 days. If treated adequately, lesions fade within days and the late manifestations of the disease are prevented. If delayed diagnosis, may have permanent neurologic or joint disabilities.

Signs and Symptoms

History—acute onset of fever, chills, myalgia, weakness, headache, and photophobia
Symptoms—local burning, itching, or pain
Physical exam:
- **Erythema chronicum migrans** (ECM) develops at site of tick bite in 75% of patients within 1 month (an expanding erythematous annular plaque with a central clearing) (see Figure 12-4).
- Usually affects the trunk, proximal extremities, axilla, and inguinal area

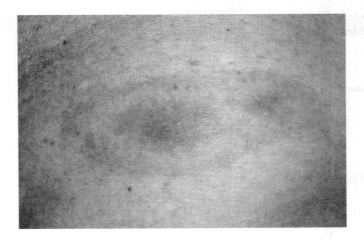

FIGURE 12-4. Erythema chronicum migrans rash of Lyme disease.
(Reproduced, with permission, from Fauci et al. *Harrison's Principles of Internal Medicine,* 14th ed. New York: McGraw-Hill, 1998: 10–47.)

- May have multiple ECM lesions if multiple tick bites present
- Fifteen percent of patients develop secondary annular lesions that resemble ECM but are smaller and migrate less.

Diagnosis

- Clinical, confirmed by serology
- IgM titers are elevated in acute disease and peak 3 to 6 weeks after exposure.
- IgG levels peak when arthritis develops.
- An elevated IgG titer in absence of an elevated IgM indicates prior exposure as opposed to recent infection.
- May have false-negative results in first 2 to 4 weeks and false-positive results with other spirochetal infection and in patients with some autoimmune disorders (systemic lupus erythematosus, rheumatoid arthritis).
- PCR can detect spirochete DNA in CSF and synovial fluid. Forty percent of skin biopsies reveal spirochetes.

Complications

- Sixty percent of untreated cases with disseminated infection develop arthritis (mediated by immune complex formation) 4 to 6 weeks following tick bite.
- May also develop neurologic (meningitis, encephalitis, or Bell's palsy) and cardiac involvement (carditis, atrioventricular block)

Treatment

Amoxicillin or doxycycline

Definition

An acute onset of superficial spreading cellulitis, arising in inconspicuous breaks in skin (see Figure 12-5)

Etiology

Group A beta-hemolytic *Streptococcus pyogenes*

Epidemiology

Increased incidence in young children and older adults

Signs and Symptoms

- Local pain and tenderness
- An erythematous, shiny area of warm and tender skin with a well demarcated and indurated advancing border
- Less edematous than cellulitis, but margins are more sharply demarcated and elevated
- Face is most commonly involved, but can affect any area, especially sites of chronic edema.

Diagnosis

Gram stain reveals gram-positive cocci in chains.

Treatment

Penicillin: If allergic, use a cephalosporin, macrolide, or vancomycin.

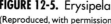

Erysipelas: High morbidity rate if untreated.

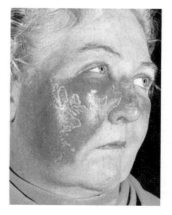

FIGURE 12-5. Erysipelas.

(Reproduced, with permission, from Fauci et al. *Harrison's Principles of Internal Medicine,* 14th ed. New York: McGraw-Hill, 1998: 10–34.)

Definition

An acute deep infection of dermis and subcutaneous tissue characterized by erythema, tenderness, and warmth of involved area.

Etiology

- *Staphylococcus aureus*
- Group A beta-hemolytic *Streptococcus pyogenes*
- *Hemophilus influenzae*

Risk Factors

- Injury to affected area such as abrasions, burns, surgical wounds, lymphadenectomy, mucosal infections, bites, tattoos, nail cutting, acupuncture, etc.
- Underlying dermatosis
- Drug and alcohol abuse
- Immunocompromised states

Signs and Symptoms

- Warmth and tenderness of infected site
- Erythematous, edematous, **shiny area of warm and tender skin** with poorly demarcated, **nonelevated** borders
- Usually overlying site of wound or trauma
- Lower leg is more frequently involved due to interdigital tinea.

Diagnosis

Confirmed by Gram stain demonstrating gram-positive cocci in clusters or chains. Culture of lesion or blood will be positive only 25% of the time.

Treatment

Penicillin: If penicillin allergic or methicillin-resistant *S. aureus* (MRSA), use vancomycin or cephalosporins. For *H. influenzae*, use cefotaxime or ceftriaxone.

Definition

- Any pressure-induced ulcer that occurs secondary to external compression of the skin, resulting in ischemic tissue necrosis
- May extend to underlying subcutaneous tissue, muscle, joints, or bones
- Fifty percent of ulcers are hospital-acquired and usually develop within the first 2 weeks of hospitalization.

Erysipelas, erysipeloid, and necrotizing fasciitis are variants of cellulitis.

Typical scenario:
A 54-year-old insulin-dependent diabetic male presents with a warm, erythematous, slightly tender rash with poorly demarcated borders that began on his calf yesterday and has now spread up his leg. *Think: Cellulitis.*

HIGH-YIELD FACTS

Dermatology

A detailed history is particularly important to reveal the portal of entry in cellulitis.

Decubitus ulcers are also called bedsores and pressure ulcers.

Etiology

Pressure induces ischemia and tissue necrosis.

Risk Factors

- Immobility, fracture
- Malnutrition
- Age > 70
- Hypoalbuminemia
- Spinal cord injury
- Fecal incontinence
- Diabetes mellitus (DM)
- Inadequate nursing care
- Decreased level of consciousness

Decubitus ulcers develop over bony prominences: sacrum, ischial tuberosities, iliac crests, greater trochanters, heels, elbows, knees, occiput. Can develop at any site that can be compressed against a hard surface.

Signs and Symptoms

- Appearance depends on extent of damage.
- Localized, blanchable erythema develops prior to ulcer formation.
- Early ulcers have irregular, ragged borders, but chronic ulcers have smooth, well-demarcated borders.
- Eschar represents devitalized tissue at the base. Purulent exudate surrounding the ulcer suggests an infection.

Stages

I—nonblanching erythema of intact skin
II—partial-thickness skin loss involving epidermis and/or dermis (superficial ulcer)
III—full-thickness skin loss involving epidermis and dermis (deep, crateriform ulcer). May involve damage to subcutaneous tissue, extending down to but not through fascia.
IV—full-thickness skin loss with extensive damage to muscle, bone, or other supporting structures

Diagnosis

- Elevated WBC and erythrocyte sedimentation rate (ESR) suggest an underlying infection (osteomyelitis, bacteremia).
- Wound culture can be used to differentiate infection from colonization.
- Culture of base detects only surface bacteria; therefore, recommend deep punch biopsy for optimal culture.
- Infection is usually polymicrobial: *S. aureus, Streptococcus, Pseudomonas, Enterococcus, Proteus, Clostridia,* and *Bacteroides.*

Complications

Osteomyelitis, bacteremia, sepsis

Treatment

Prophylaxis
- Mobilizing patients as soon as possible
- Repositioning patients every 2 hours
- Pressure-reducing devices (foam, air, or liquid mattresses)
- Correction of nutritional status.

Local Wound Care
- Proper cleansing with mild agents
- Moisturizing to maintain hydration and promote healing
- Polyurethane, hydrocolloid, or absorptive dressings, and topical antibiotics for wound
- Necrotic tissue may require surgical debridement, flaps, and skin grafts.
- Appropriate antibiotic therapy for infected ulcer

With proper treatment, stage I and II ulcers heal within 1 to 2 weeks. Stage III and IV ulcers heal within 6 to 12 weeks.

ERYTHEMA MULTIFORME

Definition

A general name used to describe an immune complex–mediated hypersensitivity reaction to different causative agents

Causes

- **Drugs** (penicillins, sulfonamides, barbiturates, NSAIDs, thiazides, phenytoin)
- **Viruses** (herpes simplex virus, hepatitis A and B)
- **Bacteria** (*Streptococcus, Mycoplasma*)
- Fungi
- Malignancy
- Radiotherapy
- Pregnancy

Fifty percent of erythema multiforme cases are idiopathic.

Epidemiology

Older children and adults

Signs and Symptoms

Although characterized by **target lesions,** multiforme refers to the wide variety of lesions that may be present, including papules, vesicles, and bullae (see Figure 12-6).

Herpes simplex virus accounts for most cases of recurrent erythema multiforme.

Treatment

- Discontinue offending agent.
- Treat any underlying infections.

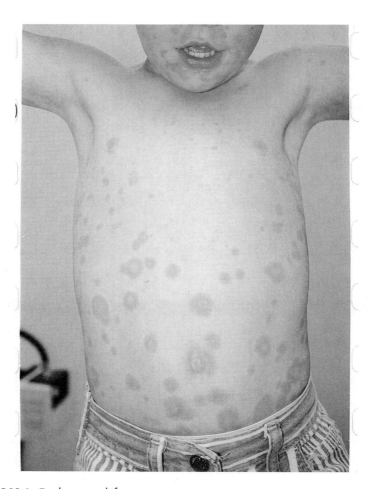

FIGURE 12-6. Erythema multiforme.
(Reproduced, with permission, from Knoop, Stack, and Storrow. *Atlas of Emergency Medicine.* New York: McGraw-Hill, 1997: 342.)

Stevens–Johnson syndrome and toxic epidermal necrolysis are severe variants of erythema multiforme that are potentially life threatening.

STEVENS–JOHNSON SYNDROME

- Erythema multiforme with systemic illness (fever, malaise) and multiple mucous membrane involvement (oral, vaginal, conjunctival) (see Figure 12-7).
- Extensive targetlike lesions and mucosal erosion covering < 10% body surface area
- Ocular involvement may result in scarring, corneal ulcers, or uveitis; 5% mortality.
- May evolve to toxic epidermal necrolysis

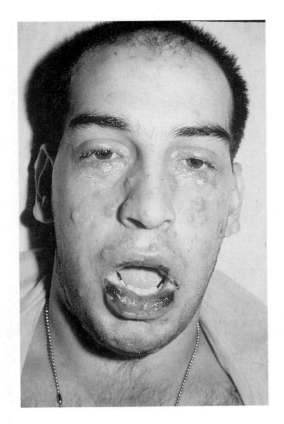

FIGURE 12-7. Stevens–Johnson syndrome.
(Reproduced, with permission, from Knoop, Stack, and Storrow. *Atlas of Emergency Medicine.* New York, NY: McGraw-Hill, 1997: 343.)

TOXIC EPIDERMAL NECROLYSIS

Definition

Widespread full-thickness necrosis of skin covering > 30% body surface area

Signs and Symptoms

- Prodrome of fever and influenzalike symptoms.
- Pruritus, pain, tenderness, and burning
- Classic targetlike lesions symmetrically distributed on dorsum of hand, palms, soles, face, and knees
- Initial **target lesions** can become confluent, erythematous, and tender, with bullous formation and subsequent loss of epidermis.
- Epidermal sloughing may be generalized, resembling a second-degree burn, and is more pronounced over pressure points.
- Positive Nikolsky's sign
- Ninety percent of cases have mucosal lesions—painful, erythematous erosions on lips, buccal mucosa, conjunctiva, and anogenital region.

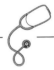

Nikolsky's sign is sloughing off of the epidermis with gentle manual pressure.

Diagnosis

Confirmed by biopsy

Complications

- Secondary skin infections
- Fluid and electrolyte abnormalities
- Prerenal azotemia
- Increased risk of death (denudation of skin results in fluid loss and infections)
- 30% mortality rate

Treatment

- Removal and/or treatment of causative agent (suppressive therapy with acyclovir to prevent recurrences of herpes simplex virus)
- Hospitalization for severe disease
- Fluid and electrolyte replacement
- Systemic corticosteroids

CUTANEOUS FUNGAL INFECTIONS

Definition

Dermatophytes are a group of noninvasive fungi that can infect keratinized tissue of epidermis, nails, and hair, resulting in a tinea infection. Clinical presentation depends on anatomic site of infection, and is thus named accordingly.

Etiology

Trichophyton, *Microsporum*, and *Epidermophyton*

Types

- Tinea pedis (Athlete's foot)
- Tinea cruris (Jock itch)
- Tinea corporis (Ringworm)
- Onychomycosis (nail infection)
- Tinea versicolor (pityriasis versicolor)

Diagnosis

- KOH preparation reveals multiple, septated hyphae. In tinea versicolor, hyphae and yeast forms are in a "spaghetti and meatballs" distribution.
- Wood's lamp reveals a bright green fluorescence of hair shaft in tinea capitis.
- Fungal culture of affected area may demonstrate dermatophyte.

Treatment

- Prevention (wearing well-ventilated shoes, cotton socks, and cotton underwear)

- Topical antifungal agents (imidazoles and terbinafine)
- Systemic antifungal agents (griseofulvin, systemic azoles, and terbinafine) if unresponsive to topical therapy or if there is involvement of nails
- Mild potency topical corticosteroids if inflammation and pruritus is severe

HERPES ZOSTER

Definition

- An acute dermatomal viral infection caused by reactivation of latent varicella-zoster virus that has remained dormant in a sensory root ganglion
- The virus travels down the sensory nerve, resulting initially in dermatomal pain, followed by skin lesions.

Etiology

Varicella-zoster virus

Epidemiology

Age > 50

Risk Factors

Age, malignancy, immunosuppression, and radiation

Signs and Symptoms

- **Prodrome of pain,** burning, itching, and paresthesia in affected dermatome precedes eruption by 3 to 5 days; accompanied by fever, headache, and malaise and heightened sensitivity to stimuli (allodynia).
- **Grouped vesicles** on an erythematous base distributed unilaterally along a dermatome
- Crust formation within 5 to 10 days
- **Some vesicles may occur outside of involved dermatome.**
- Thoracic nerves are the most commonly involved.

Diagnosis

Confirmed by **Tzanck preparation** revealing multinucleated giant cells, and culture of lesions.

Complications

- Secondary bacterial superinfection
- **Postherpetic neuralgia** (more common in the elderly and may persist for weeks to years after infection)

Patients with zoster can infect nonimmune contacts with chickenpox. Exposed nonimmune contacts should be treated with varicella-zoster immune globulin (VZIG).

- Herpes zoster ophthalmicus: Lesions on nasal tip or eye indicate zoster involvement of nasociliary branch of ophthalmic nerve, resulting in uveitis, conjunctivitis, retinitis, optic neuritis, or glaucoma. An ophthalmic consult is necessary.
- Ramsay Hunt syndrome: Lesions on external surface of ear or auditory canal indicate zoster involvement of facial and auditory nerve, resulting in facial paralysis, hearing loss, ear pain, and vertigo.

Treatment

- Moist and cool compresses to affected dermatome
- Oral acyclovir, valacyclovir, or famciclovir (accelerate healing of lesions and decrease duration of pain if started within 3 days of infection) for immunocompetent patients
- IV acyclovir for severe infections and immunocompromised individuals
- Adequate analgesia

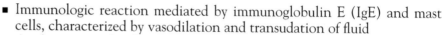

IMMEDIATE TYPE I HYPERSENSITIVITY REACTIONS (IGE MEDIATED)

- Immunologic reaction mediated by immunoglobulin E (IgE) and mast cells, characterized by vasodilation and transudation of fluid
- As the antigen binds to IgE on the mast cell surface, the mast cell degranulates and releases histamine, serotonin, heparin, leukotrienes, and prostaglandins.
- These inflammatory mediators cause vasodilation, increased capillary permeability, and smooth muscle contraction.
- Leakage of plasma into the dermis causes a swelling, characterized by a wheal.

Urticaria, angioedema, anaphylaxis, and atopic dermatitis are examples of type I hypersensitivity reactions occurring in the skin.

Urticaria (Hives)

- Characterized by **wheals:** An abrupt development of transient edematous pink papules and plaques that may be localized or generalized and are usually pruritic
- Wheals may develop after exposure to circulating antigens (drugs, food, insect venom, animal dander, pollen), hot and cold temperatures, exercise, and pressure or rubbing (dermographism).
- Wheals usually last < 24 hours and may recur on future exposure to the antigen.

Angioedema

- Describes a deeper involvement of subcutaneous tissues with less demarcated swelling, usually characterized by swelling of the eyelids, lips, and tongue (see Figure 12-8).
- A hereditary form also exists, characterized by recurrent attacks of abdominal pain, vomiting, and edema of soft tissue, caused by a deficiency of C1 esterase.

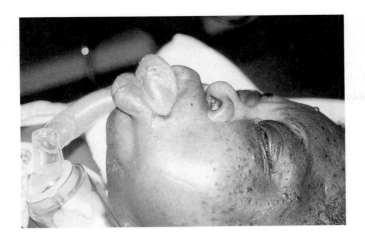

FIGURE 12-8. Angioedema.
(Reproduced, with permission, from Knoop, Stack, and Storrow. *Atlas of Emergency Medicine.* New York: McGraw-Hill, 1997: 127.)

Anaphylaxis

The most severe systemic form of type I hypersensitivity reaction, is characterized by bronchoconstriction and hypotension.

Treatment of Type I Hypersensitivity Reactions

- Airway protection
- Antihistamines
- Corticosteroids
- Epinephrine (for anaphylaxis)

ATOPIC DERMATITIS

Definition

A pruritic, type I (IgE) immediate hypersensitivity inflammatory reaction in which sensitized mast cells release pharmacologically vasoactive mediators.

Risk Factors

- Family history of atopy: Asthma, allergic rhinitis, hay fever, eczema, and increased IgE
- Exacerbating factors include scratching, stress, infection, wool, skin dehydration, pregnancy, and menstruation.

Epidemiology

- Affects all ages but onset is in first 6 months of life. Two thirds of patients outgrow the dermatitis by age 10.
- Familial predisposition

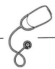

Most children have progressive improvement with increasing age, but some may evolve into adult eczema.

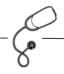

Signs and Symptoms

- Pruritus
- Lesions vary with patient's age:
  - Infantile eczema: Red, exudative, crusty, and oozy lesions primarily affecting the face and extensor surfaces; may clear by 2 years of age
  - Juvenile and adult eczema: Dry, lichenified pruritic plaques distributed over flexural areas (antecubital, popliteal, neck)

Diagnosis

Supported by a personal or family history of atopy or eczema

Complications

Secondary bacterial and viral infections with *Staphylococcus,* herpes simplex virus, and molluscum contagiosum.

Treatment

- Avoid scratching (will provoke the rash).
- Lubricate dry skin.
- Avoid wool and fragrances.
- Use mild cleansers and detergents.
- Oral antihistamines
- Oral antibiotics only if clinical signs of secondary infection (don't culture skin; 90% of atopic patients are carriers of *S. aureus*)
- Topical corticosteroids (mainstay of therapy)
- Avoid oral corticosteroids (associated with an excellent response, but patients become steroid dependent or rebound when steroids are discontinued).

IMPORTANT TYPE I HYPERSENSITIVITIES

Penicillin Allergy

- 1 to 3% of population
- Five percent of those allergic to penicillin will be allergic to cephalosporins too.
- All people have a low level of IgM against major antigenic determinant of penicillin.
- Penicillin-allergic people are usually sensitive to minor determinant.

Food Allergy

- More common in children
- Breast feeding and delayed introduction of solid foods decreases incidence.
- Eggs, cow's milk, fish, nuts most common
- Most reactions confined to GI tract and skin

Hornet Sting Allergy

- Most also allergic to yellow jacket stings
- Anaphylactic reaction possible, or just local swelling
- Most deaths in adults, less likely in kids
- No previous sting necessary
- Prophylaxis with periodic venom injection make blocking IgG Ab

TABLE 12-1. Definitions of Primary Skin Lesions

Macule	A flat, nonpalpable area of skin discoloration
Papule	An elevated, palpable solid area of skin < 0.5 cm diameter
Plaque	An elevated area of skin > 2 cm diameter that has a larger surface area compared to its elevation above the skin
Wheal	An elevated, rounded or flat topped area of dermal edema that disappears within hours
Vesicle	A circumscribed, elevated fluid-containing lesion of < 0.5 cm diameter
Bullae	A circumscribed, elevated fluid-containing lesion of > 0.5 cm diameter
Pustule	A circumscribed, elevated pus-containing lesion
Nodule	An elevated, palpable solid lesion > 0.5 cm diameter
Petechiae	A red-purple nonblanching macule < 0.5 cm diameter, usually pinpoint in size
Purpura	A red-purple nonblanching macule > 0.5 cm diameter
Teleangiectasia	A blanchable dilated blood vessel

TABLE 12-2. Definitions of Secondary Skin Lesions

Scale	An accumulation of dead, exfoliating epidermal cells
Crust	Dried serum, blood, or purulent exudate that accumulates on the skin surface (scab)
Erosion	A superficial loss of epidermis, leaving a denuded, moist surface; heals without scarring because doesn't penetrate through dermal–epidermal junction
Excoriation	A linear erosion produced by scratching
Ulcer	A loss of epidermis extending into dermis; heals with scarring because it penetrates into dermis
Scar	Replacement of normal skin with fibrous tissue as a result of healing
Atrophy	Thinning of skin
Lichenification	Thickening of epidermis with accentuation of normal skin markings

TABLE 12-3. Diagnostic Procedures Used in Dermatology

Diascopy	Pressing of a glass slide firmly against a red lesion will determine if it is due to capillary dilatation (blanchable) or to extravasation of blood (nonblanchable).
KOH preparation	Used to identify fungus and yeast. Scrape scales from skin, hair, or nails and treat with a 10% KOH solution to dissolve tissue material. Septated hyphae are revealed in fungal infections, and pseudohyphae and budding spores are revealed in yeast infections.
Tzanck preparation	Used to identify vesicular viral eruptions. Scrape the base of a vesicle and smear cells on a glass slide. Multinucleated giant cells will be identified in herpes simplex, herpes zoster, and varicella infections.
Scabies preparation	Scrape skin of a burrow between fingers, side of hands, axilla, or groin. Mites, eggs, or feces will be identified in scabies infection.
Use of Wood's lamp	Certain conditions will fluoresce when examined under a long-wave UV light ("black" lamp). Tinea capitis will fluoresce green or yellow on hair shaft.
Patch testing	Detects type IV delayed hypersensitivity reactions (allergic contact dermatitis). Nonirritating concentrations of suspected allergen are applied under occlusion to the back. Development of erythema, edema, and vesicles at site of contact 48 hours later indicates an allergy to offending agent.
Biopsy	Type of biopsy performed depends on the site of lesion, the type of tissue removed, and the desired cosmetic result. Shave biopsy is used for superficial lesions. Punch biopsy (3–5 mm diameter) can remove all or part of a lesion and provides tissue sample for pathology. Elliptical excisions provide more tissue than a punch biopsy and are used for deeper lesions or when the entire lesion needs to be sent to pathology.
Therapeutic modalities	Cryosurgery, curettage and electrodesiccation, phototherapy

Health Promotion

Barbara G. Lock

GENERAL PREVENTIVE CARE

ANNUAL EXAMS

History and Counseling

Health Maintenance
- Nutrition
- Exercise
- Weight gain/loss

Accident Prevention
- Safety belt/helmet use
- Smoke detectors
- Firearm safety

Toxic Habits
- Alcohol consumption (CAGE criteria; see Alcohol section)
- Tobacco use
- Illicit drug use

Sexuality
- Contraception
- Sexually transmitted disease (STD) prevention

Domestic Violence

Tests and Exams

Gynecologic Cancer Screening
- Pap smear and pelvic exam
- Mammogram (40+, q2y; 50+, qy)
- Breast exam

Prostate and Colon Cancer Screening
- Digital rectal exam
- Guaiac (50+)
- Sigmoidoscopy (50+, q3y)

Cardiovascular
- Lipid profile (m: 35+, f: 45+)
- Blood pressure

Age-Related Changes
- Height
- Vision and auditory screening (65+)

ADULT VACCINATIONS

Tetanus

Who: Everyone
When: DTaP series in childhood, booster q10y (or if > 5y with a dirty wound)

Hepatitis B

Who: Everyone
When: One series of three injections (each one month apart)

Influenza

Who: Health care workers, age > 65, the chronically ill
When: Annually, autumn (new vaccine each year based on prediction of prevalent strains)

Pneumococcal

Who: Age > 65, the chronically ill, recent formulation effective in children
When: Once every 5 years

Measles, Mumps, Rubella (MMR)

Who: All persons born after 1956 who lack evidence of immunity to measles
When: First one age 12 months, second booster during adulthood if not previously received

Varicella

Who: Healthy adults with no history of varicella infection or previous vaccination
When: Two doses of varicella vaccine delivered 4 to 8 weeks apart are recommended.

HEALTH PROMOTION: CANCER PREVENTION

BREAST CANCER

Epidemiology

- Second most common cause of **cancer death** in women in the United States (most common is lung CA, as in men)
- 1% of all breast CA occurs in men

Most cases of breast cancer are not associated with known gene mutations.

Etiology

10% caused by mutations in one or more of the following genes: p53 (tumor suppressor), BRCA-1, BRCA-2, erbB2 (HER-2/neu)

Risk Factors

- Age
- Prior breast CA
- Family history
- Increased estrogen exposure:
  - Early menarche
  - Late menopause
  - Nulliparity/late pregnancy
  - Oral contraceptive pills and hormone replacement therapy **do not** increase risk

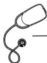

One in 9 women who live to age 80 will develop breast cancer.

Screening

Breast Exams
- Annually by physician (starting at age 20)
- Monthly self-exam (best time is 3 to 5 days after onset of menses)

Mammograms
- Age 35 baseline
- 40 to 49 years, q2y
- 50+, annually

Masses
- Cancer usually painless
- Sonography—differentiate cystic from solid
- Fine-needle aspiration cytology—high false-negative rate, can drain cystic lesions
- Excisional/open biopsy—definitive diagnosis

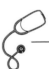

The breasts of young women contain a high proportion of fibrous tissue that is radiopaque, rendering mammograms uninterpretable. As women age, the fiber is replaced by radiolucent fat. At age 35 a woman is still at low risk for breast CA, yet has undergone fatty replacement of a substantial amount of the fiber, making it a good time for the baseline mammogram.

Treatment

- Surgical excision

- Breast conservation usually possible, mastectomy required for:
    1. Tumor > 7 cm
    2. Tumor includes nipple
    3. Extensive intraductal disease
- Adjuvant chemotherapy:
    - Unnecessary in stage I tumors (tumor < 2 cm, no nodes)
    - Battery of standard agents used:
        - Tamoxifen, an estrogen/progesterone receptor blocker, can be of use in tumors expressing these receptors
        - Postmenopausal women more likely to benefit from tamoxifen
- Radiation reduces the risk of local recurrence but **does not** improve long-term survival

OVARIAN CANCER

Epidemiology

Ovarian cancer is the fourth most common cause of death from cancer among women of all ages in the United States.

Signs and Symptoms

- Bloating
- Diffuse abdominal pain
- Ascites
- Dyspareunia
- Irregular vaginal bleeding
- Weight loss

Risk Factors

- Older age at first pregnancy
- Family history

The following appear to lower the risk of ovarian cancer (by prolonging periods of anovulation or suppressing gonadotropin levels):
- Childbearing
- Oral contraceptive use
- Breast feeding
- Tubal sterilization

Screening

There are no currently recommended screening tests.

Prognosis

Despite aggressive treatment, 5-year survival of women with ovarian cancer is only about 40%.

Definition

Cervical cancer is a STD associated with human papillomavirus (HPV) types 16, 18, 31, 45, 51, 52, and 53.

Risk Factors

- HPV
- Human immunodeficiency virus (HIV)
- Smoking
- Early age at first intercourse
- Large number of sexual partners

Signs and Symptoms

- Foul smelling vaginal discharge
- Postcoital and irregular vaginal bleeding
- Pelvic pain
- Dyspareunia
- Enlarged cervix with erosions

Screening

- Yearly Papanicolau test starting at age 18 or age at first sexual intercourse
- Counsel patients about protective effect of barrier contraceptives.

Treatment

- Colposcopic-directed cervical biopsy for carcinoma-in-situ (stage 0)
- Radical hysterectomy for disease invading cervix (stage I)
- Radiation therapy for disease that invades beyond cervix (stages II–IV)

Prognosis

Stage I and II: 5-year survival is 60%.
Stage III: 5-year survival is 40%.

PROSTATE CANCER

Definition

Adenocarcinoma of the prostatic acini

Epidemiology

- Third most common cause of **cancer** death in men in the United States

- Incidence increases with age; most cases occur after age 50.
- Higher incidence in African Americans

Signs and Symptoms

- Dysuria
- Urinary hesitancy
- Back pain
- Hematuria

Screening

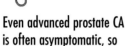

Even advanced prostate CA is often asymptomatic, so screening is important.

- Begin yearly screening at age 50; start at age 40 for African American men
- Yearly digital rectal exam to look for indurated, nodular prostate
- Yearly screening for prostate specific antigen (PSA)
- For PSA > 4.1, transrectal ultrasonography (TRUS) with biopsy of suspicious areas

Treatment

T1 Disease (Nonpalpable)
- Prostatectomy
- Consider radiotherapy

T2 (Palpable) and T3 Disease (Extracapsular Extension)
- Radical prostatectomy
- Consider androgen deprivation

Metastasis
- Radical prostatectomy
- Androgen deprivation
- Consider chemotherapy

Prognosis

Ten-year survival rates are 75% when the cancer is confined to the prostate, 55% for those with regional extension, and 15% for those with distant metastases.

TESTICULAR CANCER

Definition

Primary germ cell tumors of the testis

Epidemiology

- Common cause of cancer in men aged 20 to 40

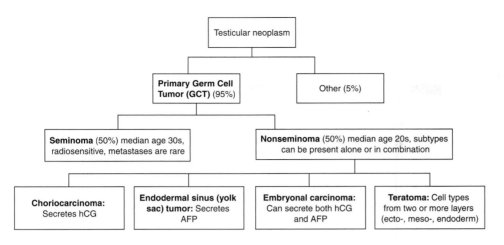

FIGURE 13-1. Classification of testicular cancer.

- Seen more frequently in whites than in African Americans
- 95% of testicular cancers are germ cell tumors

Classification

- Germ cell tumors are divided into seminomas and nonseminomas (see Figure 13-1).

Findings

- Painless testicular mass or persistent swelling
- Metastases may present as back pain (retroperitoneal) or dyspnea (lung mets).

Treatment

- Nonseminoma: Orchiectomy, retroperitoneal lymph node dissection (RPLND), chemotherapy for lymph node involvement or metastasis. Patients without lymph node involvement or metastases have a 95% cure rate.
- Seminoma: Orchiectomy, retroperitoneal radiation has 98% cure rate for nonmetastasized seminomas; chemotherapy for metastases.

HEALTH PROMOTION IN WOMEN

HORMONE REPLACEMENT THERAPY (HRT)

Benefits

Estrogen decreases risks of:
- Osteoporosis by 25%
- Coronary artery disease by 40% (controversial; new studies are inconclusive)

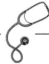

- Estrogen inhibits osteoclast bone resorption.
- Estrogen elevates high-density lipoprotein (HDL), lowers low-density lipoprotein (LDL), but raises triglycerides.

- Senile dementia
- Urinary incontinence, urinary tract infections (UTIs), and vaginal atrophy

Patient Evaluation

- Osteoporosis: Family history, bone densitometry
- Coronary artery disease: History, blood pressure, lipid profile, electrocardiogram (ECG)
- Breast cancer: History, lifetime estrogen exposure
- Ovarian cancer: History, risk factors
- Dementia: Family history, level of education (less educated are more at risk)
- Gyn surgeries: Hysterectomy, oophorectomy

Treatment

Most commonly low-dose estrogen and progesterone in constant (uncycled) dosage regimen

Risks

- Endometrial cancer: Associated with unopposed estrogen use. Can be prevented by using estrogen–progestin combination.
- Breast cancer: Women with estrogen receptor positive breast cancer may worsen with HRT.

Raloxifene mimics estrogenic effects on osteoclasts but has no effect on breast, endometrium, or lipid profile. Useful for prevention of osteoporosis in women at high risk for breast cancer. Other benefits are lost.

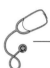

There are very few true risks of hormone replacement therapy. Women with multiple risk factors for breast cancer may be put at increased risk.

DOMESTIC VIOLENCE

Epidemiology

- Lifetime prevalence 20% for women
- In the United States, approximately 2,000 women die each year as a direct result of injuries.

Signs and Symptoms

- Frequent or unexplained injuries
- Depression/suicide attempts
- Substance abuse
- Anxiety
- Headaches
- Chronic pain

Screening

- Women should be routinely asked about domestic violence due to its high prevalence.
- Routine screening of women by physicians is thought to yield positive results in about **half** of all cases.

Domestic violence help is more commonly sought during pregnancy.

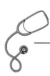

How to ask:
- "Have you ever been hit, hurt, or threatened by your partner?"
- "Have you ever been a victim of domestic violence?"
- "Many of my patients with your symptoms have experienced physical violence. Has this happened to you?"

Treatment

- Treat medical conditions.
- Assess safety of patient's current situation.
- Provide information (shelters, social agencies).
- Reassure patient that no one deserves to be abused.

DEPRESSION

Epidemiology

- Debilitating mood disorder that has a lifetime prevalence of about 15%
- Incidence higher in women
- Mean age is 40 years.

Risk Factors

- Family history of depression, suicide, substance abuse
- Presence of chronic disease
- Personal history of substance abuse
- Lack of support system

Signs and Symptoms

Depressed mood with sadness, weight loss, guilt, fatigue, insomnia or hypersomnia, anhedonia, psychomotor agitation or retardation, difficulty concentrating or suicidal ideation, for at least 2 consecutive weeks

Treatment

- All patients should be asked specifically about suicidal intent.
- Patients who are actively suicidal require inpatient evaluation by a psychiatrist.
- Evaluate for antidepressant medication.

SUBSTANCE ABUSE

ALCOHOL ABUSE

Definition

Alcohol intoxication is legally defined in most states as a blood alcohol level of 0.10 g/dL, although the clinical response to alcohol will vary between individuals. Ten percent of alcohol users develop alcohol-related problems including alcoholism.

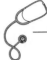

Differential diagnosis:
Depression must be distinguished from bereavement, substance abuse, hypothyroidism, medication side effect, and organic brain disease.

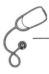

How to ask about depression:
"Have you been feeling overwhelmingly sad lately?"
"Have you lost pleasure in the things you used to enjoy?"

How to ask about suicidal intent:
"Have you ever thought that life was not worth living?"
"Have you ever thought about killing yourself?"
"Have you ever made a plan to kill yourself?"

TABLE 13-1. Systemic Effects of Alcohol Abuse

	Acute	Chronic
Central nervous system	CNS depression, amnesia, fragmented sleep	Peripheral neuropathy, Wernicke's and Korsakoff's syndromes (thiamine deficiency), cerebellar degeneration, alcoholic dementia
Cardiovascular system	Decreased myocardial contractility, peripheral vasodilation	Hypertension, cardiomyopathy, increased HDL cholesterol
Gastrointestinal system	Esophageal and gastric inflammation, acute pancreatitis	Mallory–Weiss tear, esophageal varices, portal hypertension, chronic pancreatitis
Liver	Impaired gluconeogenesis	Alcohol-induced hepatitis, cirrhosis
Hematopoietic system	Macrocytosis	Thrombocytopenia, hypersplenism, decreased platelet aggregation
Genitourinary system	Erectile dysfunction	Testicular atrophy, amenorrhea, ovarian atrophy, increased risk of spontaneous abortion, fetal alcohol syndrome

Cancers due to alcohol use:
- Head and neck cancers
- Esophageal and gastric cancers
- Pancreatic cancer
- Liver cancer
- Breast cancer

Screening

CAGE Questions

1. Have you ever tried **c**ut down your drinking?
2. Have you ever been **a**ngry/annoyed when people ask about your drinking?
3. Have you ever felt **g**uilty about your drinking?
4. Have you ever had an **e**ye-opener (drink on waking up in the morning)?

Systemic Effects

See Table 13-1.

Withdrawal Syndrome

Can range from mild anxiety and tremor, to alcohol withdrawal seizures and delirium tremens

Delirium Tremens

- Tachycardia, fever, hallucinations
- 5 to 30% mortality if untreated
- Treatment: Sedation with benzodiazepines and intensive care

TOBACCO USE

Definition

- Single largest cause of preventable death in the United States

- About 450,000 people in the United States die each year from tobacco-related disease:
  - 40% cardiovascular
  - 35% due to cancer
  - 20% respiratory
  - 5% cerebrovascular

Tobacco-Related Disease

Smoking:
- Promotes atherosclerosis, thrombosis, arrhythmias
- Reduces oxygen carrying capacity of the blood
- Reduces elasticity in the lungs and causes COPD and emphysema:
  - During pregnancy associated with increased risk of spontaneous abortion, fetal death, and sudden infant death syndrome

Smokeless tobacco products cause oral and head and neck cancers.

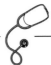

Types of
tobacco-related cancer:
Colon
A
Neck
Cervix
Esophagus
Renal
Pancreas
Lung
Urogenital (bladder)
Stomach

Smoking Cessation Counseling

Should be a primary focus of all physician encounters with smokers:
- Identify all smokers and tobacco users by routine questioning during history.
- Instruct all tobacco users to stop, giving personalized advice and support (e.g., "If you stop smoking, your cough will improve").
- Evaluate each patient for readiness and motivation. If the patient is not motivated, reinforce that support for smoking cessation will be available when the patient is ready.
- Formulate a plan with the patient, including a quit date, nicotine replacement or other pharmacologic therapy, and follow-up appointment for support.

Smoking Cessation Pharmacotherapy

- Nicotine patches are associated with a 40% quit rate.
- Bupropion is associated with a 55% quit rate.
- Combination is associated with a 66% quit rate.
- Ongoing counseling may improve abstinence.

OPIOID USE

Signs and Symptoms

- Depressed mental status
- Respiratory depression
- Pupillary constriction (or dilation with profound respiratory depression)
- Overdose can cause death.

Treatment

- Naloxone is an opioid antagonist that rapidly reverses toxicity, but is short acting (< 30 min).
- Use is both diagnostic and therapeutic.

OPIATE WITHDRAWAL SYNDROME

- Not life threatening, except in very young and very old, but may lead to relapse, using street drugs, and exposure to needle sharing with its attendant risks such as acquisition of HIV and hepatitis C.

Signs and Symptoms

- Nausea
- Vomiting
- Diarrhea
- Mydriasis
- Piloerection
- Diffuse muscle pain
- Desire for more drug

Treatment

- Long-acting opioid (e.g., methadone)
- Symptomatic relief
- Supportive care

SYMPATHOMIMETICS

Signs and Symptoms

- Syndrome of catecholamine excess
- Agitation
- Tachycardia
- Hypertension
- Hyperthermia
- Psychosis
- Seizures
- Chest pain

Treatment

- Benzodiazepines to control excess sympathetic discharge and anxiety
- Cooling measures to control hyperthermia
- Nitroglycerin and heparin to control chest pain

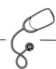

A patient on opioids for pain control has very little risk of developing opiate dependence.

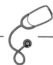

3% of all patients seen in the emergency department and 6% of all patients admitted to the hospital with cocaine chest pain will have biochemical evidence for a myocardial infarction.

Beta blockers are contraindicated in patients with cocaine use due to the risk of unopposed alpha-adrenergic tone, which may worsen vasoconstriction.

Injury Prevention

Statistics

- Cause about 30% of all deaths between ages 15 and 25
- Disproportionately affect the young, so responsible for more years of life lost than any other single cause
- Alcohol is implicated in 44% of all traffic fatalities.

Seatbelt Use

Associated with an 89% reduction in mortality, and concurrent airbag use further reduces mortality

Motorcycle Collisions

Motorcycle use is associated with a fatality rate 20 times greater than that of passenger cars.

Helmet Use

Reduces motorcycle fatalities by 37% and reduces the incidence of head injury by 67%.

Screening

- Ask all patients about seatbelt use, airbag availability, helmet use, child safety seat use, and alcohol use.
- Intervene when patients show behaviors that put others in danger (e.g., adult does not provide toddler with a child safety seat).

FALLS

Most common cause of injuries

RISK FACTORS

- Elderly
- Disability
- Alcohol intoxication

PREVENTION

- Assess gait of each patient.
- Assess vision of each patient.

- Provide corrective devices or referral for identified impairment.
- Counsel alcohol use cessation.

NUTRITIONAL DISORDERS

MALNUTRITION

Definitions

- Marasmus: Starvation
- Kwashiorkor: Protein deficiency
- Essential fatty acids: Linoleic and linolenic acids

Risk Factors

- Low socioeconomic class
- Nursing home and hospitalized patients

Complications

- Anemia
- Hypoalbuminemia
- Poor wound healing
- Weakness
- Decubitus ulcers
- Infection
- Death

OBESITY

Definition

Body mass index (BMI) greater than 30 kg/m²

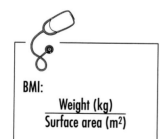

BMI:
$$\frac{\text{Weight (kg)}}{\text{Surface area (m}^2)}$$

Complications

- Atherosclerosis
- Type 2 diabetes
- Sleep apnea
- Osteoarthritis
- Gout
- Venous stasis
- Biliary disease
- Endometrial cancer
- Postmenopausal breast cancer

Treatment

- Behavior modification, exercise
- Low-calorie diet with < 25% of calories from fat
- Goal: 10% weight loss over 6 months

If the above fail, consider:
- Pharmacologic therapy
- Bariatric surgery (for BMI > 40 m^2 or > 35 m^2 with comorbid disease)

BERIBERI (THIAMINE DEFICIENCY)

Signs and Symptoms

Wet Beriberi (Beriberi Heart Disease)
- Peripheral vasodilation
- High cardiac output
- Sodium and water retention
- Right and left heart failure

Dry Beriberi
- See thiamine deficiency (Table 13-2).

TABLE 13-2. Syndromes of Vitamin Deficiency and Excess

Vitamin	Deficiency	Excess
Vitamin A	Early: Night blindness Late: Keratomalacia, blindness	Acute: GI symptoms, headache, papilledema Chronic: Joint pain, hair loss, fissured lips, anorexia, weight loss, hepatomegaly
Vitamin C	Scurvy: Petechial hemorrhage, ecchymoses, gum bleeding, poor wound healing, anemia	Uricosuria, kidney stones
Vitamin E	Areflexia, decreased proprioception, gait abnormality	Potentiates oral anticoagulants
Vitamin K	Prolonged bleeding time	Attenuates oral anticoagulants
Niacin	Pellagra: Chronic wasting, dermatitis, dementia, diarrhea	GI symptoms, flushing, pruritus, hepatotoxicity
Thiamine (vitamin B$_1$)	Beriberi Peripheral neuropathy Wernicke's encephalopathy (horizontal nystagmus followed by lateral rectus palsy, fever, ataxia, encephalopathy, death) Korsakoff's syndrome (retrograde amnesia, confabulation)	
Pyridoxine (vitamin B$_6$)	Seizures Glossitis, cheilosis GI symptoms Weakness Peripheral neuropathy	

Treatment

- Thiamine results in increased peripheral vascular resistance and some improvement in cardiac function in wet beriberi.
- Thiamine restores full function in 50% of patients with neurological signs from dry beriberi.

PELLAGRA (NIACIN DEFICIENCY)

Signs and Symptoms

- Diarrhea
- Dermatitis
- Dementia

How to remember 3 D's, niacin, and pellagra: Three doctors drank a nice Pellegrino.

ENVIRONMENTAL EXPOSURES

HEAT EXHAUSTION

- Normal core temperature, symptoms due to dehydration and salt loss
- Characterized by headache, nausea and vomiting, weakness, irritability, and cramps.
- Treat with oral or IV hydration with salt-containing fluids, and patient should rest in a cool environment.

HEATSTROKE

- Failure of thermoregulation
- Associated with elevated core temperature and central nervous system (CNS) dysfunction such as altered mental status, focal deficits, hemiplegia, and posturing
- Exertional heatstroke is a result of exercise or physical labor in a high heat-index environment
- Classic or nonexertional heatstroke is usually seen in elderly or nonacclimated patients during summer heat-waves.

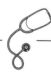

Patients who are dehydrated, disabled, or chronically ill or who are alcohol or drug users are more prone to developing heatstroke.

Treatment of Heatstroke

- Rapid cooling by cooling blanket, evaporation, ice packs to axilla and groin, or gastric or peritoneal lavage is critical to prevent rhabdomyolysis, multiorgan failure, and death.

Cooling should be halted when the patient's core temperature reaches 40°C to prevent hypothermia.

COLD-RELATED ILLNESS

Risk Factors

- Overwhelming cold exposure
- Extremes of age
- Intoxicated patients
- Homeless
- Concurrent illness
- Iatrogenic

FROSTBITE

- Caused by exposure of the skin to freezing temperatures; usually seen on the extremities, nose, and ears.
- As the body reduces cutaneous blood flow in freezing temperatures to maintain the core body temperature, capillary blood becomes more viscous, and ice crystals form in the extracellular space. This causes direct tissue injury and osmotic pressures that cause intracellular dehydration.

Frostbite is more common in diabetics due to neuropathy.

Treatment of Frostbite

- Rapid rewarming with clean water at 40 to 42°C
- Tetanus prophylaxis
- Debridement of tissues and prophylactic antibiotics remains controversial.

HYPOTHERMIA

Definition

Core (rectal) temperature:
- Mild: 35 to 32°C
- Moderate: 32 to 28°C
- Severe: < 28°C

Signs and Symptoms

- Shivering
- Poor judgment
- Paradoxical undressing
- Cardiac dysrhythmias
- Osborne wave: A convex, upward deflection of the J point on the ECG (not pathognomic).

Rewarm patients and continue cardiac resuscitation before declaring death. "You're not dead until you're warm and dead."

Treatment

Rewarming by:
- Warming blanket
- Warm packs to groin and axillae
- Infusion of warmed IV fluid

For severely hypothermic or pulseless patients:
- Warm-fluid lavage of bladder, stomach, peritoneum, and pleural space
- Extracorporeal rewarming techniques (cardiac bypass)

PRINCIPLES OF MEDICAL ETHICS

See Table 13-3.

TABLE 13-3. Principles of Medical Ethics

Principle	Definition
Autonomy	■ Ability to function independently and to make decisions about one's care free from the undue influence or bias of others ■ All patients are considered autonomous if they have the ability to understand the situation as evaluated with competency examination by psychiatrist (capacity) and are not a danger to self or others (suicidal, homicidal, demented, delirious).
Nonmalfeasance	■ The principle of *primum non nocere,* or first, do no harm
Beneficence	■ The principle of doing good ■ The practice of doing whatever is best for the patient without the consideration of the patient's wishes is called *paternalism*
Distributive justice	■ The principle of equal and fair allocation of benefit. Patients of different race, gender, and disability should be treated differently only on the basis of medical need and projected benefit.
Advance directives	■ Oral or written instructions from a patient to family members and health care professionals about health care decisions ■ May include living wills, designation of a health care proxy, specific instructions about which therapies to accept or decline including intubation, surgery or medical treatments, and Do Not Resuscitate (DNR) orders ■ A DNR order applies only to advanced cardiac life support (ACLS) resuscitation, and does not include intubation and ventilation unless specifically addressed.

PRINCIPLES OF EVIDENCE-BASED MEDICINE

Definition

- Practice of incorporating the best available evidence from the medical literature for a diagnostic test or treatment into daily patient care
- Best evidence obtained from randomized clinical trials

Steps

1. Identify a clinical problem.
2. Formulate a question.
3. Search for the best evidence.
4. Appraise the evidence.
5. Apply the information to the clinical problem.

Sources of Medical Evidence

- **Meta-analysis:** Evaluates the data of many trials that address the same question, and attempts to combine the information. These studies are best used when the clinical problem is infrequent and large randomized trials cannot be done.
- **Randomized controlled clinical trial:** The selected population is randomized to receive either the treatment in question or a placebo, and the outcome is measured. The ideal RCT is triple-blinded, meaning that both the treating physician, the patient, and the investigators, do not know which treatment has been given until the analysis is complete. These studies can establish cause and effect.
- **Cohort study:** The selected population is identified as being exposed or not exposed, and is monitored for subsequent effects. These studies are used when the exposure cannot be assigned for logistical or ethical reasons.
- **Case control study:** Populations with and without a given outcome are selected, and historical (retrospective) data is collected on exposure to a given agent or treatment.

STATISTICAL CONCEPTS

See Table 13-4.

TABLE 13-4. Statistical Concepts

Concept	Definition
Sensitivity	■ Measures the ability of a test to accurately detect true-positive results: tp/(tp + fn) (true positive test results/all patients with the disease). ■ The more sensitive a test, the less likely the test is to fail to detect a positive result. This is sometimes called a true-positive rate (TPR).
Specificity	■ Measures the ability of a test to accurately detect true-negative results: tn/(fp + tn) (true negative test result/all patients without the disease). ■ The more specific a test, the less likely the test is to fail to detect a negative result. This is sometimes called a true-negative rate (TNR).
Positive predictive value	■ Measures the chance that a patient with a positive test result in truth has the disease: tp/(tp + fp) (true positives/test positives).
Negative predictive value	■ Measures the chance that a patient with a negative test result in truth does not have the disease tn/(tn + fn) (true negatives/test negatives).
Likelihood ratio	■ Measures the fixed relationship between the chance of given test result in a patient with the disorder and the chance of the same test result in a patient without the disorder. ■ Likelihood ratio for a positive test result is expressed as: sensitivity/(1-specificity) or true-positive rate (TPR)/false-positive rate (FPR). ■ Likelihood ratio for a negative test result is expressed as: (1-sensitivity)/specificity or false-negative rate (FNR)/true-negative rate (TNR). ■ A test with known likelihood ratios can help a clinician with decision making; the pretest likelihood that a patient has a disease can be either improved with a high positive likelihood ratio (> 2) or reduced with a low negative likelihood ratio (< 0.5).
Confidence interval	■ Range around a sample mean that contains the true population mean to any desired degree of probability (frequently 95%).
Number needed to treat	■ Measures the number of patients with a given disease that a clinician would need to treat with the tested therapy in order to see one beneficial event or prevent one adverse event.

Awards and Opportunities for Students Interested in Medicine

The Paul & Daisy Soros Fellowships for New Americans

The fellowships are grants for $20,000 for up to 2 years of graduate study in the United States. The recipients are chosen on a national competitive basis. Thirty fellowships will be awarded each year.

A New American is an individual who (1) is a resident alien (i.e., holds a green card) or (2) has been naturalized as a U.S. citizen or (3) is the child of two parents who are both naturalized citizens.

The purpose of The Paul & Daisy Soros Fellowships for New Americans is to provide opportunities for continuing generations of able and accomplished New Americans to achieve leadership in their chosen fields. The program is established in recognition of the contributions New Americans have made to American life and in gratitude for the opportunities the United States has afforded the donors and their family. *Contact:* 400 West 59th Street, New York, NY 10019. Phone: 212-547-6926; Fax: 212-548-4623; *www.pdsoros.org.*

AMERICAN ASSOCIATION FOR THE HISTORY OF MEDICINE OSLER MEDAL

The medal is awarded for the best unpublished essay on a medico-historical subject written by a student in a school of medicine or of osteopathy in the United States or Canada. Essays appropriate for consideration by the committee may pertain either to the historical development of a contemporary medical problem or to a topic within the health sciences of a discrete past period. The essay should demonstrate either original research or an unusual appreciation and understanding of the problem or situation discussed. Winner will receive $500 in travel money to deliver paper at the American Association for the History of Medicine.

Ty Cobb Scholarship Program

For medical students who are legal residents of Georgia. *Contact:* Ty Cobb Foundation, Post Office Box 725, Forest Park, GA 30298, or e-mail *tycobb@ mindspring.com.*

Coe Memorial Scholarship

For medical students who are from the Auburn, New York, area. *Contact:* Norstar Trust Company, Coe Memorial Scholarship Fund, 120 Genesee St., Auburn, NY 13021.

COUNTRY DOCTOR SCHOLARSHIP PROGRAM

$10,000 annually, $40,000 aggregate

Georgia residents qualify for funding to obtain primary care medical degrees such as internal medicine, general surgery, OB-GYN, pediatrics, and family practice. In return, the student must practice in a Georgia board-approved town of 15,000 or less population. *Contact:* Joe B. Lawley, Ph.D., State Medical Education Board, 270 Washington St. SW, 7th Floor, Room 7093, Atlanta, GA 30334.

Southern Medical Association Medical Student

$500 to $2,500 awards for students who are SMA members in their first year of medical school, of superior ability with demonstrated financial need.

Olive D. Hoffman Scholarship

$5,000 scholarship for students committed to community service. *Contact:* Olive D. Hoffman Memorial Inc., 1474 North Pointe Village, Center Suite 280, Reston, VA 22094.

ILLINOIS HOSPITAL ASSOCIATION SCHOLARSHIP

$500 award for students who are Illinois residents with demonstrated financial need and academic acheievement. *Contact:* Scholarship, The Illinois Hospital Association, Center for Health Affairs, 1151 East Warrenville Rd., P.O. Box 3015, Naperville, IL 60566.

International Order of the King's Daughters and Sons

$1,000 scholarships for medical students. *Contact:* Health Careers Director, Mrs. Fred Cannon, Box 1310, Brookhaven, MS 39602-1310.

NEW YORK ACADEMY OF MEDICINE: DAVID E. ROGERS FELLOWSHIP PROGRAM

The David E. Rogers Fellowship Program is national fellowship for medical students in support of a project initiated during the summer between the first and second years of medical school. Ten fellowships of $2,500 will be awarded. The fellowship is meant to enrich the educational experiences of medical students through projects that couple medicine with the needs of underserved or disadvantaged patients or populations. For more information, contact the Rogers Fellowship at *rogers@nyam.org* or the New York Academy of Medicine. Contact your school's financial aid office for more info.

DoctorsCare Internationale Foundation Scholarships

DoctorsCare is an independent nonprofit organization created to promote scientific research, education, and medical health programs that contribute toward improving the health of mankind. The foundation has funds for annual grants for needy men and women in the field of medicine. Applications may be obtained by sending a self-addressed, stamped envelope to: Grants Department, Doctors Care Internationale Foundation, P.O. Box 1111, Houston, TX 77251-1111.

Wilderness Society Charles S. Houston Award

Award for a project proposal that is likely to result in a substantive contribution to the field of wilderness or environmental medicine. The applicant will conduct his project during the calendar year and present results at the Annual Meeting of the Society. Award: $1,500.

U.S. DEPARTMENT OF HEALTH AND HUMAN SERVICES INNOVATIONS IN HEALTH AWARD

An annual competition for innovative proposals for health promotion and disease prevention. The proposal must be concerned with disease prevention or health promotion. It could describe a community risk-reduction effort; a project for a whole community or a special population group, such as the aged or children; a health promotion program at the worksite; or a preventive approach for community education, such as primary and secondary school programs. Awards range from $250 to $3,000.

Life and Health Insurance Medical Research Fund Medical Scientist Scholarship

A five-year scholarship program for an MD/PhD student who will have completed 2 years of medical school before July and is usually not already funded. $16,000 per year.

Johnson & Johnson Student Paper

Students are invited to submit papers expressing original ideas in the broad area of engineering in medicine and biology.

American Academy of Medical Ethics William Liley Essay Contest

An essay contest for medical students and residents on a topic designated by the Academy. $250–$2,000 prizes.

PAUL W. MAYER SCHOLARSHIP IN MEDICINE AND BIOLOGY

Sponsored by the Alliance for Engineering, this is a scholarship to encourage student excellence in the field of biomedical engineering. Grant is $200. Contact your school's financial aid office for more info.

Jerry L. Memorial Pettis Scholarship

Sponsored by the American Medical Association Education and Research Foundation, this scholarship will be awarded to a junior or senior medical student with a demonstrated interest in the communication of science. Financial need of nominees will not be a consideration. *Contact:* American Medical Association Education and Research Foundation, 515 North State Street, Chicago, IL 60610. Phone: 312-464-5357; Fax: 312-464-5973; *www.ama-assn.org/med-sci/erf/toc.htm.*

Student Paper Competition in Medical Informatics

Students are invited to submit papers expressing original ideas in the broad areas of medical informatics and computer applications in medical care for the SCAMC (Symposium on Computer Applications in Medical

Care). Awards consist of the Martin N. Epstein Award of $1,000 and two cash prizes of $600 and $400 for second and third place. Contact your school's financial aid office for more info.

AMERICAN COLLEGE OF LEGAL MEDICINE SCHWARTZ AWARD

Each year the ACLM presents the Schwartz Award for the outstanding paper on legal medicine. The award provides a $1,000 honorarium, transportation, accommodations and meals at the ACLM annual meeting. Contact your school's financial aid office for more info.

Medical History Society of New Jersey Stephen Wickes Prize in the History of Medicine

Any currently enrolled undergraduate, graduate, or professional student is eligible to submit an original essay on a historical subject in the medical or allied fields. The topic may be historical aspects of a current problem, or it may deal with a specific subject in a defined period of the past. Prize: $100. Contact your school's financial aid office for more info.

Northeastern Ohio University College of Medicine William Carlos Poetry Competition

The Human Values in Medicine at Northeastern Ohio Universi-

ties College of Medicine is sponsoring this annual poetry-writing competition for students attending schools of medicine or osteopathy in the United States. Prize: $100–$300. Contact your school's financial aid office for more info.

New York Academy of Medicine:

The Paul Klemperer Fellowship in the History f Medicine and the Audrey and William H. Helfand Fellowship in the Medical Humanities

Each year the New York Academy of Medicine offers the Paul Klemperer Fellowship and the Audrey and William H. Helfand Fellowship to support work in history and the humanities as they relate to health, medicine, and the biomedical sciences. The Klemperer Fellowship supports research using the Academy Library as a historical resource. It is intended specifically for a scholar in residence in the collections of the Academy Library.

The Helfand Fellowship more broadly supports work in the humanities, including both creative projects dealing with health and the medical enterprise, and scholarly research in a humanistic discipline—other than history of medicine—as applied to medicine and health. Although residence is not obligatory, preference in the selection process will be given applicants whose projects require use of the resources of the Academy Library and who plan to spend

time at the Academy. The Helfand Fellowship and the Klemperer Fellowship each provide stipends of up to $5,000 to support travel, lodging, and incidental expenses for a flexible period between June 1, 2001, and May 31, 2002. Besides completing research or a creative project, each Fellow will be expected to make a presentation at the Academy and submit a final report on the project. Applications are accepted from anyone—regardless of citizenship, academic discipline, or academic status—who wishes to use the Academy's collections for historical research or for a scholarly or creative project in the medical humanities. *Contact:* Fellowship Program Coordinator, New York Academy of Medicine, 1216 Fifth Avenue, Room 612, New York, NY 10029. Phone: 212-822-7204; Fax: 212-996-7826.

AGENCY FOR INTERNATIONAL DEVELOPMENT INTERNSHIP

Sponsoring Agency: A.I.D. Two-week educational program (over Christmas holiday) for graduate students from the Caribbean and South and Central America, which may lead to summer placement in transnational corporations over summer. Program focuses on U.S. foreign policy and Latin American indebtedness. Travel costs to seminar in Baton Rouge paid.

Alpha Omega Alpha Essay Award

The purpose of these $500–$750 awards is to stimulate medical students to address general topics in medicine and to enable the society to recognize in a tangible way excellent and thoughtful presentations. The topic of the essay may be any nontechnical aspect of medicine including, medical education, medical ethics, philosophy as related to medicine, reflections on illness, science, and the culture and history of medicine.

American Bureau for Medical Advancement in China

Open to fourth-year students. Several university teaching hospitals in Taiwan offer clinical clerkships to qualifying students. Electives of 2 months are optimal, although shorter ones will be considered. It is expected that students will be able to provide for their own transportation and room and board, but Warner–Lambert has provided a grant to accommodate several partial scholarships.

AMERICAN COLLEGE OF NUTRITION

Award based on original scientific work in Clinical Nutrition. Award: $500 plus transportation to meeting.

American College of Preventive Medicine

$1,000 award for the best paper on preventive medicine—oriented topics; papers concerned with women's health issues encouraged.

National Council on Aging—Geriatric Fellowship

Sponsored by Travelers Insurance Aging, Inc., this program is designed to increase students' technical knowledge of geriatrics and to help sensitize them to social and personal problems facing older people. A fellowship of $3,000 will be provided.

JOSEPH AND ROSE KENNEDY INSTITUTE OF ETHICS NATIONAL HUMANITIES IN MEDICINE SEMINAR

This seminar was established to achieve three purposes: to provide selected medical students with an intensive experience in research and writing in the history of medicine, or philosophy of medicine, or literature and medicine; to encourage these students to develop programs of research and writing in a discipline of the humanities, which they will carry out during subsequent years of professional education and training and during careers as clinicians and humanists; and to link these students with other humanists in medicine across generational and disciplinary boundaries. Each student will receive a stipend of $1,200 to cover room and board. Students will be reimbursed for round-trip air fares to and from their school or home.

ACP-ASIM Medical Student Abstract Competition

Wanted: Students involved in research projects through their medical schools or community service programs they want to share with others, or who have come across as interesting case during an internal medicine rotation or through an internal medicine preceptorship program. If you are a medical student member of the ACP-ASIM, you are invited to submit an abstract to the annual Medical Student Abstract Competition. Ten winners will be awarded an expense-paid trip to the annual session. Abstracts may be submitted electronically using our online form at *www.acp.org*.

Medical Student Membership in the American College of Physicians–American Society of Internal Medicine

ACP-ASIM membership entitles you to special discounts on various college products, free attendance at ACP-ASIM annual session (the annual scientific meeting) and local chapter meetings, and a subscription to IMpact, the medical student newsletter.

AMA POLITICAL ACTION COMMITTEE (AMPAC)

AMPAC is a bipartisan group that serves to advance the interest of medicine within Congress, specifically by supporting candidates for office that are friendly to medicine. They also provide numerous programs to educate physicians, medical students, and their families on political activism. The board directs the programs and activities of this extremely important political action committee. Adding medical students to the leadership of this group will provide for better medical student representation within the group, as well as greater student involvement in this important process. Terms are for 2 years. Contact the American Medical Association for more information.

AMA Foundation Leadership Award Program

This award is an exciting opportunity to advance your leadership skills within organized medicine. Medical students who have demonstrated strong non-clinical leadership skills in medicine or community affairs and have an interest in further developing these skills within organized medicine are eligible. The objective of the award program is to encourage involvement in organized medicine and continue leadership development among the country's brightest and most energetic medical students and residents. Twenty-five medical students will be selected. Travel expenses for award winners, including airfare and 3 night's hotel, will be paid for directly by the AMA Foundation to attend the 2001 AMA National Leadership Development Conference. For applications, call 1-800-AMA-3211, ext. 4751 or 4746.

AMA-MSS Councils

The medical student section of the AMA (AMA-MSS) has several councils for which it seeks medical students. Application involves a current curriculum vitae, an essay on why you want to be a member of an AMA Council, which Council(s) you prefer, what you consider to be your major strengths and qualifications for the position, and what benefits you feel are likely to result from your participation.

- Council on Constitution and Bylaws
- Council on Ethical and Judicial Affairs
- Council on Legislation
- Council on Long-Range Planning and Development
- Council on Medical Education
- Council on Medical Service
- Council on Scientific Affairs

EDITORIAL POSITIONS WITH MEDICAL STUDENT JAMA

MS/JAMA is the 7- to 8-page medical student section of the *Journal of the American Medical Association* (JAMA) that appears in the first JAMA of every month, September through May, and is also produced each month on the MS/JAMA Web site. As a regular section of a major medical journal, pro-

duced by and for medical students, MS/JAMA represents a unique opportunity to train to become journal editors, writers, and contributors. The MS/JAMA Web site is located at *www.ama-assn.org/msjama*.

AMA-MSS Committee Application

Medical students are sought to serve on the following AMA-MSS committees:

- Committee on Computers and Technology (formerly Computer Projects Committee)
- Committee on Long-Range Planning
- Legislative Affairs Committee
- Minority Issues Committee
- Ad Hoc Committee on Community Service and Advocacy
- Ad Hoc Committee on Membership Recruitment and Retention
- Ad Hoc Committee on MSS Programs and Activities
- Ad Hoc Committee on Scientific Issues Committee (CSI)
- Ad Hoc Committee on International Health and Policy

All applications must be completed and submitted with a CV to: American Medical Association, Department of Medical Student Services, 515 North State Street, Chicago, IL 60610. Fax: 312-464-5845.

NATIONAL TAY-SACHS & ALLIED DISEASE FOUNDATION

The primary objective of these awards is to stimulate interest in the field of lysosomal storage diseases. The research may be basic, applied, or clinical and should be performed under the direction of an investigator experienced in the field. Stipend: $1,500.

New York Academy of Medicine:

The Glorney–Raisbeck Medical Student Grants in Cardiovascular Research Program

Three grants of $3,000 will be provided to support projects in either clinical or basic research initiated during the summer. Competition is open to MD candidates in a metropolitan area medical school in New York City, Long Island, Westchester County, or New Jersey. The award will be paid directly to the sponsoring medical school for distribution to the recipient. The deadline for submission of applications is March. *Contact:* Fellowship Program Coordinator, New York Academy of Medicine, 1216 Fifth Avenue, Room 612, New York, NY 10029. Phone: 212-822-7204; Fax: 212-996-7826.

New York Academy of Medicine: The Louis L. Seaman Medical Student Research Grants in Microbiology

Four grants of $2,500 will be provided to support summer research projects in the field of microbiology. Competition is open to MD students in a metropolitan area medical school in New York City, Long Island, Westchester County, or New Jersey. The award will be paid directly to the student, but is contingent on the submission of a written report on the project. *Contact:* Fellowship Program Coordinator, New York Academy of Medicine, 1216 Fifth Avenue, Room 612, New York, NY 10029. Phone: 212-822-7204; Fax: 212-996-7826.

American Medical Association Education and Research Foundation Seed Research Grants

Up to $2,500 support for medical students for small research projects, or in some instances, to provide interim funding prior to large grant approvals from other sources. Grants will be awarded in two cycles during the school year: (1) September through November and (2) January through March. *Contact:* American Medical Association Education and Research Foundation, 515 North State Street, Chicago, IL 60610. Phone: 312-464-5357; Fax: 312-464-5973; *www.ama-assn.org/med-sci/erf/toc.htm.*

WEIS CENTER FOR RESEARCH GEISINGER CLINIC

Three-month program designed to expose medical students to career opportunities in research. Primary emphasis is at the cellular/molecular level of cardiovascular function. Stipend: $800/ month.

John A. Hartford/AFAR Medical Student Geriatric Scholars Program

To encourage medical students, particularly budding researchers, to consider geriatrics as a career, the Medical Student Geriatric Scholars Program awards short-term scholarships through a national competition. The program provides an opportunity for these students to train at an acclaimed center of excellence in geriatrics. Each scholar receives a $3,000 stipend. Students in the New York Metropolitan area can apply for funding through the Farr Fox and Leslie R. Samuels Foundation/AFAR Medical Student Geriatric Scholars Program. Contact American Federation for Aging Research (AFAR), 1414 Avenue of the Americas, 18th Floor, New York, NY 10019. Phone: 212-752-2327; Fax: 212-832-2298; E-mail: *amfedaging@aol.com.*

Glenn Foundation/AFAR Scholarships for Research in the Biology of Aging

Inaugurated in 1994, this scholarship program was designed to attract potential scientists and clinicians to aging research. Provides PhD and MD students the opportunity to conduct a 3-month research project. Students will work in an area of biomedical research in aging under the auspices of a mentor. Each scholarship carries an award of $5,000. *Contact:* American Federation for Aging Research (AFAR), 1414 Avenue of the Americas, 18th Floor, New York, NY 10019. Phone: 212-752-2327; Fax: 212-832-2298; E-mail: *amfedaging@aol.com.*

MERCK/AFAR RESEARCH SCHOLARSHIPS IN GERIATRIC PHARMACOLOGY FOR MEDICAL STUDENTS

To develop a corps of physicians with an understanding of medication use in the elderly, the Merck Company Foundation and AFAR created the Merck/AFAR Research Scholarships in Geriatric Pharmacology. Medical students will have the opportunity to undertake a 2- to 3-month full-time research project in geriatric pharmacology. Up to nine $4,000 scholarships will be awarded in 2001. *Contact:* American Federation for Aging Research (AFAR), 1414 Avenue of the Americas, 18th Floor, New York, NY 10019. Phone: 212-752-2327; Fax: 212-832-2298; E-mail: *amfedaging@aol.com.*

American Oil Chemists' Society

Graduate students in any area of science dealing with fats and lipids who are doing research toward an advanced degree, and who are interested in the area of science and technology fostered by this Society, are eligible. Must be a graduate student who has not yet received his or her degree or begun employment prior to the AOCS meeting he/she is to attend. The award will provide funds equal to travel costs, hotel accommodations and stipend to permit attendance at the National Meeting of the AOCS held in the spring.

Biomedical Synergistics Institute—Ninth International Conference

Award for those individuals in training who submit the best original paper dealing with the Institute enhancement of human functioning. Papers published previously are not eligible for awards. Four student award categories with each receiving a prize of $250. The All Functioning Categories winner will receive a $1,000 prize.

AAA PRESLEY–CARL ZEISS YOUNG INVESTIGATOR AWARD

Recognizes excellence in research using light and/or electron microscopy. Must be a graduate student, medical student, postdoc (within 5 years of receiving PhD), or medical resi-

dent. $500 prize and certificate. Contact the Advisory Committee of Young Anatomists (ACYA) at 301-571-8314 or *exec@anatomy.org.*

AAA Zeiss Student Research Award

Recognizes excellence in research using state-of-the-art imaging methods, such as confocal and/or electron microscopy. Must be a graduate student or medical student. $500 prize and certificate. Contact the Advisory Committee of Young Anatomists (ACYA) at 301-571-8314 or *exec@anatomy.org.*

AAA/Genentech Student Research Award

Recognizes excellence in research using molecular biological techniques in the study of morphological changes at the cellular and/or whole animal level. Must be a graduate student, medical student, postdoc (within 5 years of receiving PhD), or medical resident. $500 prize and certificate. Contact the Advisory Committee of Young Anatomists (ACYA) at 301-571-8314 or *exec@anatomy.org.*

HELLENIC UNIVERSITY CLUB OF NEW YORK DR. FRED VALERGAKIS GRANT

Research grants to graduate students of Hellenic ancestry enrolled in an accredited university engaged in research. Minimum grants of $1,000.

Alpha Omega Alpha Research Fellowships

The purpose of the fellowships is to stimulate interest in research among medical students. Areas of research may include clinical investigation, basic research, epidemiology, and the social sciences, as related to medicine. The program is designed to stimulate students who have not had prior research experience. Fellowship is for $2,000.

American Medical Association Education and Research Foundation

Open to third- and fourth-year medical students who have completed the required clerkships in medicine, surgery, and pediatrics. The program consists of 4- to 6-week clerkships in general, pediatric, and surgical nutrition. Scholarships are only for students who do not have clinical nutrition clerkships available at their own schools. Students accepted into the program will receive a $700 award to defray living and traveling costs.

AMERICAN COLLEGE OF SPORTS MEDICINE NATIONAL STUDENT RESEARCH AWARD

The National Student Research Award recognizes the most outstanding research project of the year at the graduate/professional student level. An important consideration for the award is the extent of the student's participation in the project. Each applicant must be enrolled in a graduate or professional program in the areas of clinical or basic exercise science or sports medicine at an accredited university; be principal author of a submitted and accepted abstract for presentation at the ACSM Annual Meeting; and be a member of ACSM or one of its regional chapters at the time of application and at the time the award is presented. The New Investigator and National Student Research awards provide support for the recipients to attend the annual meeting and present their research. Registration fees, travel expenses, lodging, banquet tickets, and framed certificates (presented at the annual awards banquet) are awarded to the recipients. *Contact:* American College of Sports Medicine, Graduate

Scholarships for Minorities and Women, 401 W. Michigan St., Indianapolis, IN 46202-3233. Phone: 317-637-9200; Fax: 317-634-7817; *www.acsm.org/*.

American Academy of Allergy Asthma and Immunology Summer Fellowship Grant

Summer fellowship grants of $2,000 will be awarded to outstanding medical students who wish to pursue research in the following areas: physiology of allergic diseases, pharmacology of allergy and inflammation, basic cellular and molecular immunology, AIDS, and other topics pertinent to the understanding of allergic and immune mechanisms of disease. Elgibility: Full-time medical students residing in the United States or Canada who have successfully completed at least 8 months of medical school by the time the fellowship starts. Past Summer Fellowship Grant recipients are not eligible. *Contact:* American Academy of Allergy Asthma and Immunology, 611 East Wells Street, Milwaukee, WI 53202-3889. Phone: 414-272-6071; Fax: 414-272-6070; *www.aaaai.org/*.

SUMMER EXTERNSHIPS

Africa with Crossroads

Sponsoring Agency: Operation Crossroads Africa

For senior medical school students who would like to work on a 5- to 7-week project in Africa that might focus on one of the following themes: (1) the community health approach,

(2) diagnosis and treatment of tropical diseases, (3) preventive approaches to tropical diseases, and (4) the use of paramedics. Each project will also involve some labor. No stipend. The sponsoring agency will assist students in finding funds for transportation.

AMERICAN LIVER FOUNDATION STUDENT RESEARCH FELLOWSHIPS

To gain exposure in the research laboratory and possibly consider liver research a career option. Award is $2,500 per month for 3 months. *Contact:* American Liver Foundation, 1425 Pompton Avenue, Cedar Grove, NJ 07009. Phone: 201-857-2626; *www.liverfoundation.org/*.

Mucopolysaccharidosis Society Summer Fellowship

Eight-week summer fellowship for study of mucopolysaccharide diseases Stipend: $1,500.

Utica College of Syracuse Summer Clerkships

Both of the following programs offer students clinical experience augment their classroom university instruction, reinforce clinical skills, and create interest in their future choice of both medical specialty and geographic area of practice: The summer clerkships (2 to 8 weeks) are designed for students who have completed either 1 or 2 years of training. Preference is given to second-year students. Stipend is $250/2 weeks. The clinical electives are credit courses offered on a year-round basis in 22 specialties for third- and fourth-year medical students.

MEMORIAL SLOAN–KETTERING CANCER CENTER SUMMER FELLOWSHIP

Sponsored by National Cancer Institute and Eugene W. Kettering Education Fund

Eight-week summer fellowship offered to medical students in their first 2 years. Objective of program is the educational enrichment of medical students by offering experience in research and clinical oncology and enhancement of their knowledge of cancer and promotion of future interest in the field. *Contact:* Chuck Ferrero, Box 187, Memorial Sloan–Kettering Cancer Center, 1275 York Ave., NY 10012 (212) 639-8457

Paul Alexander Memorial Fellowship

To provide an international public health opportunity to a medical student after the third year to work with a Management Sciences for Health team for 2 to 3 months.

American Medical Student Association/Adolescent Substance Abuse Prevention

Six- to 8-week summer internships in homeless and runaway shelters to help develop programs in self-esteem, decision-making skills, health education relating to substance abuse, and abuse prevention. $250/week.

ALLEGHENY GENERAL HOSPITAL EXTERNSHIPS

For students who have completed at least 1 year of medical school. This is an 8-week summer clerkship. Stipend of $1,000 is available through the hospital. A peformance evaluation is submitted by Allegheny General Hospital to the student's medical school. (Second-year students preferred.)

Bertram Low–Beer, V.A. Memorial Fellowship for Radiation Oncology

Sponsored by University of California in San Francisco, this summer fellowship will support a medical student to spend 10 weeks in the Department of Radiation Oncology at the University of California, San Francisco. Student must have completed 2 years of medical school. During the 10-week experience, the student will spend time interviewing patients, learning and participating in physical examinations, and learning the natural history, psychosocial impact, and cancer treatment techniques. Student will participate in a small research project the findings of which will be presented to the staff and other students. Stipend is $1,000.

MAP–Reader's Digest Missionary Medicine Fellowship

The purpose of this program is to provide selected senior medical students with firsthand exposure to missionary medicine and inform them of the cultural, social, and health-related problems characteristic of developing countries. Students serve for a minimum of 8 weeks. MAP will provide 75% of least expensive round-trip air fare.

J.M. FOUNDATION SCHOLARSHIPS

One to 3-week scholarships covering tuition, room and board, travel at selected summer schools of alcohol studies.

Simon Kramer Externship in Radiation Oncology

Sponsored by the Thomas Jefferson Hospital, Philadelphia, this fellowship provides a unique opportunity for the medical student to obtain a 6-week experience in the Department of Radiation Therapy and Nuclear Medicine at Jefferson. Flexible beginning date; stipend of $1,200.

NEW YORK STATE LEGISLATIVE FELLOW

Fellows work as regular legislative staff members of the offices to which they are assigned. The work is full time, demanding, and is intended to use and develop the expertise of Fellows while offering an exclusive view of legislative procedures.

Education and Research Foundation of the Society of Nuclear Medicine Awards

The purpose of the Student Fellowship Program is to provide financial support for students wishing to spend time in clinical or basic research activities in a nuclear medicine division for a 3-month period with a stipend of $3,000.

Student Fellowship Award Foundation of the Society of Nuclear Medicine

This fellowship provides financial support for students to spend elective quarters and/or summers in departments of nuclear medicine assisting in clinical and basic research activities.

Upjohn Summer Extern Program

Students are assigned to a unit in either the Medical Affairs or Research Division to give them an opportunity to acquire first-hand experience within the pharmaceutical industry. There is also a biweekly lecture series to provide exposure to key scientists and a more comprehensive view of pharmaceutical operations.

ARTHRITIS FOUNDATION, NY CHAPTER, ALBERT GROEKOEST PRIZE

Eight-week summer research fellowship in rheumatic diseases and/or skeletal diseases. May be used at any American institution. Stipend of $3,000.

Harbor Branch Oceanographic Institute Internship

Ten-week internship for students interested in ocean engineering, marine sciences, biomedical marine research, and related fields. Aquaculture, computer science, marine biology, tumor biology, virology, microbiology, molecular biology, etc. Stipend: $260/wk.

Roswell Park Memorial Research Institute (Buffalo, NY) Summer Oncology Program

Provides direct support for students in the health professions engaged in research during the summer. Fellowships are awarded for an 8-week period. Research is restricted to topics in oncology. Participation in this program is limited to students completing their first or second year of study.

RUTGERS UNIVERSITY SUMMER SCHOLARSHIPS

Ten scholarships are available for this year's Summer School of Alcohol Studies to medical students. Award covers university fees, tuition, room, and meals ($975); weekend meals and travel are not included. However, a $200 stipend for related expenses will also be given to each scholarship recipient.

New York Academy of Medicine HIV Professional Development Project

Two-month internship in HIV-focused health care and social service settings. 35 hours/week, $10/hr.

Case Western Reserve University—Pathology

For those who have completed their sophomore year in medical school. This is a 12-month fellowship with a $12,000 stipend. The time will be divided between diagnostic pathology on the autopsy service and research related to the immunological and biochemical characterization of human cancer.

Clendening, Logan Traveling Fellowship

Sponsoring Agency: University of Kansas Medical Center

This fellowship is open to registered medical students of any recognized medical or school in the United States or Canada.

The fellowship is of the value of $1,500. Applicants may elect to travel anywhere in the world for the purpose of studying any aspect of medical history of interest to them.

COSTEP OF THE U.S. PUBLIC HEALTH SERVICE

U.S. Public Health Service offers opportunities in Indian Health Services, Health Resources, and Services Administration, NIH, Food and Drug Administration, CDC, Alcohol, Drug Abuse and Mental Health Administration, etc. U.S. citizenship and at least one year of medical school required. Positions are available all year round. $2,000/month plus travel costs. Information is available in Student Affairs; for application, call 1-800-279-1605 or 301-594-2633.

NIH Predoctoral Fellowship Awards for Medical Students

All branches of the NIH have grants for medical student summer research. *Contact: www.nih.gov.*

Cystic Fibrosis Foundation Student Traineeships

The Cystic Fibrosis Foundation announces student traineeships which are offered to introduce students to research related to CF. Applicants must be students in or about to enter a doctoral program (MD, PhD, or MD/PhD). Each applicant must work with a faculty sponsor on a research project related to CF. The award is $1,500, of which $1,200 is designated as a stipend for the trainee, and the remainder $300 may be used for laboratory expenses. For an application, write to: Office of Grants Management, Cystic Fibrosis Foundation, 6931 Arlington Road, Bethesda, MD 20814, or call 1-800-FLIGHT CF.

AMA-MSS GOVERNMENT RELATIONS INTERSHIP PROGRAM APPLICATION

The Department of Medical Student Services, in conjunction with the Washington office of the American Medical Association, is pleased to offer assistance to students seeking to increase their involvement and education in national health policy and in the national legislative activities of organized medicine.

Through the Government Relations Internship Program, stipends of $2,500 are available to assist selected students who are completing health policy internships in the Washington, DC area. To be eligible for the Program, students must be AMA members who have secured a policy internship in the Washington, DC, area. Through the program, students may also apply for an internship at the AMA's Washington office (two positions available), or at the Health Care Financing Administration in Baltimore, Maryland (one position available). Students participating in the program generally arrange their internships with Congressional offices, specialty societies, or federal agencies in the DC area.

A list of possible internship contacts is available.

The Betty Ford Center Summer Institute for Medical Students

Provides experiential education in chemical dependency and its treatment, primarily by student participation in the patient and family rehabilitation process. Five groups of 12 students will participate in the 5-day summer school program. Each session four Family Program participants follow the weekly schedule of family members, and eight students selected for the Inpatient Program are assigned to one of four inpatient treatment units. Program activities include lectures, meals, group therapy sessions, peer groups, exercise sessions, meditation, medallion ceremonies and Alcoholics and Narcotics Anonymous meetings. Students are asked to maintain a focused journal. A basic set of books and a reference manual is provided to each student. Scholarships to this very special program include the cost of all materials, lodging and meals. A travel stipend is also included. A total of 60 scholarships will be awarded. Students may apply to attend one of four summer sessions. For application information, write: Betty Ford Center Training Department, 39000 Bob Hope Drive, Rancho Mirage, CA 92270. Phone: 619-773-4108; Toll free: 1-800-854-9211, ext. 4108; Fax: 619-773-1697.

The Albert Schweitzer Fellowship

Provides complete funding for medical students who will work in Lambaréné, Gabon, as junior physicians, supervised by Schweitzer Hospital medical staff. Prior completion of clerkships in medicine, pediatrics, and surgery are required; some background or coursework in tropical medicine or parasitology is important but not a prerequisite. Because all patient encounters occur in French, a working knowledge of that language is absolutely essential. For more information, contact: The Albert Schweitzer Foundation, 330 Brookline Avenue, Boston, MA 02215.

YEAR-LONG FELLOWSHIPS

HOWARD HUGHES MEDICAL INSTITUTE RESEARCH SCHOLARS TRAINING

Students in good standing in a medical school in the United States who have completed the second year but have not yet received the MD are eligible. The program is for at least 9 months and usually 1 year at NIH. Salary program $16,800, and other benefits are included. *Contact:* 1-800-424-9924.

American Diabetes Association, Inc. Medical Scholars Program Awards

The goal of the program is to produce new leaders in diabetes research by supplying physicians-in-training the opportunity to contribute to the process of discovery in basic or clinical research laboratories. Award is $30,000 for 1 year. Eligibility: Students must have completed at least two years of medical school. *Contact:* American Diabetes Association, Inc. Research Department, 1701 North Beauregard Street, Alexandria, VA 22311. Phone: 703-549-1500, ext. 2376; Fax: 703-549-1715. *www.diabetes.org/research/*

Pew Charitable Trust/Rockefeller University Fellowships in Human Nutrition

One-year program designed to give hands-on laboratory experience and mastering of new methods in biomedical science for application to problems in human nutrition. Students should have completed their third year by July 1. Stipend: $14,700. Pierce, Chester Research Symposium.

UNIVERSITY OF PITTSBURGH PATHOLOGY FELLOWSHIP

One-year fellowship for medical students who have completed their second year and wish to spend an additional year of in-depth study of pathology in research (pathology, molecular biology, genetics, etc.) and practice before going on to the third year. The stipend is $11,000, and a scholarship for the next year of medical school (up to the state tuition rate at Pittsburgh) will be provided.

Association of Pathology Chairman Student Fellowship

Year-long full-time fellowship in participating schools for students after the second year of medical school. Intended to give students an in-depth research and/or clinical experience in pathology between the basic science and clinical years. Support varies by school, as do openings for students not from that school.

New York City Health Research Training Program

This is a practicum in public health research. The student participates in a project under the direct supervision of a preceptor. The projects are submitted by preceptors from within the Health Department or from outside agencies such as hospitals, medical schools, or other health-related institutions. A seminar series is part of the program. Work–study students are preferred. However, some alternative support is available for those not eligible for work–study. Full time in summer, part time during school year. Hourly wage of $5–$8.40.

NEW YORK CITY URBAN FELLOWS PROGRAM

Year-long program offering the opportunity and challenge of an intensive field experience in urban government. Fellows work closely with City officials on long- and short-term projects and attend weekly seminars to gain an academic perspective on the workings and problems of local government. $17,000 stipend and insurance.

National Institutes of Health Summer Research Fellowship*

With the guidance of a preceptor from one of the Institutes, students conduct research in a selected area of laboratory investigation. Program offers practical experience in research procedures and lectures and seminars designed to enhance education and investigative skills. Program runs a minimum of 8 weeks.

National Institutes of Health Clinical Electives Program

Medical students are invited to apply for clinical electives of 8 weeks with opportunities research and clinical experience with physician–scientists in Bethesda.

OSLER LIBRARY FELLOWSHIP PROGRAM

A fellowship program for historians, physicians, and students conducting research in the history of medicine. Intended to serve those who need to establish temporary residence in order to undertake research in the Osler Library.

Henry Luce Foundation Scholars Program

This program provides an intensive year-long experience in

Asia designed to broaden the scholar's professional perspectives and to sharpen their perceptions of Asia, America, and themselves. The support consists of airfare, stipend, medical insurance, etc.

Echoing Green Foundation Fellowship

One-year fellowship providing entrepreneurial people with the opportunity to develop and implement an innovative public service project (health, environment, youth service, international development, etc.). Students must develop a proposal. Stipend is $25,000 per year.

HEALTH RESEARCH GROUP MEDICAL STUDENT FELLOWSHIP

One-year fellowship in Washington researching and monitoring federal health agencies, congressional lobbying, publication of consumer-oriented educational manuals, etc.

Rosalie B. Hite Cancer Center Research Fellowship

Sponsoring Agency: University of Texas System

Fellowship open to graduate students or research workers in the area of cancer research. Selection of Fellows is on the basis of academic excellence of the candidate and applicability of the proposed program to the problems of cancer research.

Graduate work is to be under the supervision of a faculty member of a component of the University of Texas at Houston, affiliated with the Graduate School of Biomedical Sciences Sciences degree-granting program.

Charles A. Dana Foundation Clinical Research Training Program

Sponsoring Agency: University of Pennsylvania School of Medicine

Opportunity for medical students to participate in a year-long in-depth clinical research training experience under the guidance of selected faculty who are accomplished investigators in the fields of epidemiology, clinical research methodology and the delivery of health care services. Training will be provided in clinical research methods, clinical epidemiology, biostatistics, and scientific communication. Stipend of $11,000 plus expenses.

CHARLES A. AND ANNE MORROW LINDBERGH FOUNDATION

A foundation dedicated to furthering Charles and Anne Morrow Lindbergh's shared vision of a balance between technological advancement and environmental preservation. Lindbergh grants are made in the following categories: agriculture; aviation/aerospace; conservation of natural resources—including animals, plants, water, and general conservation (land, air, energy, etc.); education—including humanities/education, the arts, and intercultural communication; exploration; health—including biomedical research, health and population sciences,

and adaptive technology; and waste minimization and management. A Jonathan Lindbergh Brown Grant may be given to a project to support adaptive technology or biomedical research which seeks to re-

dress imbalance between an individual and his or her human environment. Grants are made to individuals as well as educational and publication programs. *Contact: www.lindbergh-foundation.org.*

National Medical Fellowship—Commonwealth Fund

This program is designed to encourage academically gifted minority medical students to pursue careers in academic medicine and biomedical research. Open to those students who have completed their junior year. Duration is 8 to 12 weeks. Students have the option to participate in the summer or during the academic year. Fellowship award is for $5,000 with $2,000 earmarked for mentor to offset expenses during the research period.

National Institute of Arthritis and Musculoskeletal and Skin Diseases (NIAMS)

The Minority Travel Award Program provides travel funds for minority students and faculty members from minority institutions for attendance at national scientific meetings. *Contact: www.nih.gov/niams.*

NIH PREDOCTORAL FELLOWSHIP AWARDS FOR MINORITY STUDENTS

The National Research Service Award Predoctoral Fellowship

for Minority Students will provide up to 5 years of support for research training leading to the PhD or equivalent research degree; the combined MD/PhD degree; or other combined professional degree and research doctoral degree in biomedical, behavioral sciences, or health services research. These fellowships are designed to enhance the racial and ethnic diversity of the biomedical, behavioral, and health services research labor force in the United States. Accordingly, academic institutions are encouraged to identify and recruit students from underrepresented racial and ethnic groups who can apply for this fellowship. Support is *not* available for individuals enrolled in medical or other professional schools *unless* they are also enrolled in a combined professional doctorate/PhD degree program in biomedical, behavioral, or health services research. *Contact: www.nih.gov.*

National Medical Fellowships, Inc.

NMF offers awards and fellowships to American Blacks, mainland Puerto Ricans, Mexican Americans, and American Indians who are U.S. Citizens enrolled in accredited schools of allopathic or osteopathic medi-

cine in the United States. Funding is variable, yearly, and renewable. *Contact:* National Medical Fellowships, Inc., 254 West 31st Street, 7th Floor, New York, NY 10001. Phone: 212-714-1007.

Metropolitan Life Award Program for Academic Excellence in Medicine

This program recognizes and rewards third-year minority medical students for outstanding academic achievement and demonstrated leadership. $2,500 need-based awards to underrepresented minorities. Nominated by dean's office.

AMERICAN COLLEGE OF SPORTS MEDICINE MINORITY SCHOLARSHIP

The American College of Sports Medicine annually awards graduate scholarships for minorities and females of up to $1,500 each to be used to cover college or university tuition and/or fees. The purpose of these scholarships is to provide partial support toward the education of graduate and/or medical students with outstanding promise and a strong interest in research and scholarly activities as they pursue a career in sports medicine or exercise science. Scholarships are renewable for up to 4 years based on their research and professional activities and satisfactory academic progress in full-time study toward a graduate degree. Students who are not currently ACSM members are eligible to apply. Free student membership in the American College of Sports Medicine is also provided each year of an awardee's graduate scholarship. *Contact:* American College of Sports Medicine, Graduate Scholarships for Minorities and Women, 401 W. Michigan St., Indianapolis, IN 46202-3233. Phone: 317-637-9200; Fax: 317-634-7817; *www.acsm.org/.*

Congressional Black Caucus Foundation, Inc. Scholarships

Offers grant money for doctoral study to minority students. *Contact:* Congressional Black Caucus Foundation, Inc., 1004 Pennsylvania Avenue SE, Washington, DC 20003. Phone: 1-800-784-2577 or 202-675-6730; Fax: 202-547-3806.

AMERICAN INDIAN GRADUATE CENTER GRANTS

Grants of $250–$10,000 are available for American Indian students who are members of a federally recognized American Indian tribe or Alaska Native group, or possess one-fourth degree federally recognized Indian blood with financial need after exhausting available aid at their school financial aid office. *Contact:* American Indian Graduate Center, 4520 Montgomery Blvd. NE, Suite 1-B, Albuquerque, New Mexico 87109. Phone: 505-881-4584.

Dr. Anthony Bagatelos Memorial Scholarship

Grant money available for Greek descent/Greek Orthodox faith with intentions to practice medicine within the nine-county area surrounding San Francisco Bay. Applications may be obtained by contacting: Annunciation Greek Orthodox Cathedral, 245 Valencia St., San Francisco CA 94103.

Chinese American Physicians Society (CAPS)

CAPS is offering eight to ten scholarships of $1,000 to $2,000 each annually to two categories of medical students. The first is the Dr. Lester Chen Memorial Scholarships to students of Asian descent from the San Francisco Bay area. The other is the CAPS Scholarships to all

medical students in need of financial aid regardless of their hometown, sex, race, or color. The applicants are judged according to their academic achievements, financial needs, community service records, and essays. Special credit is also given to those who are willing to serve the Chinese communities after their graduation. The deadline for submitting the completed application is usually the first Friday in October. Due to the huge number of requests for applications and our shortage of manpower, we can no longer send out the application by mail unless a self-addressed stamped envelope is enclosed with the request. Please obtain the applications from the student financial aid office of your medical school starting from April 1 each year. You can also print a copy of the published scholarship application from our

Web site. The 2000 program hasclosed. The 2001 program will start in spring. If you need more information about scholarship program, please contact Chinese American Physicians Society, Lawrence M. Ng, M.D., Executive Director, 345 Ninth Street, Suite 204, Oakland, CA 94607-4206. Phone: 510-895-5539 (voice and fax); E-mail: *scholarship@caps-ca.org.*

JAPANESE MEDICAL SOCIETY SCHOLARSHIP AWARD

$1,500–$5,000 grants to students of Japanese ancestry who are enrolled or accepted in a U.S. medical school. Applications may be obtained by contacting: Japanese Medical Society of America, Inc. Scholarship Committee, One Henry Street, Englewood Cliffs, NJ 07632.

Hellenic Medical Society of New York—Leonidas Lantzounis Research Grant

This fellowship is open to premed or medical students or science majors of Hellenic descent. Ten-week summer projects are intended to encourage, support, and assist young Greek Americans in their preparation for a scientific career in the biomedical sciences. Stipend: $2,000.

Jewish Vocational Service Academic Scholarship

For Jewish medical students living in Chicago. Applications are accepted December 1 through March 1. *Contact:* Jewish Vocational Service, One South Franklin Street, Chicago, Illinois 60606. Phone: 312-346-6700, ext. 2214.

NATIONAL HISPANIC SCHOLARSHIP FUND

$500–$1,000 awards based on academic achievement, personal strengths, leadership, and financial need for students of Mexican American, Puerto Rican, Cuban, Caribbean, Central or South American heritage. Application period is from April 1 through June 15.

Hellenic Medical Society Scholarship

Awards for medical students of Hellenic heritage from New York, New Jersey, Pennsylvania, Connecticut; Must be a second-year student enrolled at accredited U.S. school. *Contact:* Hellenic Medical Society of New York, 401 East 34th Street, New York NY 10016.

FOR WOMEN

Business & Professional Women's Clubs Grace Legendre Fellowships

For women who are residents of New York State and citizens of the United States and within 2 years of completing studies in an advanced graduate degree program. Must show evidence of scholastic ability and need for financial assistance. Scholarships are for $1,000.

AAUW EDUCATIONAL FOUNDATION INTERNATIONAL FELLOWSHIP

This is a grant for foreign students to pursue graduate studies in the United States. *Contact:* American Association of University Women, 1111 Sixteenth St. NW, Washington, DC 20036. Phone: 1-800-326-AAUW; Fax: 202-872-1425; E-mail: *info@aauw.org.*

AMWA Carroll L. Birch Award

Sponsored by the Chicago Branch of the American Medical Women's Association, the award is presented for the best original research paper written by a Student Life Member of AMWA. Women must be enrolled in an accredited U.S. medical or osteopathic medical school to apply. The recipient of the award receives a cash prize of $500 and a plaque presented at AMWA's Annual Meeting. An article noting the award winner will appear in one of the Association's publications and an abstract may be published in AMWA's journal. Contact your school's financial aid office for more info.

AMWA Bed and Breakfast Program

The program assists students who are traveling for a residency or job interview or physician members attending an out-of-town conference. Our members contact the national office with details of the trip. The national office responds by sending the traveler a listing of volunteers in the destination area. There is an administrative fee of $10.00 for students and $15.00 for physicians.

BPW Career Advancement Scholarship for Women

$500 to $1,000 grants for women over 25 in their third or fourth year of studies with critical need for assistance. *Contact:* Scholarships/Loans Business and Professional Woman's Foundation, 2012 Mass Ave. NW, Washington, DC 20036. Phone: 202-293-1200, ext. 169.

www.acponline.org/journals/ebm/ebmmenu.htm: Reviews the evidence for current medical practice.

www.ebem.org: Evidence-based emergency medicine home page.

cebm.jr2.ox.ac.uk: NHS Research and Development Centre of Evidence Based Medicine.

www.update-software.com/cochrane.htm: Web site for the Cochrane Library, the most well-known site for critically appraised topics or evidence-based reviews.

www.ebando.com: Bandolier: online publication on evidence-based health care.

www.shef.ac.uk/~scharr/ir/netting.html: Netting the evidence: A ScHARR introduction to evidence-based practice on the Internet.

www.ti.ubc.ca/pages/letter.html: Therapeutics Letter: Evidence-based review of pharmaceutical products.

www.ncbi.nlm.nih.gov/PubMed: Pub Med, a MEDLINE search engine through the National Library of Medicine.

igm.nlm.nih.gov: Grateful Med, a MEDLINE search engine through the National Library of Medicine.

www.cdc.gov: The Centers for Disease Control and Prevention: Contains full text issues of *Morbidity and Mortality Weekly Report.*

www.nejm.org: New England *Journal of Medicine.*

www.jwatch.org: Journal Watch.

www.bmj.com/index.shtml: *British Medical Journal.*

jama.ama-assm.org: Journal of *the American Medical Association.*

Index

signs and symptoms, 89
treatment, 90
Takayasu's arteritis, 206
Breast cancer
epidemiology, 337
etiology, 337
hormone replacement therapy, 342
hypercalcemia, 219
obesity, 348
risk factors, 337
screening
exams, 337
mammograms, 337
masses, 337
treatment, 337–338
Breast feeding, 338
Breast milk transmission of HIV, 294
Breath sounds, 79, 297
Bretylium, 56
Broca's aphasia, 81
Bromocriptine, 100, 247
Bronchial artery embolization, 70
Bronchiectasis
definition, 69
diagnosis, 69
etiology, 69
pathophysiology, 69
signs and symptoms, 69
treatment, 69
Bronchitis. *See* Chronic bronchitis
Bronchoalveolar lavage, 297
Bronchoconstriction, 331
Bronchodilators, 70
Bronchospasm, 164
Brush border enzymes, 117
Bruton's congenital agammaglobulinemia,
    289
Buffalo's hump, 265
Bullae, 333
Bullet presentation, 4
Bupropion, 345
Burkitt's lymphoma, 177, 181, 303
Burns
acalculous cholecystitis, 129
acute pancreatitis, 125
cellulitis, 323
hypomagnesemia, 224
toxic epidermal necrolysis, 327
toxic shock syndrome, 307
Byssinosis, 80

C

Calamine lotion, 320
Calcific disease, 30
Calcipotriene, 319
Calcitonin, 179, 186, 220, 221, 261, 270,
    272
Calcitriol, 218, 262
Calcium
chronic renal failure, 230
hypercalcemia, 219–221
hyperkalemia, 217
hyperparathyroidism, 220, 221
hyperphosphatemia, 223
hypocalcemia, 218
hypoparathyroidism, 262
hypophosphatemia, 222
osteomalacia, 268
osteoporosis, 270, 271
protein-losing enteropathy, 122
sarcoidosis, 194
scleroderma, 195

tropical sprue, 120
vertebral compression fracture, 186
Calcium channel blockers
angina, 23
atrial fibrillation, 48
cardiomyopathy, hypertrophic, 37
gastroesophageal reflux disease, 110
hypertension, 53
migraine headache, 94
scleroderma, 195
summary, 56
Torsade de pointes, 48
Wolff–Parkinson–White syndrome, 49
Calcium chloride, 209
Calcium oxalate stones, 281
Calcium pyrophosphate dihydrate (CPPD),
    198
Calciuria, 272
Cambodian people, 154
Campylobacter, 203
Cancer
acute pancreatitis, 125
adrenal insufficiency, 263
alcohol abuse, 344
back pain, lower, 184
brain, 88–90
breast, 219, 337–338, 342, 348
cervical, 279
colon, 143, 146–148, 219, 336
endometrial, 342, 348
esophageal, 110
gastric, 123
head, 344, 345
health promotion
breast cancer, 337–338
cervical cancer, 339
ovarian cancer, 338
prostate cancer, 339–340
testicular cancer, 340–341
hepatocellular, 137
hypercalcemia, 219
hypothyroidism, 255
immunocompromised patients, 290,
    291
lower GI bleeds, 116
lung, 70–73, 219
neck, 344, 345
prostate, 219
renal cell carcinoma, 165
screening and annual exams, 335–336
skin, 315–318
spontaneous pneumothorax, 79
tobacco use, 345
urethra, 274
See also Metastases; Oncology; Tumors
Candida (albicans), 39, 105, 273, 276, 278,
    288, 300
Captopril, 195, 267
Caput medusae, 132
Carbamazepine, 90, 166, 250
Carbapenem, 292
Carbidopa, 99
Carbohydrates, 117
Carbon monoxide, 59
Carboxyhemoglobin, 258
Carcinoembryonic antigen (CEA), 147
Carcinoid syndrome, 36, 139, 140
Carcinoid tumor
definition, 139
diagnosis, 140
etiology, 139
prognosis, 140

signs and symptoms, 139
treatment, 140
Cardiac enzymes, 38
Cardiology
alcohol abuse, 344
coronary artery disease, 18–28
dyslipidemia, 16–18
dysrhythmias
aortic aneurysm, 55–58
aortic dissection, 46–47
atrial fibrillation, 47–48
heart block, 49–51
hypertension, 51–53
hypertensive emergency, 53
sinus bradycardia, 51
Torsade de pointes, 46–47
ventricular fibrillation and pulseless
ventricular tachycardia, 45–46
Wolf–Parkinson–White syndrome,
    48–49
hypothyroidism, 256
Lyme disease, 321
medications, commonly used cardiac
antidysrhythmic agents, other, 56
antihypertensive agents, 57
antiplatelet agents, 57
antithrombotic agents, 57
beta blockers, 56
calcium channel blockers, 56
inotropic agents, 57
prolongs action potentials, 56
sodium channel blockers, 56
thrombolytic agents, 58
pain, causes of chest, 15
pheochromocytoma, 268
risk factors for heart disease, 16
syphilis, 275
testing, cardiac
catheterization, cardiac, 24, 25
echocardiography, 24, 25
exercise stress testing, 24
stress myocardial perfusion
imaging, 24
tobacco use, 345
uremic syndrome, 232
valvular heart disease
aortic regurgitation, 31–32
aortic stenosis, 30–31
bacterial endocarditis, 39–41
constrictive pericarditis, 44–45
dilated cardiomyopathy, 34–35
hypertrophic cardiomyopathy, 36–37
mitral regurgitation, 29–30
mitral stenosis, 28–29
mitral valve prolapse, 30
myocarditis, 38–39
pericardial tamponade, 44
pericarditis, 42–43
restrictive cardiomyopathy, 36
tricuspid regurgitation, 33–34
tricuspid stenosis, 32–33
wet beriberi, 349
Cardiomyopathy, dilated
definition, 34
diagnosis, 35
etiology
endocrine, 34
infectious, 34
metabolic, 34
toxic, 34
pathophysiology, 34
signs and symptoms, 35
treatment, 35

Podophyllin, 279
Polyarteritis nodosa (PAN)
    definition, 204
    laboratory, 204
    nephritic syndrome, acute, 234
    signs and symptoms, 204
    treatment, 204
Polyarthritis, 202
Polycystic kidney disease, 229
Polycythemia vera
    definition, 165
    diagnosis, 165
    epidemiology, 165
    etiology, 165
    signs and symptoms, 165
    treatment, 165
Polydipsia, 231, 237, 248
Polymerase chain reaction (PCR), 86, 121
Polymyositis
    definition, 199
    diagnosis, 199
    etiology, 199
    labs, 199
    prognosis, 199
    signs and symptoms, 199
    treatment, 199
Polypeptides, 117
Polyuria, 127, 237, 242, 248, 249
Porphobilinogen, 166
Porphyria, 102, 166
    See also Acute intermittent porphyria
Portal hypertension
    complications, 132
    definition, 132
    treatment, 133
Positive birefringence of crystals, 198
Positive predictive value, 354
Postherpetic neuralgia, 329
Postnasal drip syndrome
    asthma, 66
    cough, chronic, 65
    definition, 59
    etiology, 60
    pathophysiology, 60
    signs and symptoms, 60
    sinusitis, 60
    treatment, 60
Postpericardiotomy syndrome, 42
Poststreptococcal glomerulonephritis
    course, 233–234
    epidemiology, 233
    laboratory studies, 234
    pathology and pathogenesis, 233
    prognosis, 234
    signs and symptoms, 233
    treatment, 234
Potash, 68
Potassium
    acute tubular necrosis, 228
    adrenal insufficiency, 263
    asthma, 67
    diabetic ketoacidosis, 241, 242
    gastrointestinal absorption, 117
    hyperaldosteronism, 267
    hypercalcemia, 221
    hyperkalemia, 216–217
    hypertension, 53
    hypokalemia, 216–217
    laboratory studies, 207
    metabolic alkalosis, 211
    peptic ulcer disease, 111
Prazosin, 57
Predictive value, positive/negative, 354

Prednisone, 92, 95, 177–179, 181, 204
Preeclampsia, 52, 53, 193
Pregnancy
    abdominal pain, 102
    aortic dissection, 54
    aortic regurgitation, 31
    atopic dermatitis, 331
    cardiomyopathy, dilated, 34
    carpal tunnel syndrome, 196
    cholelithiasis, 127
    disseminated intravascular
        coagulation, 172
    ectopic, 102
    erythema multiforme, 325
    folate deficiency anemia, 150
    HIV (human immunodeficiency virus),
        294, 304
    laryngeal papillomatosis, 279
    lymphogranulosum venereum, 280
    ovarian cancer, 338
    pyelonephritis, 283
    respiratory alkalosis, 210
    Sheehan's syndrome, 247
    systemic lupus erythematosus, 191, 192
    thrombotic thrombocytopenic
        purpura, 171
    tobacco use, 345
    tuberculosis, 78
Preseptal cellulitis, 61
Pressure ulcers. *See* Decubitus ulcers
Preventive care, general
    annual exams, 335–336
    vaccinations, adult, 336
Priapism, 158
Primaquine, 175
Primary aldosteronism, 211
Primary amyloidosis, 36
Primary biliary cirrhosis
    definition, 132
    diagnosis, 132
    epidemiology, 132
    signs and symptoms, 132
    treatment, 132
Primary hyperaldosteronism, 52
Primary hyperparathyroidism
    definition, 220, 260
    diagnosis, 220
    epidemiology, 220, 260
    signs and symptoms, 220
Primary hypothyroidism, 255
Primary sclerosing cholangitis
    definition, 129
    treatment, 130
Primary spontaneous pneumothorax, 79
Primary syphilis, 275
Prinzmetal's angina, 23
Prisoners and tuberculosis, 76
Probenecid, 198
Procainamide, 42, 46, 49, 56, 193
Proctitis
    causes, 280
    definition, 280
    lymphogranulosum venereum, 280
    signs and symptoms, 280
    treatment, 280
Prodromal phase, rabies and, 86
Progesterone, 110, 342
Proguanil, 175
Prolactin, 245–247
Prolactinoma, 247
Propafenone, 49
Propranolol, 56, 133, 254, 259
Propylthiouracil, 253, 254

Prostaglandin, 111, 113
Prostate cancer
    definition, 339
    epidemiology, 339–340
    hypercalcemia, 219
    prognosis, 340
    screening, 336, 340
    signs and symptoms, 340
    treatment, 340
Prostatectomy, 340
Prostate specific antigen (PSA), 340
Prostatitis
    bacterial
        causes, 277
        definition, 277
        laboratory studies, 278
        signs and symptoms, 277
        treatment, 278
    cystitis, 274
    dysuria, 274
    nonbacterial
        laboratory studies, 278
        signs and symptoms, 278
        treatment, 278
Protease inhibitors, 304
Protein-losing enteropathy
    causes, 122
    diagnosis, 122
    signs and symptoms, 122
    treatment, 122
Protein(s)
    acute tubular necrosis, 228
    alcoholic cirrhosis, 131
    celiac sprue, 120
    gout, 197, 198
    hepatic encephalopathy, 134
    Kwashiorkor, 348
    Ménétrier's disease, 123
    scleroderma, 195
Proteinuria, 192, 198, 231
Proteolysis, 122
Proteolytic enzymes, 124
Proteus, 281
Proteus mirabilis, 274
Prothrombin time (PT), 120, 131, 168
Proton pump, 111
Proton pump inhibitors, 113
Protozoal diarrhea, 298–299
Proximal aortic root dissection, 31
Proximal interphalangeal pain (PIP), 188
Proximal myopathy, 304
Pruritus
    atopic dermatitis, 332
    dialysis, 231
    hypersensitivity vasculitis, 313
    pityriasis rosea, 320
    polycythemia vera, 165
    primary biliary cirrhosis, 132
    psoriasis, 319
    toxic epidermal necrolysis, 327
Pseudoaneurysm, 55
Pseudogout
    definition, 198
    etiology, 198
    positive birefringence, 197
    signs and symptoms, 198
    treatment, 198
Pseudohyperkalemia, 216, 217
Pseudohyponatremia, 213
Pseudohypoparathyroidism, 218, 223
Pseudomembranous colitis
    complications, 142–143
    definition, 142

Tinea versicolor, 328
Tinel's sign, 196
Tinnitus, 94
Tissue plasminogen activator, 58
Tobacco use
  ankylosing spondylitis, 185
  cerebrovascular accidents, 84
  cervical cancer, 339
  cessation, 345
  chronic bronchitis, 68, 69
  counseling, smoking cessation, 345
  definition, 344–345
  diseases related to, 345
  emphysema, 68, 69
  gastritis, 114
  gastroesophageal reflux disease, 110
  hyperaldosteronism, 267
  hypertension, 52
  lumbar disc herniation, 184
  lung cancer, 72
  metabolic alkalosis, 211
  osteoporosis, 269
  peptic ulcer disease, 110
  pharmacotherapy, smoking cessation, 345
  polycythemia vera, 165
  spontaneous pneumothorax, 79
Tonic–clonic seizures, 90
Tophi, 197
Torsade de pointes
  definition, 46
  etiology, 46–47
  signs and symptoms, 47
  treatment, 47
  ventricular fibrillation and pulseless ventricular tachycardia, 45
Total iron-binding capacity (TIBC), 156
Total parenteral nutrition (TPN), 222
Toxic epidermal necrolysis
  complications, 328
  definition, 327
  diagnosis, 327
  signs and symptoms, 327
  treatment, 328
Toxic shock syndrome (TSS)
  definition, 307
  diagnosis, 307
  epidemiology, 307
  etiology, 307
  signs and symptoms, 307
Toxoplasma, 38, 229, 288
Toxoplasmosis
  AIDS (acquired immune deficiency syndrome), 298
  central nervous system, 297
  clinical presentation, 298
  diagnosis, 298
  treatment, 298
Transaminases, 192
Transesophageal echo (TEE), 85
Transient hyperthyroidism, 251
Transient ischemic attack (TIA), 47, 81, 85
Transjugular intrahepatic portacaval shunt (TIPS), 133
Transplantation
  bone marrow, 155, 158, 290
  heart, 35
  immunocompromised patients
    fever, 291
    infection, 290
  kidneys, 206, 221
  liver, 138–139
  lungs, 70
Transrectal ultrasonography (TRUS), 340

Transudative pleural effusions, 73
Trauma/injury
  acalculous cholecystitis, 129
  acute pancreatitis, 125
  adult respiratory distress syndrome, 65
  aortic aneurysm, 55
  aortic dissection, 54
  avascular necrosis of the hip, 200
  back pain, lower, 184
  bacterial meningitis, 87
  carpal tunnel syndrome, 196
  cellulitis, 323
  costochondritis, 200
  decubitus ulcers, 324
  diabetic ketoacidosis, 241
  disseminated intravascular coagulation, 172
  domestic violence, 342
  epilepsy, 90
  myxedema coma, 257
  osteoarthritis, 190
  pericardial tamponade, 44
  pleural effusions, 73
  prevention
    falls, 347–348
    motor vehicles, 347
  psoriasis, 318
  tension pneumothorax, 80
  thyroid storm, 252
  vertebral compression fracture, 186
  wounds, 91, 307, 324, 325, 348
Treponema pallidum, 274, 275
Trichinella, 38
Trichomonas, 279
Trichomonas vaginalis, 273, 278
Trichophyton, 328
Tricuspid regurgitation
  diagnosis, 34
  etiology, 33
  signs and symptoms, 33
  treatment, 34
Tricuspid stenosis
  diagnosis, 32
  etiology, 32
  signs and symptoms, 32
  treatment, 32
Triglycerides, 117, 232, 256
Trihexyphenidyl, 99
Trimethoprim-sulfamethoxazole (TMP-SMZ), 61, 274, 278, 297, 299
Tripeptides, 117
Trophermyma whippleii, 121
Tropical sprue
  cobalamin deficiency, 151
  definition, 120
  diagnosis, 120
  folate deficiency anemia, 150
  pathology, 120
  signs and symptoms, 120
  treatment, 120
Troponin, 20, 38
Trousseau's sign, 218
Trousseau's syndrome, 72
True aneurysm, 55
Trypanosoma cruzi, 38
Trypsin, 117
Tubal sterilization, 338
Tuberculosis
  adrenal insufficiency, 262
  anemia of chronic inflammation, 156
  bronchiectasis, 69
  cell-mediated immunodeficiency, 288
  definition, 76

  diagnosis, 77
  epidemiology, 76, 299
  erythema nodosum, 313
  HIV (human immunodeficiency virus), 299
  hypercalcemia, 219
  isoniazid, 193
  mediastinitis, 71
  pathophysiology, 76
  pleural effusions, 74
  prevention, 78
  purified protein derivative skin test, 77
  signs and symptoms, 76–77
  syndrome of inappropriate antidiuretic hormone, 249
  toxicity of medication
    ethambutol, 79
    isoniazid, 78
    rifampin, 78–79
  treatment, 78
Tuberculosis bacillus, 187
Tubes and chest radiograph, 5
Tubulointerstitial diseases, 227
Tumor calcinosis, 223
Tumor lysis syndrome, 218, 225, 228
Tumor necrosis factor (TNF), 146
Tumors
  adenomas, 246, 250, 251, 261, 266
  carcinoid, 139–140
  cauda equina syndrome, 188
  cell-mediated immunodeficiency, 288
  cholangitis, ascending, 129
  cholecystitis, 128
  hypopituitarism, 247
  melanoma, malignant, 318
  pituitary, 245–247, 265, 266
  pleural effusions, 73, 74
  proximal, 318
  spinal metastasis, 187–188
  syndrome of inappropriate antidiuretic hormone, 250
  See also neoplasms *under* Brain
Turner's syndrome, 31, 54
Tyrosine, 125
Tzanck preparation, 277, 329, 334

U

Ulcer, 333
  See also specific type, 333
Ulcerative colitis (UC)
  complications, 144
  definition, 143
  diagnosis, 144
  epidemiology, 143
  pathology, 144
  signs and symptoms, 144, 145
  treatment
    specific therapy, 145–146
    support care, 144
Ulnar deviation, 188
Ultrasound
  abdominal aortic aneurysms, 103
  acute pancreatitis, 126
  acute renal failure, 226
  aortic aneurysm, 55
  breast cancer, 337
  cholangitis, ascending, 129
  cholecystitis, 128
  cholelithiasis, 127
  chronic renal failure, 230
  prostate cancer, 340
  renal, 284